Methamphetamine Addiction

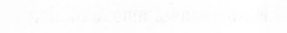

Methamphetamine Addiction
From Basic Science to Treatment

Edited by

John M. Roll
Richard A. Rawson
Walter Ling
Steven Shoptaw

The Guilford Press
New York   London

© 2009 The Guilford Press
A Division of Guilford Publications, Inc.
72 Spring Street, New York, NY 10012
www.guilford.com

Printed in the United States of America

This book is printed on acid-free paper.

Last digit is print number: 9   8   7   6   5   4   3   2   1

The authors have checked with sources believed to be reliable in their efforts to
provide information that is complete and generally in accord with the standards
of practice that are accepted at the time of publication. However, in view of the
possibility of human error or changes in medical sciences, neither the authors,
nor the editor and publisher, nor any other party who has been involved in the
preparation or publication of this work warrant that the information contained
herein is in every respect accurate or complete, and they are not responsible for
any errors or omissions or the results obtained from the use of such information.
Readers are encouraged to confirm the information contained in this book with
other sources.

Library of Congress Cataloging-in-Publication Data

Methamphetamine addiction: from basic science to treatment / editors,
John M. Roll ... [et al.].
       p. cm.
    Includes bibliographical references and index.
    ISBN 978-1-60623-252-1 (hardcover: alk. paper)
    1. Methamphetamine abuse. 2. Methamphetamine abuse—Treatment.
3. Methamphetamine. I. Roll, John M.
    RC568.A45M483   2009
    616.86′4—dc22
                                                            2009003203

With thanks to Marshall, MaryAnn, and Joy
—J. M. R.

To Maya and Jackson
—R. A. R.

For my mother
—W. L.

For all those affected by this disorder
—S. S.

About the Editors

John M. Roll, PhD, is Professor and Associate Dean for Research at Washington State University College of Nursing in Spokane, and the Director of its Program of Excellence in the Addictions. He has held postdoctoral fellowship positions at the University of Vermont and the University of Michigan and faculty appointments at Wayne State University and the University of California, Los Angeles. In 2006, Dr. Roll was elected a Fellow of the American Psychological Association. He is President of the American Psychological Association's Division on Psychopharmacology and Substance Abuse and was a vice-chairman of the Washington State Governor's Council on Substance Abuse. He has received research funding from federal, state, and local sources as well as foundation and industry support. Dr. Roll has served as a member of the editorial boards of the *Journal of the Experimental Analysis of Behavior* and the *Journal of Applied Behavior Analysis.*

Richard A. Rawson, PhD, is Associate Director of the UCLA Integrated Substance Abuse Programs, one of the foremost substance abuse research groups in the United States and worldwide, and Professor-in-Residence in the Department of Psychiatry and Biobehavioral Sciences at the David Geffen School of Medicine at the University of California, Los Angeles. Dr. Rawson oversees clinical trials on pharmacological and psychosocial addiction treatments. He has led addiction research and training projects for the United Nations, the World Health Organization (WHO), and the U.S. State Department that export science-based knowledge to many parts of the world. Dr. Rawson's research on methamphetamine is extensive, and from 1996 to 1999 he was a member of the Federal Methamphetamine Advisory Group for former U.S. Attorney General Janet Reno. He is currently principal investigator of both the Pacific Southwest Addiction Technology Transfer Center funded by the Substance Abuse and Mental Health Services Administration and the UCLA Drug Abuse Research Training Grant funded by the National Institute on Drug Abuse (NIDA). Dr. Rawson has published 2 books, 30 book chapters, and more than 200 peer-reviewed articles and has conducted over 1,000 workshops, presentations, and training sessions.

Walter Ling, MD, is a board-certified neurologist and psychiatrist, a Professor-in-Residence of Psychiatry at the David Geffen School of Medicine at the University of California, Los Angeles, and Director of the UCLA Integrated Substance Abuse Programs. He is a consultant for numerous local, national, and international private and public agencies. Dr. Ling serves as Principal Investigator of the Pacific Node of the NIDA Clinical Trials Network, designed to bring cutting-edge findings from treatment research to practice in community treatment programs throughout the United States. He also does consulting and collaborative work with the U.S. Department of State, the United Nations Office of International Narcotics Affairs, and the WHO.

Steven Shoptaw, PhD, is Professor of Family Medicine and of Psychiatry and Biobehavioral Sciences at the David Geffen School of Medicine at the University of California, Los Angeles. Dr. Shoptaw's research involves developing and implementing efficacious treatments for individuals with various drug dependence problems, particularly for those with stimulant dependence and risks for HIV infection and other health care problems. He has published over 120 scientific articles on these topics, including a 2006 treatment manual coauthored with Cathy Reback and Richard A. Rawson, *Getting Off: A Behavioral Treatment Intervention for Gay and Bisexual Male Methamphetamine Users.* In addition to clinical and research work, Dr. Shoptaw also volunteers as Executive Director for Safe House, a facility he started that provides high-tolerance emergency, transitional, and permanent housing for 26 persons living with HIV/AIDS, mental illness, and/or chemical dependency, who are also homeless or at risk for homelessness.

Contributors

Nathan M. Appel, PhD, Division of Pharmacotherapies and Medical Consequences of Drug Abuse, National Institute on Drug Abuse, Bethesda, Maryland

Michelle A. Bholat, MD, Department of Family Medicine, David Geffen School of Medicine, University of California, Los Angeles, Los Angeles, California

Ahmed Elkashef, PhD, Division of Pharmacotherapies and Medical Consequences of Drug Abuse, National Institute on Drug Abuse, Bethesda, Maryland

David Farabee, PhD, UCLA Integrated Substance Abuse Programs, Semel Institute for Neuroscience and Human Behavior, David Geffen School of Medicine, University of California, Los Angeles, Los Angeles, California

Annette E. Fleckenstein, PhD, Pharmacology and Toxicology Department, College of Pharmacy, University of Utah, Salt Lake City, Utah

Suzette Glasner-Edwards, PhD, UCLA Integrated Substance Abuse Programs, Semel Institute for Neuroscience and Human Behavior, David Geffen School of Medicine, University of California, Los Angeles, Los Angeles, California

Glen R. Hanson, DDS, Pharmacology and Toxicology Department, College of Pharmacy, University of Utah, Salt Lake City, Utah

Angela Hawken, PhD, UCLA Integrated Substance Abuse Programs, Semel Institute for Neuroscience and Human Behavior, David Geffen School of Medicine, University of California, Los Angeles, Los Angeles, California

Keith Heinzerling, MD, MPH, Department of Family Medicine, David Geffen School of Medicine, University of California, Los Angeles, Los Angeles, California

Chris-Ellyn Johanson, PhD, Department of Psychiatry and Behavioral Neurosciences, Wayne State University, Chicago, Illinois

William D. King, MD, Department of Family Medicine, David Geffen School of Medicine, University of California, Los Angeles, Los Angeles, California

Evan Landstrom, Department of Family Medicine, David Geffen School of Medicine, University of California, Los Angeles, Los Angeles, California

Sarah Lefkowith, Department of Family Medicine, David Geffen School of Medicine, University of California, Los Angeles, Los Angeles, California

Walter Ling, MD, UCLA Integrated Substance Abuse Programs, Semel Institute for Neuroscience and Human Behavior, David Geffen School of Medicine, University of California, Los Angeles, Los Angeles, California

Edythe D. London, PhD, UCLA Neuropsychiatric Institute, David Geffen School of Medicine, University of California, Los Angeles, Los Angeles, California

Jane C. Maxwell, PhD, Addiction Research Institute, University of Texas at Austin, Austin, Texas

Larissa Mooney, MD, UCLA Integrated Substance Abuse Programs, Semel Institute for Neuroscience and Human Behavior, David Geffen School of Medicine, University of California, Los Angeles, Los Angeles, California

Jagoda Pasic, MD, PhD, Department of Psychiatry and Behavioral Sciences, University of Washington at Harborview Medical Center, Seattle, Washington

Doris Payer, BS, UCLA Neuropsychiatric Institute, David Geffen School of Medicine, University of California, Los Angeles, Los Angeles, California

Richard A. Rawson, PhD, UCLA Integrated Substance Abuse Programs, Semel Institute for Neuroscience and Human Behavior, David Geffen School of Medicine, University of California, Los Angeles, Los Angeles, California

Richard Ries, MD, Department of Psychiatry and Behavioral Sciences, University of Washington at Harborview Medical Center, Seattle, Washington

John M. Roll, PhD, College of Nursing, Washington State University, Spokane, Washington

Craig R. Rush, PhD, College of Medicine, University of Kentucky, Lexington, Kentucky

Beth A. Rutkowski, MPH, UCLA Integrated Substance Abuse Programs, Semel Institute for Neuroscience and Human Behavior, David Geffen School of Medicine, University of California, Los Angeles, Los Angeles, California

Charles R. Schuster, PhD, Department of Psychiatry and Behavioral Neurosciences, Wayne State University, Chicago, Illinois

Steven Shoptaw, PhD, Department of Family Medicine, David Geffen School of Medicine, University of California, Los Angeles, Los Angeles, California

Sharon Sowell, BA, Department of Clinical Psychology, Washington State University, Spokane, Washington

William W. Stoops, PhD, Department of Behavioral Science, College of Medicine, University of Kentucky, Lexington, Kentucky

Linda J. Thompson, MA, Greater Spokane Substance Abuse Council, Spokane Valley, Washington

Gregory D. Victorianne, BA, Department of Family Medicine, David Geffen School of Medicine, University of California, Los Angeles, Los Angeles, California

Frank J. Vocci, PhD, Friends Research Institute, Baltimore, Maryland

Matthew Worley, BA, Department of Family Medicine, David Geffen School of Medicine, University of California, Los Angeles, Los Angeles, California

Contents

Chapter 1

Introduction

John M. Roll, Richard A. Rawson, Steven Shoptaw,
and Walter Ling

As a drug of abuse methamphetamine (MA) has received tremendous press, much of which has been inaccurate. For example people do not become addicted to MA after one exposure; it is not inherently more reinforcing than other drugs with abuse potential. Moreover, treatment for MA addiction *can be effective*; in fact it often appears to be as effective as treatment for cocaine addiction (e.g., Copeland & Sorensen, 2001; Luchansky et al., 2007).

That is not to say, of course, that MA is benign. It is an incredibly dangerous drug. Those who use it, even once, put themselves at tremendous risk for a variety of deleterious consequences, including legal sanctions, physical injury, increased susceptibility to illness and victimization, and damage to their property. Moreover, regular users often neglect their families, friends, and communities, and become burdens to society instead of contributing members.

Users of MA also support the criminal elements that manufacture and distribute the drug. Although some users manufacture their own drugs, recent legislation and efforts at local, state, and federal levels have severely limited access to the precursor chemicals needed to produce MA, which has greatly curtailed local manufacture. Although manufacturers are finding new ways to produce the drug, local production remains low relative to historic highs. This is a bright spot in the "war against methamphetamine," as manufacture poses very serious risks to those in proximity (e.g., chemical exposures, burns, and, in the case of children, severe neglect and abuse). Notably, these consequences are not limited to the individuals actually making the drug but also affect others

1

in the environment, including first responders. Manufacture also results in significant environmental degradation and property contamination as the precursors and byproducts are introduced into homes and the outdoors.

Concerned individuals from many social strata have contributed to efforts to prevent initial use of MA, curtail its production and use, treat addiction, and formulate sensible policies to address the problems caused by MA abuse. These concerned individuals represent families, communities, counties, state governments, federal governments, and worldwide bodies such as the United Nations and the World Health Organization. All share the goal of preventing new MA use and successfully treating those currently addicted. An observation that has emerged from these efforts is that a transdisciplinary approach incorporating treatment providers, scientists, community members, prevention specialists, members of the criminal justice system, and policy makers has the greatest likelihood of success.

This book has been designed to provide a cutting-edge review of current knowledge about many aspects of MA, ranging from cellular effects to the drug's effect on communities. In addition, we hope that the contents will serve as a foundation for future efforts. The chapters are arranged in such a way that they can be read sequentially or individually. Reading the entire book will result in a very good working knowledge of the basics of many aspects of MA. The information will be useful to many different professions united by the common goal of removing the scourge of MA addiction from among us. This would include scientists whose work spans the spectrum from neuropharmacology to treatment and prevention. Also included are those who provide service to addicts and others touched by MA (e.g., teachers, social workers, treatment providers, physicians, nurses, those in the criminal justice system, and clergy). Finally the book may interest readers on whose lives MA has had a direct impact. Parents whose children are addicted may glean an understanding of the effects of the drug on the user's brain and modify their interactions with, and expectations of, their children accordingly. Others may encounter, for the first time and in the face of so much inaccurate press, the data demonstrating that treatment for MA addiction can work—that addicts have significant recovery potential and can, in fact, reclaim their lives.

The book begins with a comprehensive review in Chapter 2 of the epidemiology of MA use (Rutkowski and Maxwell). This sets the stage for subsequent chapters by providing the reader with an understanding of who is using MA and how they are using it.

Chapter 3 describes, in exquisite detail, the basic neuropharmacology of MA (Hanson and Fleckenstein). The authors present complex material in an accessible fashion, providing the reader with an understanding of how MA exerts its effects. This chapter provides the reader with a foundation that will support a greater appreciation of the behavioral effects of MA and the challenges inherent in treating addiction.

Human behavior arises from interactions between a person and his or her environment and, to a large extent, this interaction is regulated by the person's brain. Chapter 4 (Payer and London) describes our nascent understanding of the impact of MA on a user's brain, which is essential if one is to fully appreciate the allure of the drug and the difficulties inherent in initiating and maintaining abstinence from it. Making use of data collected with cutting-edge technology, Payer and London introduce the reader to this complex and fascinating area of inquiry.

The observable output of the interaction of an MA-affected brain with the environment is generally aberrant behavior. Rush, Stoops, and Ling (Chapter 5) provide a thorough review of behavioral pharmacology data demonstrating how MA affects behavior in controlled laboratory settings, as well as how behavior in a person's natural environment can often result in signs and symptoms of psychopathology. Left unanswered is the intriguing question about the directionality of the relationship between MA use and psychiatric comorbidity: which comes first, the psychiatric condition or the addiction? It is likely that each exacerbates the other. As our understanding of genetics and epigenetics increases, we may be able to answer this question, which will likely have important implications for treatment.

Mooney, Glasner-Edwards, Rawson, and Ling (Chapter 6) describe the impact of MA on major body systems. Understanding the common medical conditions that arise as a result of MA addiction is important for those providing support or treatment to addicted individuals. Understanding medical effects is crucial for developing pharmaceutical treatment approaches to address MA addiction. To the extent that the drug produces cardiac, pulmonary, or hepatic toxicity, the potential agents available for treatment of MA addiction or common co-occurring psychiatric conditions is limited due to potentially dangerous side effects.

In addition, given that MA addiction is driven by the drug's reinforcing potential and that this potential is influenced by available alternative sources of reinforcement in a user's environment, it is important to understand the medical conditions that may limit the users' access to these other sources of reinforcement. For example, consider an addicted individual whose primary method of administration was smoking and as a result had incurred pulmonary disability. It might not be appropriate to tell this person to combat his drug use by engaging in strenuous aerobic exercise. Although exercise can be an important component of some treatments, in this individual's case it would be counterproductive.

Chapter 7 (Shoptaw, King, Landstrom, Bholat, Heinzerling, and Roll) builds on our understanding of the epidemiology, action, and medical effects of MA use by discussing important associated public health issues. Primary among these are HIV, hepatitis, and sexually transmitted diseases. To the extent that the transmission of these diseases is mediated or moderated by MA addiction it becomes imperative to address MA use in our public health policies governing our responses to these types of diseases. Moreover, some treatment strategies (e.g., HAART [highly active antiretroviral therapy] for HIV/AIDS) require strict adherence to complex treatment regimens. Failure to comply may result in the development of drug-resistant strains of the disease organism. When an individual is under the influence of MA, it is unlikely he or she will have the wherewithal to adhere to these treatment regimens, further increasing the public health imperative to include MA treatment strategies in the management of these conditions.

MA use is against the law. Those who manufacture the drug or use it are overloading some criminal justice jurisdictions. Farabee and Hawken (Chapter 8) discuss the contributions of MA to criminal behavior. The authors detail the unique opportunities for collaboration between the criminal justice system and treatment providers to address the pernicious criminal behavior often perpetuated by MA-addicted individuals.

In Chapter 9 Thompson, Sowell, and Roll describe, from a community activist point of view, how MA affects not only individuals and their families but entire communities. A focus is placed on addressing community-level challenges by engaging in dynamic problem solving with stakeholders from throughout the community. This chapter provides a hopeful message that through combined, somewhat novel, partnerships, communities can take local action to address the effects of MA.

The remaining three chapters address treatment issues. Chapter 10 (Shoptaw, Rawson, Worley, Lefkowith, and Roll) details the early results showing great promise for the use of behavioral and psychosocial approaches to treating MA addiction. Given the efficacy of these approaches in treating cocaine addiction, it is not surprising that they are the most effective treatments currently available for treating MA addiction. Chapter 11 (Vocci, Elkashef, and Appel) details the exciting search for a pharmacological agent. Although no drug has current approval of the Food and Drug Administration (FDA) for the treatment of MA addiction, an international cadre of researchers is closing in on likely candidates. Finally Pasic and Ries (Chapter 13) address the treatment of MA addiction that co-occurs with serious mental illness. Like other types of addiction, MA addiction is frequently encountered in users who have other psychiatric conditions. This group poses unique treatment challenges involving medication management and psychosocial intervention. Even with these challenges, data suggest that MA addiction among this group can be treated.

Taken together, all of the chapters equip the reader to be a critical consumer of media reports concerning MA. In addition, the informed individuals can be justifiably skeptical of "quick-fix" schemes promoted by some for the rapid treatment of MA addiction. Finally this volume should provide readers with the requisite knowledge to seek further information on specific topics and to formulate their own questions about MA for further scientific inquiry. While MA was developed in hopes of improving the human condition (cf. Anglin et al., 2000), it has fallen far short of initial expectations. Instead, it has become a drug of abuse that has fueled grievous addiction and destroyed many lives. However, individuals who are addicted have significant recovery potential. It is our hope that this book will play a role in ending the scourge of MA addiction.

References

Anglin MD, Burke C, Perrochet B, et al. (2000). History of the methamphetamine problem. *J Psychoactive Drugs* 32(2):137–141.

Copeland AL, Sorensen JL. (2001). Differences between methamphetamine users and cocaine users in treatment. *Drug Alcohol Depend* 62(1):91–95.

Luchansky B, Krupski A, Stark K. (2007). Treatment response by primary drug of abuse: Does methamphetamine make a difference? *J Subst Abuse Treat* 32(1):89–96.

Chapter 2

Epidemiology of Methamphetamine Use

A Global Perspective

Beth A. Rutkowski and Jane C. Maxwell

This chapter summarizes the latest international epidemiological reports on the use of methamphetamine (MA) and amphetamine, which reflect a growing concern because of substantial increases in production and consumption and ensuing harm related to the use of these drugs (Degenhardt et al., 2008). Some data sources differentiate between the two drugs, others use terms such as "meth/amphetamine," some use the term "amphetamine" to mean both amphetamine and MA, others use the term "amphetamine" to apply only to diverted pharmaceuticals, and still others use the term amphetamine-type stimulants (ATS).[1] Information is drawn from a wide range of sources, including, but not limited to, historical accounts, research projects, population surveys, and treatment data.

The primary focus of the chapter is a description of MA and amphetamine use in North America, with a secondary, more limited discussion of the patterns and trends of MA and amphetamine use in other countries throughout the world. The data generally encompass the time period of 1992 to 2007.

---

[1] Amphetamine-type stimulants (ATS) include amphetamines (MA and amphetamine), Ecstasy (MDMA and related substances), and other synthetic stimulants (methcathinone, phentermine, fenetylline, etc.)

The European Monitoring Centre for Drugs and Drug Addiction (EMCDDA) and the United Nations Office on Drugs and Crime (UNODC) have summarized the trends in the use of MA and amphetamine:

- The largest production sources are in Southeast Asia and North America, and the majority of MA users reside in these areas. The highest MA prevalence rates worldwide have been reported from the Philippines.
- Amphetamine production is primarily located in Europe, and use of this form is more common there. MA use is more limited, but has been reported in the Czech Republic, and more recently in the Slovak Republic. According to EMCCDA, qualitative and seizures data from the United Kingdom, Norway, France, Latvia, Denmark, and Bulgaria suggest increases in seizures and/or use.
- South Africa is emerging as a market for both MA and methcathinone ("khat").

Major Data Sources in the United States

This chapter evaluates data from a number of sources to identify national and regional trends and patterns of use of MA and amphetamine. The data are arrayed in such a way to present a somewhat cohesive picture of who tends to use MA or amphetamine, the trends in use, and the consequences of their use. The following data sources are discussed in detail, and will be referred to hereafter by their abbreviated acronyms.

The *Monitoring the Future Survey (MTF)* is conducted by the University of Michigan's Institute for Social Research and is funded by the National Institute on Drug Abuse (NIDA). The annual U.S.-based survey tracks illicit drug use and attitudes toward drugs by approximately 50,000 8th, 10th, and 12th graders, as well as follow-up questionnaires mailed to a sample of each graduating class for a number of years after their initial participation. The data presented in this chapter covers 8th, 10th, and 12th graders, college students, and young adults ages 19–28. MTF reports can be accessed at *monitoringthefuture.org*.

The *National Survey on Drug Use and Health (NSDUH)*, formerly called the National Household Survey on Drug Abuse (NHSDA), is a multistage area probability sample of 67,802 individuals in 2006 conducted by the Office of Applied Studies of the Substance Abuse and Mental Health Services Administration. NSDUH collects information on the prevalence, patterns, and consequences of alcohol, tobacco, and illegal drug use and abuse in the U.S. civilian noninstitutionalized population, ages 12 and older. The survey reports can be found at *www.oas. samhsa.gov/nsduh.htm*.

The *Drug Abuse Warning Network (DAWN)* has two components: U.S.-based emergency department (ED) data and mortality data reported by medical examiners and coroners (ME/C). The ED component provides statistical estimates of drug-related visits to EDs for selected metropolitan areas as well as for the nation. The ME/C component includes deaths associated with substance abuse and drug misuse, both unintentional and accidental. Unlike the ED component, the ME/C component is not a sample and it does not provide statistical estimates for the nation as a whole; it simply collects data voluntarily reported by medical examiners. DAWN is conducted by the Office of Applied Studies of the Substance Abuse and Mental Health Services Administration (SAMHSA). The reports can be accessed at *dawninfo.samhsa.gov*.

The *Treatment Episode Data Set (TEDS)* collects information on individuals admitted to substance abuse treatment facilities that are licensed or certified by the 50 state substance abuse agencies. In 2006, over 1.8 million treatment admissions were reported. TEDS is conducted by the Office of Applied Studies of SAMHSA. The reports are available at *www.oas.samhsa.gov/dasis.htm#teds2*.

The *Community Epidemiology Work Group (CEWG),* sponsored by NIDA, is composed of 22 researchers from across the nation who meet twice per year to report on drug abuse patterns and trends and emerging problems in their local areas. Members use quantitative statistics and qualitative techniques such as focus groups and key informant interviews to monitor drug trends. The full reports of the CEWG can be accessed at *www.nida.nih.gov/about/organization/cewg/ Reports.html*.

Major International Data Sources

In addition to detailing the domestic trends and patterns of MA and amphetamine use and U.S. at-risk populations, this chapter highlights available data from other regions of the world differentially impacted by MA and amphetamines (i.e., Mexico, Canada, Central and South America, the Caribbean, Europe, Africa, Asia, and Oceania). Data and main findings from peer-reviewed journal articles and national survey reports are included, and are supplemented with the following major international data sources from the EMCDDA and UNODC.

- European Monitoring Centre for Drugs and Drug Addiction (EMCDDA) Annual Report (2006), *www.emcdda.europa.eu/*; *www.emcdda.europa.eu/index.cfm?LanguageISO=EN*.
- International Narcotics Control Board Annual Report (2006)—United Nations, *www.incb.org*; *www.incb.org/incb/annual_report_2006.html*.
- World Drug Report (2007)—UNODC, *www.unodc.org*; *www.unodc.org/unodc/en/data-and-analysis/WDR.html*.
- Patterns and Trends of Amphetamine-Type Stimulants (ATS) and Other Drugs of Abuse in East Asia and the Pacific (2006)— UNODC Regional Centre for East Asia and the Pacific, *www.apaic.org*.

MA and Amphetamine Use in North America

MA and amphetamine use in North America is characterized by geographic variations, with different types of the drug and different types of users at various times (UNODC, 2007b). According to national household surveys, the annual prevalence for "speed" use in Canada was 0.8% in 2004 (Adlaf et al., 2005), 0.1% for "amphetamine" use in Mexico in 2002 (UNODC, 2007b), and 1.4% for "stimulant" use in the United States in 2006 (SAMHSA, 2007c).

The United States

Amphetamine tablets were available in the United States without a prescription until 1951; inhalers containing amphetamine were available over the counter until 1959 (Anglin et al., 2000; Ling et al., 2006). Initially, the illicit amphetamine market consisted of diverted pharmaceutical amphetamine (Anglin et al., 2000), but in 1970, the drug was rescheduled to the more restrictive Schedule II, which lessened its availability. Illicit manufacturers began making MA using the "P2P" method. In the 1980s, two simpler production methods were developed: the "Nazi" method, which used ephedrine or pseudoephedrine, lithium, and anhydrous ammonia, and the "cold" method which used ephedrine or pseudoephedrine, red phosphorus, and iodine crystals (Maxwell, 2004). At the same time, large quantities of a smokable and highly pure form of d-methamphetamine hydrochloride ("ice, crystal") began to be imported into Hawaii from Far Eastern sources (Joe-Laidler & Morgan, 1997). From Hawaii, use of "ice" moved to the West Coast.

In the 1990s in the United States, the first stage of the MA epidemic was characterized by production of powder MA in California and Mexico, with delivery elsewhere in the country via overnight express. During this phase, crack cocaine was the primary problem drug in urban areas (SAMHSA, 1996). "Ice" use spread among gay men, and its use gradually moved east toward the end of the 1990s (Kurtz & Inciardi, 2003).

The middle stages of the epidemic saw the increase in small-time "cooks" in the United States who used over-the-counter cold medications and readily available chemicals to produce MA. Although MA was a problem in the rural areas in the Midwest and South and most of those entering treatment were white, crack cocaine was still the primary drug of abuse in urban areas (Israel-Adams & Topolski, 2003). As the number of laboratories in these areas declined with the limitation on precursor chemicals beginning in 2004, there was a commensurate increase in the amount of Mexican MA which was trucked into the urban areas to replace the less pure and less available product produced by small local laboratories.

The later stage of the epidemic, which has occurred in many westerns states, is characterized by MA being the primary drug problem for individuals seeking treatment (U.S. Department of Health and Human Services [US DHHS], 2007). Its use spread to other racial and ethnic groups; smoking was the dominant route of administration; and the supply of powder MA decreased with the increase in "ice."

Beginning in 1989, efforts were made to regulate ephedrine and pseudoephedrine through various federal laws passed in 1989, 1995, 1996, and 1997 (Cunningham & Liu, 2005). In 2004, in response to the proliferation of local laboratories, various U.S. states began to limit access to over-the-counter pseudoephedrine products and in September, 2006, federal legislation imposed limits nationwide,[2] which resulted in a decline in clandestine laboratories and items seized and examined in forensic laboratories (Figure 2.1; National Clandestine Laboratory Database [NCLD], 2007; Office of Diversion Control, 2008). As of 2007, domestic production of MA was mainly concentrated in the Midwestern and Southern states. The 11 states with the highest number of seized laboratories (in order from highest to lowest) are Missouri, Indiana,

---

[2] See *The Combat Methamphetamine Epidemic Act of 2005,* Title VII of Public Law 109-177, for the federal legislation; for the status of legislation in each state, see The Office of National Drug Control Policy, *Pushing Back against Meth: A Progress Report on the Fight against Methamphetamine in the United States,* published November 30, 2006. Accessed July 26, 2007 at *www.whitehousedrugpolicy.gov/publications/pdf/pushing-back_against_meth.pdf.*

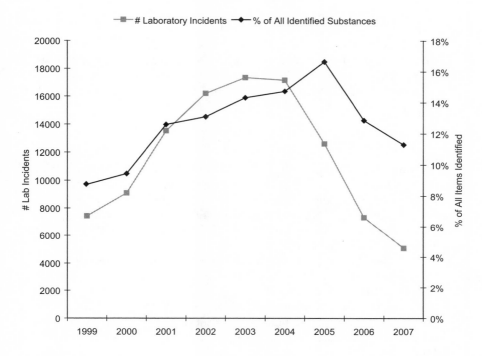

FIGURE 2.1. Number of all MA clandestine laboratory incidents and percentage of all substances identified that were MA in the United States: 1999–2007. Data from NCLD (2007) and Office of Diversion Control (2008).

Tennessee, Illinois, Kentucky, Arkansas, California, Michigan, North Carolina, Iowa, and Mississippi (NCLD, 2008). The decreased supply has resulted in an 84% increase in the average price per pure gram of all domestic MA purchases from $152.39 to $280.06, and a 26% decrease in purity from 57% to 42% between January and December 2007 (Drug Enforcement Administration [DEA], 2008).

Based on the changing supply pattern, at the June 2007 meeting of the National Institute on Drug Abuse's Community Epidemiology Work Group, 20 of the 22 correspondents from metropolitan areas across the United States reported that MA indicators in their areas were "stable" or "down," and there was a "wait and see" consensus as to the future direction of the epidemic and the impact of additional high purity MA from Mexico (Maxwell & Rutkowski, 2007).

Emergency Department Reports

In 2005, DAWN estimated that stimulants (including MA and amphetamine) were involved in about 8.5% of the drug misuse/abuse ED visits, following cocaine, marijuana, and heroin. Sixty-five percent of the stimulant-related ED visits were male and 58% were white (SAMHSA, 2008b).

Treatment Admissions

According to substance abuse treatment admissions statistics from TEDS, between 1992 and 2006, the proportion of clients admitted to treatment with a primary problem with MA or amphetamine increased from 1% to nearly 9%, and the routes of administration changed as "ice" became more dominant (Figure 2.2; SAMHSA, 2005b, 2007d, 2008c; US DHHS, 2007).

The characteristics of the users entering treatment for a primary MA/amphetamine problem have also changed, with the proportion who were white decreasing from 91% in 1992 to 68% in 2006, and the proportion of Hispanics increasing from 9% to 19%. In 2006, 3.2% were Native American or black. The proportion of clients who were male remained consistent at 54%–55% (SAMHSA, 2006b, 2008c; US DHHS, 2007).

The impact of MA/amphetamine on the rate of treatment admissions in individual states is shown by the fact that in 1992, only one state (Oregon) had a rate higher than 50 per 100,000 population. By 2005, 21 states had population adjusted rates of 50 or more per 100,000 (SAMHSA, 2007e). Regional/ spatial variations in the epidemic were also seen in treatment data. Generally, the highest rates were seen in

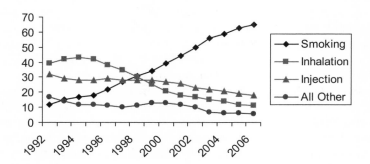

FIGURE 2.2. Route of administration of MA admissions: U.S. TEDS, 1992–2006. Data from SAMHSA (2008c).

TABLE 2.1 Demographics and Route of Administration among Primary MA Treatment Admissions in Selected U.S. States: 2006

	Hawaii	California	Washington	Iowa	Florida	New York	National
% of all admissions	34	36	18	16	2	0.2	9
% Male	57	57	47	49	39	76	54
% Hispanic	3	38	8	3	7	13	23
% Smoke	97	75	64	66	62	43	66
% Inhale	1	12	1	9	13	26	11
% Inject	2	11	24	24	14	17	18

Note. Data run at *www.icpsr.umich.edu/gi-bin/SDA/SAMHDA/hsda3* and SAMHSA (2008c).

the Pacific and Mountain States (SAMHSA, 2008a). In Hawaii, the rate of treatment admissions per 100,000 went from 33 in 1992 to 244 in 2005, while in California, it went from 49 to 218 per 100,000 during the same time period. The use of MA/amphetamine increased within certain southern states of the United States, as well, with the rate in Georgia going from 2 in 1992 to 77 in 2005 (SAMHSA, 2007d, 2008a). The route of administration and sociodemographic characteristics of the clients differed by location (see Table 2.1).

Among all MA treatment admissions in 2004, 33% were treated in large central metropolitan areas, 21% in large fringe metropolitan areas, 31% in small metropolitan areas, 9% in nonmetropolitan areas with a city, and 6% in nonmetropolitan areas without a city (rural) (SAMHSA, 2006a). The percentage that smoked the drug was highest in the most urbanized areas (62%) and lowest in the most rural areas (48%) (SAMHSA, 2006a), while the percentage that injected was lowest in large metropolitan areas (between 14% and 15%) and highest in small and nonmetropolitan areas (between 24% and 25%), which reflects the presence of "ice" in the metropolitan areas and powder in the smaller and nonmetropolitan areas (SAMHSA, 2006a).

Deaths

MA-induced and MA-related deaths continued to be geographically concentrated in the Midwest and West. According to the 2003 DAWN report on drug-related mortality, stimulants (reported as either amphetamine or MA) were listed among the top 5 most frequently mentioned drugs in 5 of 32 reporting metropolitan areas, including Minneapolis, Minnesota, Ogden-Clearfield, Utah, Phoenix, Arizona, San Diego, California, and San Francisco, California, and among the top 10 drugs in the states of New Mexico and Utah. The patterns seen in stimulant-related mortality coincide with other known patterns of MA use and abuse, where abuse is most concentrated in the western United States, but spreading to several cities in the midwestern and southeastern United States (SAMHSA, 2005a).

Survey Findings

The 2007 MTF survey reported that past-year use of MA was 1.7% for 12th graders, which represented a significant decrease from the percentage reported in 2006 (2.5%); past year use of "ice" was 1.6% (Johnston et al., 2008). Further, past year use of MA decreased significantly among 8th graders (from 1.8% in 2006 to 1.1% in 2007) and remained relatively stable among 10th graders (from 1.8% in 2006 to 1.6% in 2007) (Johnston et al., 2008).

NSDUH in 2006 estimated that 5.8% of persons ages 12 and older had used MA at least once in their lifetime. This estimate was up slightly (but not significantly) from the adjusted 2005 estimate of 5.2% (SAMHSA, 2007c). Past year and past month percentages of MA use were 0.8% and 0.3%, respectively (SAMHSA, 2007c). The number of recent new users of MA was 259,000 in 2006, which did not differ significantly from the estimate in each year between 2002 and 2005. And in 2006, 277,000 persons ages 12 and older were estimated to be dependent on stimulants, as compared with 273,000 in 2005.

Between 2002 and 2005, persons in nonmetropolitan areas (0.8%) and metropolitan (0.7%) areas were more likely to have used MA in the past year than persons in large metropolitan areas (0.5%) (SAMHSA, 2007a). In 2006, persons in the West (1.6%) were more likely to have used MA in the past year than persons in the South (0.7%), Midwest (0.5%), and Northeast (0.3%) (SAMHSA, 2007c).

In 2006, past-year MA users reported their sources as "from friend or relative for free" (53.6%), "bought from a friend or relative" (21.4%), or "bought from dealer or stranger" (21.1%) (SAMHSA, 2007c). From 2002 to 2005, Native Americans and Alaska Natives were significantly more likely than members of other racial groups to report past year use of MA (2.0% vs. 1.2%) (SAMHSA, 2007b).

Until 2006, when questions about the use of illicitly produced MA were added, the NSDUH stimulant questions were asked as part of the module on nonmedical use of prescription-type drugs, which was appropriate when diverted pharmaceutical amphetamine was the major problem. With the emergence of illegally produced MA, there has been concern about the underestimation of stimulant users in the NSDUH. This underestimation is illustrated by the findings of the National Longitudinal Study of Adolescent Health (Add Health) of persons ages 18–26, which reported past-year use of crystal MA in 2001–2002 at 2.8% (Iritani et al., 2007). This past-year prevalence rate from Add Health was higher than the 2001 NSDUH estimate of past-year MA use among 18- to 25-year-olds (1.7%) (Iritani et al., 2007), and higher than the 2001 MTF estimate of use of crystal MA among 19- to 28-year-olds (1.1%) (Johnston et al., 2002).

U.S. Populations at High Risk

The NSDUH has documented that Native Americans are more likely to report past-year use of MA, and the TEDS treatment data show that the proportion of Native Americans admitted to treatment is greater for MA than for any other substance, except inhalants and alcohol. The Indian Health Service-affiliated outpatient primary care clinics reported that the number of MA-related encounters increased by nearly 250% between 2000 and 2005. In certain areas on the Navajo Nation, MA arrests now exceed alcohol-related arrests (U.S. Department of the Interior, 2007).

Another population at risk is the homeless. A study of urban homeless adults in Los Angeles found that over one-quarter of the overall sample (60% of whites and 10% of blacks) reported lifetime use of MA. Approximately one-tenth of respondents reported current MA use, half used it daily, and almost 90% of current users shared straws to snort MA (Nyamathi et al., 2008).

The use of MA is embedded in many urban gay communities. It is especially sexually arousing and disinhibitory (Paul et al., 1993; Semple et al., 2002; Zule & Desmond, 1999) and is strongly associated with sexual behaviors that put men at risk for HIV infection (Kurtz & Inciardi, 2003; Mansergh et al., 2006). A U.S. survey of young men newly diagnosed with HIV in the southeastern United States found that the number using club drugs (MA, Ecstasy, or other stimulants) increased from 12% in 2000 to 22% in 2005. Being diagnosed with early-stage HIV infection was more likely among those reporting club drug use (OR = 2.44) and men who have sex with men were more likely to be club drug users (OR = 2.28) (Hurt et al., 2007).

In another study of HIV-positive men who have sex with men (MSM), MA users were more than twice as likely to report unprotected receptive anal sex with a partner whose HIV serostatus was negative or unknown and were four times more likely to report that behavior with HIV-positive partners in the past 3 months. HIV-positive MSM may be more likely than HIV-negative MSM to use MA, and some MSM MA users may be more likely than other MA users to use it during sex (Mansergh et al., 2006).

Among heterosexuals, noninjecting MA users engaged in multiple sexual risk behaviors (Molitor et al., 1998) and HIV-negative heterosexuals who had become dependent on MA used the drug to get high, to get more energy, and to party. They reused syringes, shared needles, drank alcohol daily, used other drugs, had unprotected sex, had multiple sex partners (average of 9.4 in the past 2 months), and engaged in "marathon" sex (Semple et al., 2004). An ongoing study in Tijuana suggests that one of the main drugs of choice among female sex workers is MA (Patterson et al., 2005).

Except for studies about using MA for sexual encounters, the literature is still developing about other user groups and their reasons for use. Women are more likely to start using MA to lose weight (von Mayrhauser et al., 2002). There is also evidence that some individuals may use MA in the workplace. This is especially the case for long-distance truck drivers (Hartley & Arnold, 1996; Hartley et al., 1997a, 1997b; Mabbott & Hartley, 1999; McCartt et al., 2000; Williamson et al., 2000). Use by workers was shown in the results of workplace drug testing. The incidence of positive drug tests among general U.S. workforce employees attributed to amphetamines rose from 0.34% in 2002 to 0.48% in 2005 and dropped to 0.42% in 2006 (Quest Diagnostics, 2007). Between 2005 and 2007, there was a 50% decline in the rate of persons testing positive specifically for MA, from 28 per 10,000 in 2005 to 14 per 10,000 in 2007 (Quest Diagnostics, 2008). MA use in the workplace remains an area of concern that warrants further examination.

MA is also a growing problem among Hispanic users (Maxwell et al., 2006). The increase in treatment admissions in Mexico and among Hispanics in the United States may reflect use by migrants and day laborers and men and women in maquiladoras working multiple jobs and long hours.

Mexico

In the 1990s, the use of synthetic drugs, primarily in the form of MA ("cristal"), re-emerged among young people in Mexico (Medina-Mora et al., 1993). Since then, the proportion of persons admitted to treatment nationwide with a primary amphetamine/MA problem has increased from 2% in 1996 to 14% in 2003 (Maxwell et al., 2006).

The 2002 Mexican National Comorbidity Survey estimated that nationwide 0.3% of males and 0.4% of females had ever used "anfetaminas" (98,592 males and 140,496 females), and 0.1% of males and <0.1% of females had used "metanfetaminas" (46,274 males and 9,252 females). In the northern region of the country, overall lifetime use of "anfetaminas" was 0.3% and use of metanfetaminas was 0.1%. In contrast, in the central region, overall lifetime use of "anfetaminas" was 0.4% and use of "metanfetaminas" was <0.1%. Lastly, in the southern region of Mexico, overall lifetime use of "anfetaminas" was 0.1% and use of metanfetaminas was <0.1% (Instituto Nacional de Psiquiatría, 2007).

Data from school surveys in the states of Baja California (across from California) and Sonora (across from Arizona) reported the percentages of students in grades 7–9 who experimented five or fewer times with drugs in 1991 and 2006. In Baja, the rate for amphetamine/MA experimentation by boys increased from 2.6% to 4.6% in this period, while in Sonora, it increased from 2.6% to 6.2%. Surveys on lifetime drug use were conducted in family homes in Tijuana and Ciudad Juarez among persons ages 12 to 65 in 1998 and 2005. Use of amphetamine/MA by males in Tijuana increased from 0.7% to 1.6%, and use by males in Juarez increased from 0.1% to 2.0% (Villatoro et al., 2006).

The increased use of amphetamine/MA in Mexico was partially due to the role of the country in the trafficking and production of illicit drugs. Drugs are stockpiled in Mexican border towns before delivery to the United States, and this has increased the problem with "spillage" (Maxwell, 2003), which has contributed to higher rates of local drug consumption in northern border cities compared with the rest of Mexico (Brouwer et al., 2006). Local residents traffic in drugs by walking quantities across the border. These couriers are often paid in drugs rather than in cash, and the ease of access contributes to the high rates of local drug consumption on both sides. In addition, the perceived availability of drugs has increased and has been associated with increased experimentation and continued use in Mexican adolescents (Villatoro et al., 1998).

In the states on both sides of the U.S.–Mexico border, the proportion of MA/amphetamine admissions has increased. It went from 7% in 1996 to 25% in 2003 in the Mexican border states, and from 12% to 27% in the U.S. border states. In the Mexican border states, the proportion of treatment clients smoking the drug increased from 45% to 74%, while those inhaling MA dropped from 38% in 1997 to 21% in 2003. Only 2% injected MA in 2003 (Maxwell et al., 2006).

MA is the dominant drug on the Pacific Ocean end of the border. In Baja California, 44% of all treatment admissions in 2003 were for MA, as were 31% of all admissions in California. On the Gulf of Mexico side of the border, the proportion of MA admissions in the Mexican states opposite Texas comprised 0% to 1% of all admissions, while in Texas, 8% of admissions in 2003 were for MA. Cocaine was the major drug for which clients entered treatment in 2003 on both sides of the Texas–Mexico border (Maxwell et al., 2006).

Canada

In 2004, the Canadian Addictions Survey (CAS) of persons ages 15 and older asked about the use of "speed." Some 6.4% of all respondents reported lifetime use of "speed," and 0.8% used "speed" in the previous year. Lifetime "speed" use was particularly high among young adults, where 8.3% of 15- to 19-year-olds and 11.2% of 20- to 24-year-olds reported using "speed" at least once in their lives. Among adults (ages 25 or older), the lifetime rate of "speed" use was highest among 45- to 54-year-olds (8.9%). Lifetime use of "speed" was highest in Quebec (8.9%), British Columbia (7.3%), Alberta (6.1%), and Ontario (5.5%) (Adlaf et al., 2005).

Only Manitoba and Ontario have asked about MA use on provincial student surveys, and 2.7% of adolescents in Manitoba in 2001 and 3.3% of students in Ontario in 2003 reported past-year use of MA (Deguire, 2005). A convenience sample of street youths and young adults ages 14 to 30 in 2000 in Vancouver found 71% had tried an ATS at least once in their lifetime, and 57% had used ATS more than ten times (Buxton, 2003). And according to the results of the 2004 "Sex Now" survey of gay men in British Columbia, 9.0% of respondents had used crystal MA; respondents who reported having unprotected sex were 2.6 times more likely to have used crystal MA than respondents who reported engaging only in safe sex (Trussler et al., 2006).

The Western Canadian Summit on Methamphetamine in 2005 concluded that MA use was increasing among certain subpopulations of inhabitants. A low prevalence of use was reported for the general population, but an increase in use was identified among street-involved youth, gay men, and young adults in the club scene. Contrary to the results of the household survey, summit participants thought the highest prevalence of use and production to be in Western Canada, with movement from west to east. Indicators of hospital admissions, police contacts, clients seeking treatment, and number of clandestine labs seized were increasing (Vancouver Coastal Health, 2005).

MA and Amphetamine Use
in Central and South America and the Caribbean

In South America, some 0.7% of the population reported past-year use of amphetamine or MA in 2005 (UNODC, 2007b). In recent years, the trafficking of the precursor chemicals has become problematic in both Central America and the Caribbean. Controlled precursor ingredients, including ephedrine and pseudoephedrine, are legally imported into countries in the region, and are then transported into either North or South America where they are used in the illicit production of MA (International Narcotics Control Board [INCB], 2006). In Guatemala, MA/amphetamine is ranked as the second most prevalent drug, while it is ranked between third and sixth in prevalence in other countries in this area (UNODC, 2007b). Insignificant quantities of the drug have been seized throughout South America, but drug use surveys of residents have shown that stimulant use is becoming more prevalent in some countries, including Peru and Argentina (INCB, 2006).

MA and Amphetamine Use in Europe

According to the EMCDDA (2006), injection of amphetamines has been a long-term problem in Europe. Recently, however, more European countries have reported either seizures or use of MA. Table 2.2 shows that the level of past-year use among persons ages 15 to 64 is 0.5% (0.7% in Western and Central Europe, 0.2% in Southeast Europe, and 0.2% in Eastern Europe) (UNODC, 2007b).

MA ("pervitin") is the most prevalent problem drug in the Czech Republic (Griffiths et al., 2008). The number of problem MA users in the Czech Republic nearly doubled that of problem opiate users (20,500 vs. 11,300) (Zabransky, 2007). It is also the number one drug among

TABLE 2.2. Annual Prevalence of Amphetamine/MA Use, 2005, or Latest Year Available

	Number of users	% use in population 15–64 years	Seizures of amphetamines by region[a]
Europe	2,750,000	0.5	
West and Central Europe	2,220,000	0.7	5,949
Southeast Europe	180,000	0.2	1,411
Eastern Europe	350,000	0.2	123
Americas	5,710,000	1.0	
North America	3,790,000	1.3	6,300
South America	1,920,000	0.7	
Asia	13,700,000	0.5	16,128
Oceania	620,000	2.9	328
Africa	2,100,000	0.4	3,460
Global	24,890,000	0.6	

Note. Data from UNODC (2007b).
[a]Amphetamine, MA, and related stimulants in kilogram equivalents.

individuals seeking treatment in Slovakia and in some subpopulations in Hungary (EMCDDA, 2006). In the Czech Republic, Slovakia, Finland, and Sweden, amphetamine and MA account for between 25% and 50% of all treatment admissions, and anywhere from one- to two-thirds of these users inject the drug (EMCDDA, 2006). It is also an increasing problem in Latvia and Lithuania, and it is the second most common drug reported in possession cases in Poland, where treatment episodes are increasing (Reference Group to the United Nations on HIV and Injecting Drug Use, 2008). In the Russian Federation, frequent MA and amphetamine use has been found to be a strong predictor of HIV infection (Koslov et al., 2006).

In Austria, use is increasing (Reference Group to the United Nations on HIV and Injecting Drug Use, 2008); in Belgium, 11% of calls to phone drug help lines were about MA or amphetamine (Reference Group to the United Nations on HIV and Injecting Drug Use, 2008); in Germany, treatment admissions for the drug have increased, and smoking and inhaling were the most common routes of administration (Reference Group to the United Nations on HIV and Injecting Drug Use, 2008). In Denmark, there is evidence of increased treatment need among young adults using this drug (Reference Group to the United Nations on HIV and Injecting Drug Use, 2008); in Italy, population surveys show increasing use; in the Netherlands, use is common among school dropouts and juvenile detainees, and it tends to be snorted or swallowed (Reference Group to the United Nations on HIV and Injecting Drug Use, 2008). In the UK, MA use was reported as low and stable, but injected amphetamine sulphate has been a longstanding part of the "drugs scene" (Advisory Council on the Misuse of Drugs, 2005). MA use was reported to be limited in France, Greece, and Ireland. Ireland's National Drug Trend Monitoring System (DTMS) Pilot Study reported the primary route of administration was ingestion (43%), followed by inhalation (40%), injection (3%), or a combination of ingestion/injection (2%) (O'Gorman et al., 2007).

Griffiths et al. (2008) have speculated that the lower levels of MA use in Europe may be due to the nature of the stimulant market in Europe and the lack of any current popular appeal for the drug. In some countries, amphetamine is widely available for injection, and cocaine consumption in Europe is rising and the price has fallen (Griffiths et al., 2008).

MA and Amphetamine Use in Africa

In Africa, 0.4% of the population reported past-year use of amphetamine or MA in 2005 (Table 2.2; UNODC, 2007b). The stimulant khat is widely used in some African countries, with MA being a problem primarily in South Africa. The South African Community Epidemiology Network on Drug Use (SACENDU) reported admissions for primary MA abuse were very low (or nonexistent) in all provinces except for Cape Town. In the second half of 2006, 52% of Cape Town treatment patients reported a primary or secondary MA (a.k.a., "tik"), and the number of patients increased from 1,551 in the second half of 2002 to 2,798 in the second half of 2006 (Parry et al., 2007; Pluddemann et al., 2007). The majority of MA patients in Cape Town were young, male (72%) and Colored (90%), with 8% white, 1% Indian/Asian, and 1% Black/African (Parry et al., 2007; Pluddemann et al., 2007).

MA and Amphetamine Use in Asia

Southeast Asia, along with North America, is a leading producer of MA. This area experienced an MA epidemic in the period 1997–2001. Since then, the situation has stabilized in many countries, but trafficking and use are still increasing in parts of the Mekong region, and there is evidence of large-scale manufacturing in Cambodia, Indonesia, Malaysia, and the Philippines. In this region, MA is usually smoked, but it is also ingested (Mcketin et al., 2008). The forms of MA produced vary by country. Myanmar and Thailand together accounted for 83% of seizures of the MA pill "yaba" in 2006. In 2005 and 2006, China accounted for more than 70% of all seizures of crystal MA ("shabu") in the region and, along with the Philippines in 2004 and Indonesia in 2006, made 92% and 86% respectively, of all regional seizures of "shabu" during those years (UNODC, 2007a).

According to the UNODC 2007 World Drug Report, Brunei, Cambodia, Japan, Lao PDR, Philippines, and Thailand cited MA as the leading drug of concern. The crystal form of the drug ("shabu") was the only form of MA seen in Brunei, Japan, and the Philippines, while in Cambodia, Lao PDR, and Thailand, "yaba" or "yama" pills are the common form of the drug. Only Thailand and China cited abuse of both the pill and crystal forms of MA (UNODC, 2007a). In Asia, 0.5% of the population reported past-year use of amphetamine in 2005 (Table 2.2; UNODC, 2007b).

Since the late 1990s, Cambodia has been both an MA manufacturing site and major transshipment area, and MA pills are the leading drug of abuse. Abuse of both crystal MA and the powder form are increasing (UNODC, 2007a). And although heroin is the leading drug of abuse in China, crystal MA and MA pills are the second- and third-largest drug problems (INCB, 2006). The number of MA and ecstasy pills seized during 2006 was nearly double the amount seized during the previous year (UNODC, 2007a).

In Hong Kong, abuse of crystal MA ("ice") was first noted during the early 1990s, and law enforcement officials believe that the number of MA abusers has been relatively stable for the past few years (UNODC, 2007a); use of ketamine and Ecstasy are more common (McKetin et al., 2008). In India, while MA/amphetamine is not a leading drug problem at present, abuse appears to be increasing in some parts (INCB, 2006) and the seizure of clandestine laboratories during the past several years suggest that the potential for abuse or trafficking of the drug should be monitored (INCB, 2006).

MA/amphetamine is not the leading drug of abuse in Indonesia, but increased use has been reported. The quantity of crystal MA seized more than tripled between 2005 and 2006, and the number of MA pills almost doubled (UNODC, 2007a). Likewise, the drug is not a major problem in Malaysia, but the number of "yaba" tablets seized went from 92,549 in 2004 to 193,764 in the first half of 2006 (Tsay, 2006).

The major drug of abuse in Japan in 2006 was crystal MA, as it has been for many decades. Since 2000, 80% to 90% of all drug-related arrests involved MA, and injection is the preferred route of administration (UNODC, 2007a).

In the Republic of Korea, 68% of treatment admissions were for MA use (Tsay, 2006). "Shabu" is the major form abused in the Philippines, with, 81% of all treatment admissions in 2005 reporting use of "shabu" (Tsay, 2006). In Taiwan, 94% of treatment admissions in 2006 reported problems with heroin, with 30% also reported problems with MA (Tsay, 2006). Over one-half of admissions in Singapore in 2006 were for MA. In these countries, the drug is usually smoked.

MA pills are the leading drug problem in Lao PDR (UNODC, 2007a), where the drug is typically smoked. Despite the high levels of MA production in Myanmar, heroin and opium are the leading drugs of abuse (McKetin et al., 2008). The leading drugs of concern in Thailand were "yaba" pills and "crystal" ("ice") (UNODC, 2007a), and smoking was the primary route of administration. In Vietnam in 2006, there has been an increase in the abuse of MA pills, which are usually swallowed (UNODC, 2007a).

MA and Amphetamine in Oceania

There are indications that Oceania may be developing into a significant transit area and a potential consumption area for MA (INCB, 2006). Organized criminal groups use the region as a transshipment area for ATS, including MDMA and MA (INCB, 2006).

The 2004 Australian National Drug Strategy Survey reported that 9.1% of Australians ages 14 and older had ever used amphetamine or "speed" for nonmedical purposes, and 3.2% had used in the past year. Of the respondents, 74% used powder MA, 41% used "crystal" ("ice"), 27% used the more moist form of the drug, which is called "base," "paste," or "pure," and 11% used a tablet form of MA (Australian Institute of Health and Welfare, 2005a, 2005b). Use of crystal MA has increased to the levels of use of "speed" powder (O'Brien et al., 2007). There has been an increase in both importation and local manufacturing of the drug, and while use of powder MA remains low and stable, there are increases in use of crystal MA among regular drug users (Degenhardt et al., 2008).

In New Zealand, an increasing number of people receiving treatment for drug abuse are identifying MA as their primary drug of abuse. It is the third most commonly abused drug, following alcohol and cannabis (INCB, 2006), and, in 2004, 10% of treatment episodes involved this drug (Adamson et al., 2006). "Ice" in New Zealand is known as "pure" or "P." The illicit manufacture of MA is increasing in New Zealand, where 204 laboratories were dismantled in 2005, compared with 182 in 2004 (INCB, 2006).

In Guam, crystal MA ("Shabu") poses a serious illicit drug threat. Half of the individuals admitted for substance abuse treatment in 1997 and 1998 were MA users. "Shabu," typically smoked in a glass pipe or vial, is readily available because of a steady supply of the drug from the Philippines, as well as from Hong Kong, China, Taiwan, and South Korea (U.S. Department of Justice, 2003).

MA has recently supplanted marijuana as the most serious drug threat in American Samoa. Local law enforcement authorities point to rising MA abuse as the cause of a rise in violent crime in the territory. Powdered MA use is limited, as most users prefer to smoke "ice" (U.S. Department of Justice, 2001).

Acknowledgments

This research was supported by the Center for Substance Abuse Treatment Cooperative Agreement UD1 TI13423 to the Gulf Coast Addiction Technology Transfer Center and Cooperative Agreement UD1 TI13594 to the Pacific Southwest Addiction Technology Transfer Center.

References

Adamson S, Sellman D, Deering D, et al. (2006). Alcohol and drug treatment population profile: A comparison of 1998 and 2004 data in New Zealand. *New Zealand Med J* 119(1244), 287.
Adlaf EM, Begin P, Sawka E (Eds). (2005). *Canadian Addiction Survey (CAS):*

A national survey of Canadians' use of alcohol and other drugs: Preva-lence of use and related harms: Detailed report. Ottawa, Ontario: Cana-dian Centre on Substance Abuse.

Advisory Council on the Misuse of Drugs. (2005) Author. *Methamphetamine review 2005: Executive summary.* London: Retrieved, September 4, 2007, from *drugs.homeoffice.gov.uk/publication-search/acmd/ACMD-meth-exec-summ-Nov-2005?view=Binary.*

Anglin MD, Burke C, Perrochet B, et al. (2000). History of the methamphet-amine problem. *J Psychoact Drugs* 32(2):137–141.

Australian Institute of Health and Welfare. (2005a). *2004 National Drug Strat-egy Household Survey: First Results.* Canberra, ACT: Author.

Australian Institute of Health and Welfare. (2005b). *2004 National Drug Strat-egy Household Survey: Detailed Findings.* Canberra, ACT: Author.

Brouwer KC, Case P, Ramos R, et al. (2006). Trends in production, trafficking, and consumption of methamphetamine and cocaine in Mexico. *Subst Use Misuse* 41(5):707–727.

Buxton J. (2003). Vancouver drug use epidemiology. Vancouver site report for the Canadian Community Epidemiology Network on Drug Use. Vancou-ver, BC: Canadian Community Epidemiology Network on Drug Use.

Cunningham JK, Liu LM. (2005). Impacts of federal precursor chemical regula-tions on methamphetamine arrests. *Addiction* 100:479–488.

Degenhardt L, Baker A, Maher L. (2008). Methamphetamine: Geographic areas and populations at risk, and emerging evidence for effective interventions. *Drug Alcohol Rev* 27(1):217–219.

Degenhardt L, Roxburgh A, Black E, et al. (2008). The epidemiology of meth-amphetamine use and harm in Australia. *Drug Alcohol Rev* 27(1):243–252.

Deguire A-E. (2005). *Fact Sheet on Methamphetamine.* Ottawa, ONT: Cana-dian Centre on Substance Abuse. Retrieved July 27, 2007, from *www.ccsa.ca/2005%20%CCSA%20DOCUMENTS/ccsa-011134-2005.pdf*

Drug Enforcement Administration. (2008). *System to Retrieve Information on Drug Evidence* (STRIDE) Database, March 12, 2008.

European Monitoring Centre for Drugs and Drug Addiction [EMCDDA]. (2006). *The state of the drugs problem in Europe: Annual report 2006.* Luxembourg: Office for Official Publications of the European Communi-ties.

Griffiths P, Mravcik V, Lopez D, et al. (2008). Quite a lot of smoke but very limited fire. The use of methamphetamine in Europe. *Drug Alcohol Rev* 27(3):236–242.

Hartley LR, Arnold PK. (1996). *Management of fatigue in the road transport industry. Recommendations from the Second International Conference on Fatigue in Transport.* Fremantle: Western Australian Department of Transport.

Hartley LR, Arnold PK, Penna F, et al. (1997a). *Fatigue in the Western Aus-tralian transport industry Part 1: The principle and comparative findings.* (Institute for Research in Safety and Transport Report No. 117). Freman-tle: Western Australian Department of Transport.

Hartley LR, Penna F, Corry A, et al. (1997b). *Comprehensive review of fatigue research*. (Institute for Research in Safety and Transport Report No. 226).

Hurt C, Green K, Torrone E, et al. (2007, July). *Methamphetamine and club drug use is frequent among recently infected HIV-positive young men who have sex with men in North Carolina, United States*. Poster exhibition: 4th International AIDS Society, Sydney, Australia. Conference on HIV Pathogenesis, Treatment and Prevention.

Instituto Nacional de Psiquiatría. (2002). *Mexican National Comorbidity Survey*. Special data run: prevalencias de anfetaminas, received September 24, 2007.

International Narcotics Control Board [INCB]. (2006). *The Report of the International Narcotics Control Board for 2006* (E/INCP/2006/1). Vienna, Austria: United Nations.

Iritani BJ, Hallfors DD, Bauer DJ. (2007). Crystal methamphetamine use among young adults in the USA. *Addiction* 102:1102–1113.

Israel-Adams H, Topolski J. (2003). *Patterns and trends in drug abuse in St. Louis: Epidemiologic trends in drug abuse, Vol. II*. (Proceedings of the Community Epidemiology Work Group, June 2003). Bethesda, MD: National Institute on Drug Abuse.

Joe-Laidler K, Morgan P. (1997). Kinship and community: The "ice" crisis in Hawaii. In H Klee (Ed), *Amphetamine misuse: International perspectives on current trends* (pp. 113–134). Amsterdam: Harwood Academic.

Johnston LD, O'Malley PM, Bachman JG. (2002). *Monitoring the Future national survey results on drug use, 1975–2001. Vol. II: College students and adults ages 19–40* (NIH Publication No. 02-5107). Bethesda, MD: National Institute on Drug Abuse.

Johnston LD, O'Malley PM, Bachman JG, et al. (2008). *Monitoring the Future national results on adolescent drug use: Overview of key findings, 2007* (NIH Publication No. 08-6418). Bethesda, MD: National Institute on Drug Abuse.

Kozlov AP, Shaboltas AV, Toussova OV, et al. (2006). HIV incidence and factors associated with HIV acquisition among injection drug users in St Petersburg, Russia. *AIDS* 20(6):901–906.

Kurtz SP, Inciardi JA. (2003). Crystal meth, gay men, and circuit parties. *Law Enforce Exec Forum* 3:97–114.

Ling W, Rawson R, Shoptaw S. (2006). Management of methamphetamine abuse and dependence. *Curr Psychiatry Rep* 8:345–354.

Mabbott NA, Hartley LR. (1999). Patterns of stimulant drug use on Western Australian heavy transport routes. *Transport Res* Part F2(2):115–130.

Mansergh G, Purcell DW, Stall R, et al. (2006). CDC consultation on methamphetamine use and sexual risk behavior for HIV/STD infection: Summary and suggestions. *Pub Health Rep* 121:127–132.

Maxwell JC. (2003). Profiles of methamphetamine users as seen in various data sets. *Law Enforce Exec Forum* 3(3):77–88.

Maxwell JC. (2004). Substance abuse trends in Texas, June 2004. Austin, TX: Gulf Coast Addiction Technology Transfer Center. Retrieved July 27, 2007, from *www.utexas.edu/research/cswr/gcattc/Trends/trends604.pdf*.

Maxwell JC, Cravioto P, Galvan F, et al. (2006). Drug use and risk of HIV/ AIDS on the Mexico-US border: A comparison of treatment admissions in both countries. *Drug Alcohol Depend* 82(Suppl. 1):S85–S93.

Maxwell JC, Rutkowski BA. (2007). Authors' Community Epidemiology Work Group meeting notes dated June 15, 2007.

McCartt AT, Rohrbaugh JW, Hammer MC, et al. (2000). Factors associated with falling asleep at the wheel among long-distance truck drivers. *Accident Anal Prevent* 32:493–504.

McKetin R, Kozel N, Douglas J, et al. (2008). The rise of methamphetamine in Southeast and East Asia. *Drug Alc Rev* 27(3):220–228.

Medina-Mora ME, Rojas E, Juarez F, et al. (1993). Consumption of psychotropic substances in a Mexican junior and senior high school population. *Salud Mental* 16(3):2–8.

Molitor F, Truax S, Ruiz J, et al. (1998). Association of methamphetamine use during sex with risky sexual behaviors and HIV infection among non-injection drug users. *Western J Med* 168:93–97.

National Clandestine Laboratory Database [NCLD]. (2007). *Maps of methamphetamine lab incidents, 1999–2006.* Washington, DC: U.S. Drug Enforcement Administration.

National Clandestine Laboratory Database [NCLD]. (2008). *Maps of methamphetamine lab incidents, 1999–2007.* Washington, DC: U.S. Drug Enforcement Administration.

Nyamathi A, Dixon E, Shoptaw S, et al. (2008). Profile of lifetime methamphetamine use among homeless adults in Los Angeles. *Drug Alcohol Depend* 92(1–3):277–281.

O'Brien S, Black E, Degenhardt L, et al. (2007). *Australian drug trends 2006: Findings from the Illicit Drug Reporting System (IDRS).* Sydney: National Drug and Alcohol Research Centre.

Office of Diversion Control. (2008). *National Forensic Laboratory Information System: Year 2007 Annual Report.* Washington, DC: U.S. Drug Enforcement Administration.

O'Gorman A, Doyle M, Crean D, et al. (2007). *National Drug Trend Monitoring System pilot study: Summary report.* Dublin, Ireland: National Advisory Committee on Drugs.

Parry C, Pluddemann A, Bhana A. (2007). *Alcohol and drug abuse trends: July–December 2006 (Phase 21).* Tygerberg, South Africa: Medical Research Council, South African Community Epidemiology Network on Drug Abuse.

Patterson TL, Semple SJ, Bucardo J, et al. (2005, June). *A comparison of drug use patterns and HIV/STD prevalence among female sex workers in two Mexican–U.S. border cities.* Paper presented at the 67th annual meeting of the College on Problems of Drug Dependence, Orlando, FL.

Paul JP, Stall R, Davis F. (1993). Sexual risk for HIV transmission among gay/ bisexual men in substance abuse treatment. *AIDS Ed Prevention* 5(1):11–24.

Pluddemann A, Myers B, Parry C. (2007). *Fact Sheet—Methamphetamine.* Tygerberg, South Africa: Medical Research Council, South African Community Epidemiology Network on Drug Abuse.

Quest Diagnostics. (2007). *Amphetamines use declined significantly among US workers in 2005, according to Quest Diagnostics' drug testing.* Retrieved July 1, 2007, from *www.questdiagnostics.com/employersolutions/dti/2007_03/dti_index.html.*

Quest Diagnostics. (2008). *Monthly trends in workplace drug testing, through December 2007.* Retrieved May 7, 2008, from *www.whitehousedrugpolicy.gov/news/press08/quest_data.pdf.*

Reference Group to the United Nations on HIV and Injecting Drug Use, (2008). *The global epidemiology of meth/amphetamine injection.* Sydney: National Drug and Alcohol Research Centre, University of New South Wales.

Semple SJ, Patterson TL, Grant I. (2002). Motivations associated with methamphetamine use among HIV+ men who have sex with men. *J Sub Abuse Treat* 22(3):149–156.

Semple SJ, Patterson TL, Grant I. (2004). The context of sexual risk behavior among heterosexual methamphetamine users. *Addict Behav* 29:807–810.

Substance Abuse and Mental Health Services Administration [SAMHSA]. (1996). *Substance abuse in states and metropolitan areas: Model-based estimates from the 1991–1993 National Household Surveys on Drug Abuse.* (Office of Applied Studies Analytic Paper, DHHS Publication No. SMA 96-3095). Rockville, MD. Retrieved September 15, 2007, from *oas.samhsa.gov/96state/ch3.htm#Ex3.2A.*

Substance Abuse and Mental Health Services Administration [SAMHSA]. (2005a). *Drug Abuse Warning Network, 2003: Area profiles of drug-related mortality.* (DAWN Series D-27, DHHS Publication No. SMA 05-4023). Rockville, MD: Office of Applied Studies, U.S. Department of Health and Human Services.

Substance Abuse and Mental Health Services Administration [SAMHSA]. (2005b). *The Drug and Alcohol Services Information System (DASIS) Report, smoked methamphetamine/amphetamines: 1992–2002.* Retrieved from *www.oas.samhsa.gov/2k4/methSmoked/methSmoked.pdf.*

Substance Abuse and Mental Health Services Administration [SAMHSA]. (2006a). *The DASIS Report: Methamphetamine/amphetamine treatment admissions in urban and rural areas, 2004.* Rockville, MD: Office of Applied Studies, U.S. Department of Health and Human Services.

Substance Abuse and Mental Health Services Administration [SAMHSA]. (2006b). *Treatment Episode Data Set (TEDS). Highlights–2005. National admissions to substance abuse treatment services* (DASIS Series: S-36, DHHS Publication No. SMA 07-4229). Rockville, MD: Office of Applied Studies, U.S. Department of Health and Human Services.

Substance Abuse and Mental Health Services Administration [SAMHSA]. (2007a). *The NSDUH Report: Methamphetamine use.* Retrieved July 27, 2007, from *www.oas.samhsa.gov/2k7/meth/meth.htm.*

Substance Abuse and Mental Health Services Administration [SAMHSA]. (2007b). *The NSDUH Report: Substance use and substance use disorders among American Indians and Alaska Natives.* Retrieved January 19, 2007, from *www.oas.samhsa.gov/2k7/AmIndians/AmIndians.pdf.*

Substance Abuse and Mental Health Services Administration [SAMHSA]. (2007c). *Results from the 2006 National Survey on Drug Use and Health:*

National findings (Office of Applied Studies, NSDUH Series H-32, DHHS Publication No. SMA 07-4293). Rockville, MD: Office of Applied Studies, U.S. Department of Health and Human Services.

Substance Abuse and Mental Health Services Administration [SAMHSA]. (2007d). Special data run: Primary methamphetamine/amphetamine admissions by state or jurisdiction: 2005. Data downloaded on June 29, 2007.

Substance Abuse and Mental Health Services Administration [SAMHSA]. (2007e). *Treatment Episode Data Set (TEDS): 1995–2005. National admissions to substance abuse treatment services* (DASIS Series: S-37, DHHS Publication No. SMA 07-4234). Rockville, MD: Office of Applied Studies, U.S. Department of Health and Human Services.

Substance Abuse and Mental Health Services Administration [SAMHSA]. (2008a). *The DASIS Report: Geographic differences in substance abuse treatment admissions for methamphetamine/amphetamine and marijuana: 2005.* Rockville, MD: Office of Applied Studies, U.S. Department of Health and Human Services.

Substance Abuse and Mental Health Services Administration [SAMHSA]. Drug Abuse Warning Network. (2008b). *National estimates of drug-related emergency department visits, 2005.* Rockville, MD: Office of Applied Studies, U.S. Department of Health and Human Services.

Substance Abuse and Mental Health Services Administration [SAMHSA]. (2008c). *Treatment Episode Data Set (TEDS). Highlights—2006. National admissions to substance abuse treatment services* (DASIS Series: S-40, DHHS Publication No. SMA 08-4313). Rockville, MD: Office of Applied Studies, U.S. Department of Health and Human Services.

Trussler T, Marchand R, Gilbert M. (2006). *Sex now, numbers rising: Challenges for gay men's health.* Vancouver, BC: Community-Based Research Centre.

Tsay W. (2006). *Highlights of AMCEWG meeting 2006.* Taipei: Taiwan National Bureau of Controlled Drugs.

United Nations Office on Drugs and Crime [UNODC] Regional Centre for East Asia and the Pacific. (2007a). *Patterns and trends of amphetamine-type stimulants (ATS) and other drugs of abuse in East Asia and the Pacific 2006.* Bangkok, Thailand: United Nations. Retrieved September 2, 2007, from *www.apaic.org.*

United Nations Office on Drugs and Crime [UNODC]. (2007b). *World drug report, 2007.* Vienna, Austria: UNODC Research and Analysis Section. Retrieved July 27, 2007, from *www.unodc.org/pdf/research/wdr07/WDR_2007.pdf.*

U.S. Department of Health and Human Services [US DHHS], Substance Abuse and Mental Health Services Administration [SAMHSA]. (2007). *Treatment Episode Data Set (TEDS), 1992–2005.* Concatenated data [Computer file]. Original data prepared by Synectics for Management Decisions, Incorporated. ICPSR ed. Ann Arbor, MI: Inter-university Consortium for Political and Social Research [producer and distributor]. Data downloaded June 30, 2007.

U.S. Department of the Interior. (2007). *Safe Indian communities: Departmental highlights, DH 43-46.* Retrieved August 29, 2007, from *www.doi.gov/budget/2008/08Hilites/DH43.pdf.*

U.S. Department of Justice, National Drug Intelligence Center. (2001). *American Samoa drug threat assessment,* Product No. 2001-S0388AS-001, Jonestown, PA.

U.S. Department of Justice, National Drug Intelligence Center. (2003). *Guam drug threat assessment,* Product No. 2003-S0388GU-001. Jonestown, PA.

Vancouver Coastal Health. (2005). *Western Canadian summit on methamphetamine: Bringing together practitioners, policy makers and researchers, Consensus panel report.* Vancouver, BC: Author. Retrieved July 27, 2007, from *www.sfu.ca/dialogue/Meth_Booklet_2005_Final.pdf.*

Villatoro JA, Medina-Mora ME, Juarez F, et al. (1998). Drug use pathways among high school students of Mexico. *Addiction* 93(10):1577–1588.

Villatoro JA, Medina-Mora ME, Gutierrez-Lopez D, et al. (2006). *Drug use among 7th–9th grade students in Baja California and Sonora and general population trends in drug use in Tijuana and Ciudad Juarez: 1998–2005* (Border Epidemiology Work Group Proceedings). Bethesda, MD: National Institute on Drug Abuse.

von Mayrhauser C, Brecht M, Anglin M. (2002). Use ecology and drug use motivations of methamphetamine users admitted to substance abuse treatment facilities in Los Angeles: An emerging profile. *J Addict Dis* 21(1):45–60.

Williamson A, Feyer A, Friswell R, et al. (2000). *Demonstration project for fatigue management in the road transport industry: Summary of findings.* Consultant Report CR192, Canberra: Australian Transport Safety Bureau.

Zabransky T. (2007). Methamphetamine in the Czech Republic. *J Drug Iss* 37(1):155–180.

Zule WA, Desmond DP. (1999). An ethnographic comparison of HIV risk behaviors among heroin and methamphetamine injectors. *Am J Drug Alcohol Abuse* 25(1):1–23.

Chapter 3

Basic Neuropharmacological Mechanisms of Methamphetamine

Glen R. Hanson and Annette E. Fleckenstein

Methamphetamine (MA), first synthesized in the late 19th century, was, and to a limited degree continues to be, prescribed for a variety of medical and emotional purposes such as attention-deficit/hyperactivity disorders or narcolepsy (Westfall & Westfall, 2006). Superimposed on these clinical issues is the fact that, when not managed properly or if persistently self-administered (especially via smoking, snorting, or intravenous routes) for recreational or nonmedical purposes, this drug often leads to severe psychological and physical dependence that can damage critical brain systems (Chang et al., 2007). The outcomes of such neuropathology may compromise cognitive functions and damage decision-making capacity (Wang, Volkow, et al., 2004; Volkow et al., 2001a, 2001b), leading to destructive behaviors and devastating personal and social consequences. These issues are discussed at length in other chapters of this book and consequently will not be elaborated here other than to note that the why, how, and when of MA influences on these systems is based on how and why this potent stimulant/sympathomimetic agent influences basic cellular mechanisms and neurotransmitter/neuromodulator or hormonal functions. The basic pharmacological effects of MA on these systems are the principal topics of this chapter. To assist the reader this chapter has been divided according to the pre- and postsynaptic impact of both the immediate and long-term consequences of using/abusing MA. The first section discusses how MA influences monoamine presynaptic systems relative to its direct pharmacology as well as its persistent neurotoxicological consequences. The second section focuses on the downstream impact of MA use (both direct and long term) and addresses the postsynaptic consequences of this potent psychostimulant in the central nervous system and throughout the body.

Presynaptic Monoaminergic Pharmacology

Monoamine Synthesis and Metabolism

MA administration rapidly alters the function of several proteins that serve as key regulators of intra- and extraneuronal monoamine concentrations. Among these is tyrosine hydroxylase (TH), the rate-limiting enzyme in the synthesis of dopamine (DA). Three decades ago Gibb and coworkers (Kogan et al., 1976; Koda & Gibb, 1973) demonstrated in a rodent model that repeated high doses of MA, administered in regimens designed to mimic binge use in humans, decrease the activity of striatal TH, thus decreasing DA levels, as assessed during the first hours and days following MA treatment. In contrast, a single MA exposure did not affect (Haughey et al., 1999; Bakhit & Gibb, 1981) or increase (Haughey et al., 1999) TH activity in the caudate and/or globus pallidus, as assessed early after treatment. It is noteworthy that the effects of MA can be brain region–specific, as evidenced by findings that a single MA injection acutely and concurrently decreased and increased TH activity in the core and shell of the rat nucleus accumbens, respectively (Haughey et al., 1999).

In addition to effects on dopaminergic systems, MA treatment rapidly decreases the activity of tryptophan hydroxylase (TPH; Bakhit & Gibb, 1981; Peat et al., 1985; Stone et al., 1989a; Fleckenstein et al., 1997a; Haughey et al., 1999), the enzyme that catalyzes the conversion of tryptophan to 5-hydroxytryptophan, thus contributing to the formation of 5-hydroxytryptamine (serotonin, 5-HT), as assessed in numerous rat brain regions. Reactive oxygen species produced as a consequence of MA treatment (described below) likely contribute to this inhibition, as evidenced by findings that this decrease in TPH activity caused by MA or a related compound, methylenedioxymethamphetamine (MDMA) can be restored *in vitro* by incubation in a reducing environment (Stone et al., 1989a, 1989b; Fleckenstein et al., 1997a).

The effects of MA are not limited to dopaminergic and serotonergic systems. For example MA-induced decreases in norepinephrine (NE) content have also been reported (Morgan & Gibb, 1980).

Adding to the complexities of effects on monoaminergic systems, MA decreases the activity of monoamine oxidase (Suzuki et al., 1980; Kitanaka et al., 2003); an enzyme that contributes to the degradation of DA, 5-HT, and NE.

Plasmalemmal Monoamine Transporters

Plasmalemmal monoamine transporters including the DA transporter (DAT) are other important regulators of monoamine disposition, as these are responsible for the reuptake of extraneuronal monoamines, such as DA, into nerve terminals. Thus amphetamine analogues such as MA are a substrate for the DAT (Zaczek et al., 1991; Sonders et al., 1997; Sitte et al., 1998; Xie et al., 2000). Not surprisingly, this protein is the conduit through which these agents cause DA release (Raiteri et al., 1979; Fischer & Cho, 1979; Liang & Rutledge, 1982; Kahlig et al., 2005; for a review, see Fleckenstein et al., 2007), thereby contributing to its reinforcing properties.

The impact of MA on DAT is not, however, restricted to its releasing properties. For example a single *in vivo* injection of MA rapidly (within 1 hour) and reversibly (within 24 hours) decreases the V_{max} of rat striatal DA uptake (Fleckenstein et al., 1997b), as assessed in synaptosomes prepared from treated rats. This phenomenon is not caused by residual MA introduced by the original parenteral injection (Fleckenstein et al., 1997b; see also Kokoshka et al., 1998a, 1998b). A similar phenomenon has been reported after *in vitro* MA application (Sandoval et al., 2001). Notably, neither of these *in vitro* nor *in vivo* effects are associated with a decrease in binding of the DAT ligand, WIN35428 (Kokoshka et al., 1998a; Sandoval et al., 2001). Neither administration of DA antagonists nor prevention of MA-induced hyperthermia inhibits the single injection-induced deficit (Metzger et al., 2000). One possible explanation for this seeming disconnect between uptake via and binding to the DAT may be that MA causes internalization of the DAT, as has been reported *in vitro* after amphetamine application (Saunders et al., 2000; Sorkina et al., 2003).

Elegant studies by Vaughan and colleagues (Cervinski et al., 2005) indicate that phosphorylation contributes to the effects of MA on DAT. In particular, MA administration to rats increases DAT phosphorylation. MA application *in vitro* to rat DAT LLC-PK(1) cells or striatal tissue increases DAT phosphorylation as well. Both MA-induced phosphorylation of the DAT and a concurrent decrease in DA transport *in vitro* are protein kinase C (PKC)-dependent, a finding reminiscent of previously reported data (Sandoval et al., 2001).

In contrast to effects of a single injection and as noted above, many studies have focused on the acute impact of repeated administrations of MA over the course of many hours in an attempt to mimic the "runs" wherein human abusers binged on these agents. As after a single MA injection, these regimens rapidly decrease DAT function, an effect attributable to a reduced V_{max} (Kokoshka et al., 1998a). Neither residual drug introduced by the original subcutaneous injections nor an acute loss of striatal DAT protein appears to contribute to this phenomenon (Kokoshka et al., 1998a); instead, this decrease is both DA-receptor and reactive oxygen species–mediated (Metzger et al., 2000). It is worth noting that the magnitude of the deficit induced by repeated MA injections is greater than after a single injection, only partially reversed 24 hours after treatment, and associated with a decrease in the B_{max} of WIN35428 binding, suggesting that the decrease resulting from repeated injections may comprise more than one phenomenon (Kokoshka et al., 1998a; for a review, see Fleckenstein et al., 2000).

In addition to the decrease in uptake described above, Baucum et al. (2004) reported that repeated administrations of MA promote formation of higher-molecular-weight (>170 kDa) DAT-associated protein complexes. As with deficits in DA uptake, both hyperthermia and DA contribute to this formation. Sulfhydryl bridges likely contribute to complex formation because coincubation with the reducing agent, beta-mercaptoethanol, converts some complexes from a greater-than 170 kDa to a 70 kDa species.

Reminiscent of its interaction with DAT, MA is also a substrate for the 5-HT transporter (SERT; Johnson et al., 1998) and causes 5-HT release (Kuczenski et al., 1995). Also redolent of effects on DAT, a single MA injection rapidly decreases 5-HT transport, a phenomenon independent of MA-induced DA receptor activation or hyperthermia (Haughey et al., 2000a). Yet another similarity to effects on DAT is that repeated MA injections decrease 5-HT transport via DA receptor- and hyperthermia-dependent mechanisms. However—and unlike the ability of multiple MA administrations to rapidly decrease DAT ligand binding—repeated high-dose MA injections do not rapidly alter binding of the SERT ligand paroxetine (Haughey et al., 2000a).

Finally amphetamine, and presumably MA, is a substrate for the NE transporter (NET; Schwartz et al., 2005) and causes NE release (Kuczenski et al., 1995). However, and in contrast to the DAT and SERT, NET function is not affected by MA treatment once it is "washed" from the tissue preparation (Haughey et al., 2000b).

Vesicular Transporters

In addition to the DAT, the vesicular monoamine transporter-2 (VMAT-2) is a critical mediator of amphetamine- and MA-induced DA release (for an excellent review, see Sulzer et al., 2005). It is widely accepted that the weak base properties of amphetamine and its analogs contribute to DA release. In particular, these agents enter neurons via both diffusion and transporters. These drugs then diffuse into and accumulate in vesicles, thus disrupting the proton electrochemical gradient required for DA sequestration and promoting increased cytoplasmic DA accumulation. DA is then released via the DAT as noted above (for a review, see Sulzer et al., 2005; Fleckenstein et al., 2007; see also Johnson, 1988; Sulzer & Rayport, 1990; Sulzer et al., 1993, 1995; but see also Floor & Meng, 1996).

In addition to disrupting DA sequestration, MA treatment appears to alter the distribution of VMAT-2, and presumably associated vesicles, within nerve terminals. Evidence for this trafficking arises from studies by Brown et al. (2000), who reported that repeated high-dose injections of MA to rats rapidly (within 1 hour) decrease cytoplasmic vesicular DA uptake. This effect persists for at least 24 hours. Concurrently, Sonsalla and coworkers (Hogan et al., 2000) reported that MA administration decreases both DA uptake and binding of the VMAT-2 ligand dihydro-tetrabenazine (DHTBZ), as assessed in mice 24 hours after treatment in a purified vesicular preparation. However, DHTBZ binding is not altered in whole striatal homogenates at this point. These data were the first to highlight the disparity between homogenates and vesicle preparations and provided an important clue suggesting VMAT-2 trafficking. Subsequently Riddle et al. (2002) reported that repeated high-dose MA administrations rapidly redistribute rat striatal VMAT-2 immunoreactivity from synaptic vesicle-enriched nonmembrane (presumably cytoplasmic) subcellular fractions to a location not retained in the preparation of the synaptosomes.

Recent studies by Eyerman and Yamamoto (2007) suggest a mechanism underlying the acute effect of repeated MA injections on VMAT-2. In particular, MA treatment not only rapidly decreases cytoplasmic VMAT-2 immunoreactivity but also increases nitrosylation of synaptosomal VMAT-2 protein; the former effect is attenuated by administration of a neuronal nitric oxide synthase inhibitor.

Of relevance are findings that neither vesicular glutamate (GLU), acetylcholine, nor GABA transporter immunoreactivity appear altered acutely after amphetamine treatment (Riddle et al., 2007). However, there is evidence to suggest that the vesicular GLU transporter-1 (VGLUT1) is affected hours after MA treatment. In particular, MA treatment increases striatal VGLUT1 protein in subcellular fractions, cortical VGLUT1 mRNA, and the V_{max} of striatal vesicular GLU uptake, as assessed several hours after treatment. The MA-induced increases in cortical VGLUT1 mRNA, as well as striatal VGLUT1 are mediated via GABA-A receptors (Mark et al., 2007).

Reactive Oxygen and Nitrogen Species

Both *in vivo* and *in vitro* MA exposure can promote formation of reactive oxygen species (Cubells et al., 1994; Giovanni et al., 1995; Fleckenstein et al., 1997a; Yamamoto & Zhu, 1998; for review, see also Hanson et al., 2004; Cadet et al., 1998, 2003; Brown & Yamamoto, 2003; Yamamoto & Bankston, 2005). Cubells et al. (1994) was among the first to demonstrate this formation. In particular, these investigators provided *in vitro* data suggesting that MA treatment rapidly alters vesicular DA sequestration that in turn promotes aberrant accumulation of intraneuronal DA and the generation of reactive oxygen species. In addition, studies by LaVoie and Hastings (1999) indicate that oxidation of DA contributes to MA-induced toxicity to DA terminals. In addition to reactive oxygen species, reactive nitrogen species are formed after MA treatment and probably contribute to MA-induced deficits (Anderson & Itzhak, 2006; Imam et al., 2001; Itzhak & Ali, 1996).

Metabolic Consequences

One important contributor to the pharmacological effects of MA is its ability to alter intraneuronal energy balance. In particular, MA treatment depletes striatal ATP content in mice (Chan et al., 1994); MA-induced inhibition of mitochondrial function was subsequently demonstrated (Burrows et al., 2000a). Metabolic inhibitors enhance MA- and amphetamine-induced damage to DA systems, and substrates of energy metabolism attenuate this toxicity (Albers et al., 1996; Burrows et al., 2000b; Stephans et al., 1998; Wan et al., 1999). Interestingly, striatal dopaminergic terminals appear to be more vulnerable than 5-HT terminals are to damage caused by metabolic stress (Burrows et al., 2000b).

Synaptogenesis, Sensitization, and Tolerance

Repeated administration of psychostimulants over a period of weeks produces persistent alterations in dendritic structure (Robinson & Kolb, 1997; Li et al., 2003). For example one such MA regimen increased the number of mushroom and thin spines on medium spiny neurons in the dorsolateral striatum, as assessed 3 months later (Jedynak et al., 2007). In contrast, MA treatment decreased mushroom spines in the dorsomedial striatum in this same study. Robinson and colleagues have suggested that these structural alterations may result from changes in glutamatergic innervation of these striatal subregions and that this may affect the development of stimulus–response habits (Jedynak et al., 2007).

It is likely that structural modification of neuronal networks is involved in behavioral sensitization, a phenomenon characterized by long-lasting hypersensitivity to the drug after cessation of repeated (often daily) exposures. It is important to note that repeated MA treatment can cause behavioral sensitization. This phenomenon is accompanied by an increase in dopaminergic transmission (Nishikawa et al., 1983; Kazahaya et al., 1989).

Repeated MA administration causes not only sensitization but also tolerance, depending on the drug regimen employed. For example, the persistent dopaminergic and/or serotonergic deficits caused by a neurotoxic MA regimen can be attenuated by pretreatment with MA (Stephans & Yamamoto, 1996; Danaceau et al., 2007; Johnson-Davis et al., 2003, 2004; Schmidt et al., 1985a; Gygi et al., 1996). A variety of mechanisms contribute to this phenomenon, including alterations in brain MA distribution, VMAT-2 function, and MA-induced hyperthermia.

Neurotoxic Consequences

It is well established that high-dose MA administration causes persistent reductions in striatal DA content, DAT density, and/or activity of TH in rodents (Hotchkiss et al., 1979; Wagner et al., 1980; Guilarte et al., 2003; see also Gibb et al., 1994; Brown & Yamamoto, 2003; Marshall et al., 2007; Volz et al., 2007) and nonhuman primates (Woolverton et al., 1989). Dopaminergic deficits have been observed in chronic human MA users as well (Wilson et al., 1996; Volkow et al., 2001a; Sekine et al., 2001). Notably, younger rats appear less vulnerable to dopaminergic deficits than older animals do (Cappon et al., 1997; Pu & Vorhees, 1993; Kokoshka et al., 2000; see also Truong et al., 2005).

The deficits induced by MA are not, however, limited to DA neurons, as MA causes persistent serotonergic deficits. This is evidenced by findings of persistent deficits in SERT levels, the activity of TPH, and/or 5-HT levels (Hotchkiss et al., 1979; Haughey et al., 1999; Ricaurte et al., 1980; Guilarte et al., 2003; see also Gibb et al., 1994).

Several phenomena contribute to the persistent monoaminergic deficits caused by MA treatment. For example MA-induced hyperthermia contributes to this damage, as hypothermia prevention attenuates these long-term deficits (Albers & Sonsalla, 1995; Bowyer et al., 1993, 1994; see also Farfel & Seiden, 1995). This effect may be due, in part, to the contribution of hyperthermia to MA-induced reactive species formation (Fleckenstein et al., 1997a; LaVoie & Hastings, 1999).

Studies utilizing an array of strategies, including quantifying formation of reactive species (see references above), administering antioxidants/radical scavengers (Wagner et al., 1985; DeVito & Wagner, 1989), and/or administering MA to superoxide dismutase transgenic mice (Cadet et al., 1994) indicate that reactive species contribute to persistent deficits in monoaminergic neuronal function (for a review, see Brown & Yamamoto, 2003). DA also contributes, most likely by promoting reactive species formation, as MA-induced deficits are prevented by pretreatment with the TH inhibitor, alpha-methyl-p-tyrosine (Gibb & Kogan, 1979; Wagner et al., 1983; Schmidt et al., 1985b; see also Axt et al., 1990). Related to this, aberrant VMAT-2 function likely contributes to the deficits caused by MA by promoting cytoplasmic DA accumulation and reactive species formation (Fumagalli et al., 1999; for a review, see Fleckenstein et al., 2003).

Notably, studies indicate that MA promotes the formation of autophagic granules, especially in neuronal varicosities and cell bodies of dopaminergic neurons (Larsen et al. 2002).

Dopamine D_1 receptors have long been implicated in mediating the persistent monoaminergic deficits caused by MA. For example pretreatment of rats with the D_1 receptor antagonist SCH23390 prevents the dopaminergic and serotonergic deficits caused by the stimulant (O'Dell et al., 1993; Sonsalla et al., 1986; Xu et al., 2005). This protective effect on dopaminergic neurons is, at least in part, likely unrelated to any potential D_1 antagonist-induced inhibition of MA-induced hyperthermia (Xu et al., 2005; see also Albers & Sonsalla, 1995). D_2 receptors have been implicated in contributing to the persistent dopaminergic deficits caused by MA as well, as evidenced by findings that pretreatment with D_2 antagonists prevent the persistent damage caused by the stimulant (Buening & Gibb, 1974; Sonsalla et al., 1986; O'Dell et al., 1993; Xu et al., 2005), an effect that, at least in part, is independent of its ability to prevent hyperthermia (Xu et al., 2005; see also Broening et al., 2005).

GLU is yet another likely contributor to the persistent deficits caused by MA treatment, as evidenced by findings that administration of the NMDA antagonist MK801 prevents monoaminergic deficits (Bowyer et al., 2001; Sonsalla et al., 1989; Pu & Vorhees, 1995; Ali et al., 1994). One confound to these studies is that MK801 prevents MA-induced hyperthermia, and this may contribute to the neuroprotection (although see Bowyer et al., 2001).

An additional mechanism contributing to MA-induced DA deficits has been proposed by Yamamoto and colleagues (Mark et al., 2004). In particular, these investigators have suggested that MA increases D_1-mediated striatonigral GABA-ergic transmission. This in turn activates $GABA_A$ receptors in the substantia nigra pars reticulata. This activation causes a decrease in GABA-ergic nigrothalamic activity and an increase in corticostriatal GLU release, leading to long-term dopaminergic deficits.

Notably, many of the toxic processes described above (i.e., reactive species formation, altered VMAT-2 function, etc.) begin during the course of the MA treatment. Interestingly and despite these early toxic insults, evidence suggests that the neurotoxic effects of MA can be reversed by posttreatment with a variety of pharmacological interventions, including administration of lobeline (Eyerman & Yamamoto, 2005), amfonelic acid (Marek et al., 1990), or methylphenidate (Sandoval et al., 2003). Accordingly, events occurring later (i.e., 8–24 hours after treatment), and perhaps triggered by these initial insults, must also be linked to the persistent DA deficits caused by MA. Among the delayed events that may contribute to the persistent effects of MA is activation of microglia (Thomas et al., 2004).

Postsynaptic Pharmacology

As discussed at the beginning of the chapter, the direct effects of MA alter the cellular management of monoamine amine neurotransmitters and hormones. Typically, although not universally, the ultimate outcome of such effects is to increase the extracellular concentrations of dopamine, 5-HT, and NE (John & Jones 2007; Fleckenstein et al. 2007; Yui et al. 2004). As discussed earlier, these effects are caused by the efflux of monoamines through reversal of VMAT-2 and plasmalemmal monoamine transporters and by interfering with enzymatic inactivation of these neurotransmitter substances via monoamine oxidase metabolism (Fleckenstein et al., 2003, 2007; Tekes & Magyar, 2000). The immediate consequences of the elevated extracellular monoamines are concentration dependent and principally mediated by the specific receptor targets of these critical messenger substances. It is not possible to provide an exhaustive discussion of all the postsynaptic consequences of MA-induced elevation of extracellular monoamine amines in a single chapter; however, we will provide a broad overview of systems affected while dealing in some detail with a few postsynaptic systems to provide the reader an appreciation of how this stimulant works and what can be expected from its pharmacology both by the patient using MA for prescribed medical purposes as well as by the MA-dependent person who is abusing or addicted to this potent stimulant.

Dose-Dependent Nature of Pharmacological Response

MA has been shown to have a dose-dependent impact on extracellular monoamine concentrations (Kuczenski et al., 1995; Pereira et al., 2006; Melega et al., 1995). The outcome of this response is that the pattern of postsynaptic consequences (e.g., postsynaptic receptor activation) can be quite different in those using MA for prescribed medical purposes versus that associated with high doses often seen in severe addiction. Thus the high monoamine efflux consequent to high-dose bingeing by smoking or intravenous injection of MA will likely result in neurotoxicity and extremely high extracellular concentrations of these neurotransmitters interacting with their respective postsynaptic receptors (10- to 50-fold increase; Stephans & Yamamoto, 1994) in a manner distinct from that which occurs following low doses of MA seen during properly managed therapy (100–300% increase; Pereira et al., 2006). This is partially explained by the fact that the various monoamine postsynaptic receptor subtypes vary according to their affinity for the respective neurotransmitter. For example the DA system is responsible for many of the addictive and therapeutic properties of MA (Vollm et al., 2004; Baumann et al., 2002). Two types of DA receptors linked to MA effects are D_1 and D_2 subtypes. It is thought that in the dorsal striatum the D_2 receptors have the higher affinity, are more likely activated by lower increases in DA release, and are selectively associated with the striatopallidal indirect feedback projections for the basal ganglia systems (Castel et al., 1994; Hamada et al., 2004). In contrast, the D_1 DA receptor has a lower affinity for DA and is somewhat selectively linked to the striatonigral direct feedback pathway for these same basal ganglia systems and thus more likely to be stimulated by higher DA activation (Surmeier et al., 2007; Castel et al., 1994; Hamada et al., 2004; Richfield et al., 1989). In addition, D_2 receptors are typically viewed as inhibitory, with a direct effect to reduce the activity of adenylate cyclase while D_1 receptors are characterized as stimulatory and enhance adenylate cyclase activity (Hutson & Suman-Chauhan, 1990). Thus it has been reported that high doses of MA cause effects that are dominated by D_1 receptor activation, while low-dose use appears to effect CNS changes dominated by D_2 receptor mechanisms. It is likely that similar dose–response patterns of MA effects on DA receptors occur in both the basal ganglia and limbic systems (Alburges et al., 2001a, 2001b; Hanson et al., 1991, 1995). Because D_1- and D_2-mediated effects can be opposite in mechanism and impact, effects of high doses of MA are not just an enhanced expression of low doses, but can be completely distinct, if not antagonistic (Alburges et al., 2001a, 2001b; Hanson et al., 2002; Frankel et al., 2005). Although the details of how this occurs and the functional consequences have not been completely resolved, it is important to appreciate that the cellular pharmacologies of high- and low-dose MA use can be very different. A clinical implication of this difference is that the neurotoxicity commonly associated with severe MA dependence likely does not occur with therapeutic management of relatively low doses. As we describe some of the postsynaptic pharmacological effect of MA, we refer back to this critical point of differential dose-dependent MA actions when relevant.

It could be argued that similar dose–response considerations also would apply to MA-induced release of 5-HT and NE. However because this issue has not been investigated in these monoamine systems, the possibility will only be proposed without additional discussion.

Temporal Considerations of MA Postsynaptic Effects

Another important outcome when considering the effects of MA on postsynaptic systems relates to the duration of exposure as well as the temporal patterns of drug administration. MA is frequently used over long periods of time both as a therapy (e.g., long-term treatment of chronic conditions such as attention-deficit/hyperactivity disorder) as well as a consequence of addiction. The fact that MA is often taken for months or even years in both low and high doses raises the possibility that repeated exposures to MA may alter postsynaptic responses. This is probably the case in the processes of tolerance and sensitization reported to be caused by repeated administrations of MA. The expression and nature of MA-induced tolerance and sensitization appear to be related to both dosing and temporal factors (i.e., escalating doses and how often the drug is administered; Danaceau et al., 2007; O'Neil et al., 2006; Segal & Kuczenski 2006; Davidson et al., 2005; Ishikawa et al., 2005; Brady et al., 2005; Comer et al., 2001). Although the exact mechanisms of these MA-induced phenomena are not well established, it is thought they might involve glutamatergic D_1 receptor or pharmacokinetic mechanisms (Suzuki et al., 2003; Moriguchi et al., 2002; Schmidt et al., 1985a), and contribute to the addiction process and side effects of this potent stimulant (Comer et al., 2001). One intriguing suggestion has been that long-term changes such as sensitization may have to do with plastic processes such as synaptogenesis (Ujike et al., 2002), described above; however determining whether and how remodeling of synaptic contacts is involved with the impact of persistent MA use requires additional research. The temporal nature of MA effects has been minimally studied owing to their complexity. The vast majority of laboratory animal research has focused on the pharmacology of single or multiple MA administrations in adult male animals during a relatively short period of time. There are no reported studies examining MA exposures that more accurately represent the chronic condition because months, if not years, of drug administration would be necessary in order to match the typical clinical situation. Understandably, such extensive longitudinal research would be extremely expensive and difficult to accomplish. Consequently, we know little about how such MA experiences affect monoamine and other related systems, with the exception of apparent long-term mono-amine deficits reported in animal models exposed to a neurotoxic regimen of MA (Cadet et al., 2007; Hanson et al., 2004) and apparently replicated in MA addicts (Scott et al., 2007; Wang, Volkow, et al., 2004; Volkow 2001a, 2001b).

Response of Specific Postsynaptic Systems to MA

As explained earlier, MA influences downstream events principally through activation of monoamine postsynaptic receptors due to the dramatic release of the related transmitter substances. Again for the sake of brevity, this chapter focuses principally on the dopamine systems because of their well-established role in the addictive and therapeutic impact of MA use. However, although this is not discussed in detail, the reader is reminded that serotonergic and noradrenergic systems may also make significant contributions to both short- and long-term consequences of MA exposure (for a review see Fleckenstein et al., 2000). In order to develop an appreciation for the many elements of MA pharmacology, this chapter provides some detail as to how MA administration influences the relationships that exist between DA pathways and linked glutamate, GABA, cholinergic, and neuropeptide systems. Because other chapters in this book deal more with the functional outcomes of MA, this chapter focuses more on the CNS neurobiological consequences of this drug.

Glutamatergic

Glutamate pathways are ubiquitous throughout the extrapyramidal and limbic systems of the brain and universally exert an excitatory input to most projections associated with these structures. Consequently, changes in DA activity following MA administration certainly affect both basal as well as stimulated glutamate activity. Although the precise mechanisms of these interactions are complicated and appear to involve glutamatergic receptors (Mark et al., 2007), related processes associated with these MA-induced glutamate functions likely include linkages of extrapyramidal and limbic DA systems with glutamatergic projections from the frontal cortex, thalamus, hippocampus, and various feedback loops (Stephans & Yamamoto, 1994; Burrows & Meshul, 1999; Tata & Yamamoto, 2007; Raudensky & Yamamoto, 2007; Mark et al., 2004; Miyamoto et al., 2004). Much of the research has suggested that the MA-induced changes in glutamatergic functions are related to D_1 receptor activation (Mark et al., 2004). In fact, the administration of the NMDA antagonist MK801 has been shown to block several D_1-linked effects of MA on neuropeptide systems of both extrapyramidal and limbic structures (Hanson et al., 1995; Singh et al., 1992). There also exists some evidence that DA D_2 receptors might also contribute to the responses of glutamate to psychostimulants (Liu et al., 2006). An important role for glutamatergic mechanisms in MA abuse and the development of dependence has been suggested by the research of Kalivas and colleagues (Kalivas, 2007; Cornish & Kalivas, 2001) and others (Mark et al., 2004; Yamamoto et al., 1999), suggesting that medications with glutamatergic mechanisms may have some therapeutic value in dealing with MA. This intriguing theory remains to be substantiated.

GABA-ergic

Like glutamatergic projections, GABA-ergic neurons are ubiquitous and are thought to represent the most prominent inhibitory system in the brain. These projections are associated with throughput loops in both the extrapyramidal and limbic systems and are closely linked with associated DA pathways (Galvan & Wichmann, 2007; Tisch et al., 2004; Viggiano et al., 2003). Consequently, it is not surprising that exposure to MA probably has both excitatory (likely via D_1 receptors) and inhibitory (likely via D_2 receptors) effects on GABA activity (Mark et al., 2004; Zhang et al., 2006). These MA-mediated changes in GABA function are likely related to pass-through, projection feedback, and interneuronal systems (Mark et al., 2004; Bustamante et al., 2002; Burrows & Meshul, 1999; Floran et al., 1997; Zhu et al., 2006a, 2006b). Due to the broad influence of these inhibitory pathways, it has been suggested that modulation of GABA systems may have value in treatment of MA dependence (Brody et al., 2005), although it is not clear what the overall impact of MA on GABA-ergic activity is, nor what specific effect drugs that modulate this system would have on MA-related effects.

Cholinergic

Basal ganglia and limbic cholinergic systems are for the most part associated with interneurons (Selden et al., 1994). When released, the neurotransmitter acetylcholine acts on families of nicotinic and muscarinic receptors that can have either excitatory or inhibitory functions, depending on the system. The effect of MA on acetylcholine release and ultimately its impact on nicotinic or muscarinic receptors has not been well studied. It has been reported that low doses of MA increase the release of acetylcholine in the dorsal and ventral striatum (Taguchi et al., 1998), while high doses can alter nicotinic receptors (Garcia-Rates et al., 2007) and perhaps damage cholinergic interneurons (Zhu et al., 2006a, 2006b;

Kish et al., 1999; Ikarashi et al., 1997); however the functional impact of this effect is not known, and there is no indication that blockade of either cholinergic receptor type has much of an influence on MA-medicated actions.

Neuropeptidergic

It is interesting that the effects of MA on DA-related neuropeptides systems linked to the basal ganglia and nucleus accumbens are some of the most thoroughly studied of the postsynaptic responses to this stimulant. These neuropeptides include neurotensin, substance P, dynorphin, and metenkephalin, and they are found in striatal and nucleus accumbens efferent feedback projections (Gygi et al., 1993; Matorana et al., 2003; Adams et al., 2001; Ikemoto et al., 1995; Castel et al., 1994; Horner & Keefe 2006; Gerfen et al., 1984, 1991; Zahm et al., 1996). Although many details are lacking, in general it is believed that, overall, substance P, neurotensin, dynorphin, and metenkephalin have inhibitory feedback influence on nigrostriatal and mesolimbic DA pathways. Following acute exposure to high doses of MA, the tissue levels of neuropeptides generally are elevated (Hanson et al., 1991, 2002; Gygi et al., 1994), and the expression of the precursor mRNA (Smith & McGinty, 1994; Merchant et al., 1994; Adams et al., 2000, 2003) is also increased. However, much less is known about the functional significance of these MA-induced neuropeptide changes. Microdialysis has been used to evaluate the impact of MA treatment on the extracellular content of neurotensin and substance P. Surprisingly, despite dramatic changes in peptide tissue levels and mRNA expression, high doses of MA do not appear to significantly alter the release of either neurotensin or substance P in extrapyramidal and limbic structures (Frankel et al., 2005; Wagstaff et al., 1996; Hanson et al., 2002). The functional relevance of this finding is not clear.

In contrast, these findings revealed that low doses of this drug approximately double the release of both neurotensin and substance P in the caudate, substantia nigra, globus pallidus, and nucleus accumbens. This increase is blocked by both a DA D_1 and D_2 antagonist, demonstrating that these neuropeptide changes are mediated by a combination of the activation of these two DA receptors. With the use of selective receptor antagonists and antibodies, it was determined that the neurotensin response to low-dose MA has a dampening effect on the DA release being caused by MA as well as MA-induced locomotor and rearing activity (Wagstaff et al., 1994). Interestingly, the substance P studies suggest a similar inhibitor feedback function on DA projections as the neurotensin (Gygi et al., 1993; Wang, Boules, et al., 2004). These findings are a little surprising because both neurotensin and substance

P have excitatory properties when applied directly onto caudate and nucleus accumbens neurons (Reid et al., 1990; Chapman et al., 1992); consequently, these two neuropeptide systems may exert their inhibitory influence indirectly on DA function by activating an inhibitory system that releases GABA (Ferraro et al., 1998). Regardless of the mechanism, in general it appears that low-dose MA-related activation of these neuropeptide systems serves to mitigate the DA response to this stimulant, whereas these neuropeptide functions are not evident after administering high doses of MA.

In other studies examining the impact of low (therapeutically relevant) MA doses on neuropeptide responses it has been found that both DA D_1 and D_2 receptors have distinct roles. As mentioned earlier, it might be expected that, because D_2 receptors have a higher affinity than D_1 receptors do for DA, low doses of MA would cause neuropeptide changes that appear to selectively reflect an increase in D_2 activity. Although this has not been thoroughly researched, support for this theory has been reported in that striatal neurotensin, metenkephalin and substance P levels decrease after 0.5 mg/kg MA (Alburges et al., 2001a, 2001b; Wagstaff et al., 1996), an effect also observed following administration of a selective D_2 agonist (Singh et al., 1992). In contrast, as mentioned earlier, high doses of MA (drug doses comparable to what is observed in addiction) elevate both neurotensin and metenkephalin levels in this structure, much like selective D_1 agonists (Singh et al., 1992). The potential clinical significance of this observation is that the mechanisms of MA as a therapy likely differs from those responsible for its use in the addiction process.

Although most of the research on the neuropeptide responses to MA has been short term, one study did examine the long-term impact of high doses of MA on neuropeptides. The only neuropeptide changes that appeared to persist after such a treatment were observed in caudate substance P levels (Chapman et al., 2001). Changes in substance P tissue levels in the caudate nucleus were still observed as long as 6 weeks after MA exposure. Little is known as to the functional significance of this long-term substance P change; however, it is believed that it likely reflects a persistent postsynaptic consequence of MA neurotoxicity on the nigrostriatal DA pathway (see above for details).

Other CNS Systems

While much of the CNS effects of MA are thought to be associated with the impact of this drug on extrapyramidal and mesolimbic functions, it is also reported that exposure to MA changes other brain regions that are associated with monoamine pathways such as the frontal cortex, hypothalamus, and hippocampus. In summary, the effects of MA on these systems reflect increases in extracellular DA, norepinephrine, or 5-HT caused by this stimulant. The postsynaptic functional consequences of these effects on the monoamine systems include the following.

FRONTAL CORTEX

It is speculated that much of the therapeutic benefit of low doses of MA in the treatment of ADHD reflects the ability of this drug to increase DA activity in the frontal cortex (Arnsten, 2006). The precise postsynaptic mechanism of this effect is not known, although it may involve glutamate and/or GABA functions to manage subcortical brain activities, such as that which occurs in the caudate nucleus (Diaz et al., 2003; Carlsson, 2001; Viggiano et al., 2003). Generally, it is thought that MA therapy helps to reestablish the balance between DA functions of the mesocortical and nigrostriatal systems, resulting in appropriate management (both inhibition and activation) of behavior tracks by the prefrontal cortex.

HYPOTHALAMUS

As with the other two brain regions, the hypothalamus includes DA, 5-HT, and noradrenergic projections that are activated by MA administration. The precise postsynaptic MA-induced consequences by these monoaminergic systems have not been not been well studied. However, it is thought that the ability of MA to release DA, 5-HT, and noradrenaline almost certainly contributes to the effect of amphetamine-like drugs on stress response (Rotllant et al., 2007; Harris et al., 2006; Smith et al., 2004), autonomic functions (Klemfuss & Adler, 1986), and possibly immune suppression (In et al., 2005; Ligueiro-Olivera et al., 2004). All of these possibilities have been suggested but require additional investigation.

HIPPOCAMPUS

Although it is well established that MA administration can have profound effects on the hippocampal monoaminergic systems, the functional relevance of the associated postsynaptic impact has not been identified. Because the hippocampus is an emotional center, some of the changes in stress responses, emotions, and memory associated with MA use may reflect the hippocampal changes caused by this drug (Tata & Yamamoto, 2007; Gasbarri et al., 1997).

Postsynaptic Long-Term Consequences

As explained earlier, multiple high doses of MA have neurotoxic potential on some monoamine systems. These presynaptic monoaminergic deficits are probably responsible for the long-term changes observed in striatal and substantia nigral substance P tissue levels discussed earlier. However others have also reported that these high-dose MA exposures may also result in postsynaptic apoptosis in the interneurons of the caudate nucleus (Thiriet et al., 2005). These effects are thought to be associated with neuropeptide Y–related interneurons in the caudate and possibly mediated by the effects of MA on substance P systems (Zhu et al., 2006a). This possibility remains to be confirmed and linked to a functional correlation.

Blood–Brain Barrier

High doses of MA are known to disrupt the blood–brain barrier, especially in the limbic regions, and possibly are linked to MA-mediated neurotoxicity (Bowyer & Ali, 2006). It has been suggested that the breakdown of the blood–brain barrier may be related to MA-induced hyperthermia and its pro-oxidative properties (Sharma et al., 2007); however, the duration and long-term consequences of the phenomenon are unknown.

Cardiovascular System

MA use can cause vasoconstriction and elevated blood pressure that result in significant cardiac damage and compromise the function of the heart, leading to arrhythmias, ischemic episodes, and hemorrhaging. In extreme conditions this can be fatal. These problems are more likely to occur in users who have a history of cardiovascular disease and in those who abuse MA by self-administering high doses for long periods of time (Kaye et al., 2007). Some of the chronic damage to the heart may also be a consequence of long-term inflammatory processes induced by the drug (Varner et al., 2002).

Conclusion

This chapter has dealt with the pharmacological effect of MA. This information should help the reader appreciate the tremendous complexity of this potent stimulant and its capacity to cause profound short- and long-term effects to the user. When used properly, MA's effects can be managed and help control mental health problems such as ADHD. When not properly supervised, self-administration of this drug can escalate, resulting in persistent CNS damage to extrapyramidal and limbic functions as well as long-term toxicity reflected in aberrant sleep, memory, and cognitive functions (Cadet et al., 2007), as well as potentially life-threatening cardiovascular consequences (Varner et al., 2002).

References

Adams DH, Hanson GR, Keefe KA. (2000). Cocaine and methamphetamine differentially affect opioid peptide mRNA expression in the striatum. *J Neurochem* 75:2061–2070.

Adams DH, Hanson GR, Keefe KA. (2001). Differential effects of cocaine and methamphetamine on neurotensin/neuromedin N and preprotachykinin messenger RNA expression in unique regions of the striatum. *Neuroscience* 102:843–851.

Adams DH, Hanson GR, Keefe KA. (2003). Distinct effects of methamphetamine and cocaine on preprodynorphin messenger RNA in rat striatal patch and matrix. *J Neurochem* 84:87–93.

Albers DS, Sonsalla PK. (1995). Methamphetamine-induced hyperthermia and dopaminergic neurotoxicity in mice: Pharmacological profile of protective and nonprotective agents. *J Pharmacol Exp Ther* 275:1104–1114.

Albers DS, Zeevalk GD, Sonsalla PK. (1996). Damage to dopaminergic nerve terminals in mice by combined treatment of intrastriatal malonate with systemic methamphetamine or MPTP. *Brain Res* 718:217–220.

Alburges ME, Keefe KA, Hanson GR. (2001a). Unique responses of limbic met-enkephalin systems to low and high doses of methamphetamine. *Brain Res* 905:120–126.

Alburges ME, Keefe KA, Hanson GR. (2001b). Contrasting responses by basal ganglia met-enkephalin systems to low and high doses of methamphetamine in a rat model. *J Neurochem* 76:721–729.

Ali SF, Newport GD, Holson RR, et al. (1994). Low environmental temperatures or pharmacologic agents that produce hypothermia decrease methamphetamine neurotoxicity in mice. *Brain Res* 658:33–38.

Anderson KL, Itzhak Y. (2006). Methamphetamine-induced selective dopaminergic neurotoxicity is accompanied by an increase in striatal nitrate in the mouse. *Ann NY Acad Sci* 1074:225–233.

Arnsten AF. (2006). Fundamentals of attention-deficit/hyperactivity disorder: circuits and pathways. *J Clin Psychiatry* 67(Suppl. 8):7–12.

Axt KJ, Commins DL, Vosmer G, et al. (1990). Alpha-methyl-p-tyrosine pretreatment partially prevents methamphetamine-induced endogenous neurotoxin formation. *Brain Res* 515:269–276.

Bakhit C, Gibb JW. (1981). Methamphetamine-induced depression of tryptophan hydroxylase: recovery following acute treatment. *Eur J Pharmacol* 76:229–233.

Baucum AJ, Rau KS, Riddle EL, et al. (2004). Methamphetamine increases dopamine transporter higher molecular weight complex formation via a dopamine- and hyperthermia-associated mechanism. *J Neurosci* 24:3436–3443.

Baumann MH, Phillips JM, Ayestas MA, et al. (2002). Preclinical evaluation of GBR12909 decanoate as a long-acting medication for methamphetamine dependence. *Ann N Y Acad Sci* 965:92–108.

Bowyer JF, Gough B, Slikker W, Jr, et al. (1993). Effects of a cold environment or age on methamphetamine-induced dopamine release in the caudate putamen of female rats. *Pharmacol Biochem Behav* 44:87–98.

Bowyer JF, Holson RR, Miller DB, et al. (2001). Phenobarbital and dizocilpine can block methamphetamine-induced neurotoxicity in mice by mechanisms that are independent of thermoregulation. *Brain Res* 919:179–183.

Bowyer JF, Ali S. (2006). High doses of methamphetamine that cause disruption of the blood-brain barrier in limbic regions produce extensive neuronal degeneration in mouse hippocampus. *Synapse* 60:521–532.

Bowyer JF, Davies DL, Schmued L, et al. (1994). Further studies of the role of hyperthermia in methamphetamine neurotoxicity. *J Pharmacol Exp Ther* 268:1571–1580.

Brady AM, Glick SD, O'Donnell P. (2005). Selective disruption of nucleus accumbens gating mechanisms in rats behaviorally sensitized to methamphetamine. *J Neurosci* 25:6687–6695.

Brody JD, Figueroa E, Laska EM, et al. (2005). Safety and efficacy of gammvinyl GABA (GVG) for the treatment of methamphetamine and/or cocaine addiction. *Synapse* 55:122–125.

Broening HW, Morford LL, Vorhees CV. (2005). Interactions of dopamine D_1 and D_2 receptor antagonists with D-methamphetamine-induced hyperthermia and striatal dopamine and serotonin reductions. *Synapse* 56:84–93.

Brown JM, Hanson GR, Fleckenstein AE. (2000). Methamphetamine rapidly decreases vesicular dopamine uptake. *J Neurochem* 74:2221–2223.

Brown JM, Yamamoto BK. (2003). Effects of amphetamine on mitochondrial function: Role of free radicals and oxidative stress. *Pharmacol Exp Ther* 99:45–53.

Buening MK, Gibb JW. (1974). Influence of methamphetamine and neuroleptic drugs on tyrosine hydroxylase activity. *Eur J Pharmacol* 26:30–34.

Burrows KB, Gudelsky G, Yamamoto BK. (2000a). Rapid and transient inhibition of mitochondrial function following methamphetamine or 3,4-methylenedioxymethamphetamine administration. *Eur J Pharmacol* 398:11–18.

Burrows KB, Meshul CK. (1999). High-dose methamphetamine treatment alters presynaptic GABA and glutamate immunoreactivity. *Neuroscience* 90:833–850.

Burrows KB, Nixdorf WL, Yamamoto BK. (2000b). Central administration of methamphetamine synergizes with metabolic inhibition to deplete striatal monoamines. *J Pharmacol Exp Ther* 292:853–856.

Bustamante D, You ZB, Castel MN, et al. (2002). Effect of single and repeated methamphetamine treatment on neurotransmitter release in substantia nigra and neostriatum of the rat. *J Neurochem* 83:645–654.

Cadet JL, Brannock C. (1998). Free radicals and the pathobiology of brain dopamine systems. *Neurochem Int* 32:117–131.

Cadet JL, Jayanthi S, Deng X. (2003). Speed kills: Cellular and molecular bases of methamphetamine-induced nerve terminal degeneration and neuronal apoptosis. *FASEB J* 17:1775–1788.

Cadet JL, Krasnova IN, Jayanthi S, et al. (2007). Neurotoxicity of substituted amphetamines: Molecular and cellular mechanisms. *Neurotox Res* 11:183–202.

Cadet JL, Sheng P, Ali S, et al. (1994). Attenuation of methamphetamine-induced neurotoxicity in copper/zinc superoxide dismutase transgenic mice. *J Neurochem* 62:380–383.

Cappon GD, Morford LL, Vorhees CV. (1997). Ontogeny of methamphetamine-induced neurotoxicity and associated hyperthermic response. *Brain Res Dev Brain Res* 103:155–162.

Carlsson ML. (2001). On the role of prefrontal cortex glutamate for the antithetical phenomenology of obsessive compulsive disorder and attention deficit hyperactivity disorder. *Prog Neuropsychopharmacol Biol Psychiatry* 25:5–26.

Castel MN, Morino P, Nylander I, et al. (1994). Differential dopaminergic regulation of the neurotensin striatonigral and striatopallidal pathways in the rat. *Eur J Pharmacol* 262:1–10.

Cervinski MA, Foster JD, Vaughan RA. (2005). Psychoactive substrates stimulate dopamine transporter phosphorylation and down-regulation by cocaine-sensitive and protein kinase C-dependent mechanisms. *J Biol Chem* 280:40442–40449.

Chan P, Di Monte DA, Luo JJ, et al. (1994). Rapid ATP loss caused by methamphetamine in the mouse striatum: Relationship between energy impairment and dopaminergic neurotoxicity. *J Neurochem* 62:2484–2487.

Chang L, Alicata D, Ernst R, et al. (2007). Structural and metabolic brain changes in the striatum associated with methamphetamine abuse. *Addiction* 102(Suppl. 1):16–31.

Chapman DE, Hanson GR, Kesner RP, et al. (2001). Long-term changes in basal ganglia function after a neurotoxic regimen of methamphetamine. *J Pharmacol Exp Ther* 296:520–527.

Chapman MA, See RE, Bissette G. (1992). Neurotensin increases extracellular striatal dopamine levels in vivo. *Neuropeptides* 22:175–183.

Comer SD, Hart CL, Ward AS, et al. (2001). Effects of repeated oral methamphetamine administration in humans. *Psychopharmacology* 155:397–404.

Cornish JL, Kalivas PW. (2001). Cocaine sensitization and craving: Differing roles for dopamine and glutamate in the nucleus accumbens. *J Addict Dis* 20(3):43–54.

Cubells JF, Rayport S, Rajendran G, et al. (1994). Methamphetamine neurotoxicity involves vacuolation of endocytic organelles and dopamine-dependent intracellular oxidative stress. *J Neurosci* 14:2260–2271.

Danaceau JP, Deering CE, Day JE, et al. (2007). Persistence of tolerance to methamphetamine-induced monoamine deficits. *Eur J Pharmacol* 559:46–54.

Davidson C, Lee TH, Ellinwood EH. (2005). Acute and chronic continuous methamphetamine have different long-term behavioral and neurochemical consequences. *Neurochem Int* 46(3):189–203.

DeVito MJ, Wagner GC. (1989). Methamphetamine-induced neuronal damage: A possible role for free radicals. *Neuropharmacology* 28:1145–1150.

Diaz HR, Kolb B, Forssberg H. (2003). Can a therapeutic dose of amphetamine during preadolescence modify the pattern of synaptic organization in the brain? *Eur J Neurosci* 18:3394–3399.

Eyerman DJ, Yamamoto BK. (2005). Lobeline attenuates methamphetamine-induced changes in vesicular monoamine transporter 2 immunoreactivity and monoamine depletions in the striatum. *J Pharmacol Exp Ther* 312:160–169.

Eyerman DJ, Yamamoto BK. (2007). A rapid oxidation and persistent decrease in the vesicular monoamine transporter 2 after methamphetamine. *J Neurochem* 103(3):1219–1227.

Farfel GM, Seiden LS. (1995). Role of hypothermia in the mechanism of protection against serotonergic toxicity. II. Experiments with methamphetamine, p-chloroamphetamine, fenfluramine, dizocilpine, and dextromethorphan. *J Pharmacol Exp Ther* 272:868–875.

Ferraro L, Antonelli T, O'Connor WT, et al. (1998). The striatal neurotensin receptor modulates striatal and pallidal glutamate and GABA release: Functional evidence for a pallidal glutamate-GABA interaction via the pallidal-subthalamic nucleus loop. *J Neurosci* 18:6977–6989.

Fischer JF, Cho AK. (1979). Chemical release of dopamine from striatal homogenates: Evidence for an exchange diffusion model. *J Pharmacol Exp Ther* 208:203–209.

Fleckenstein AE, Gibb JW, Hanson GR. (2000). Differential effects of stimulants on monoaminergic transporters: Pharmacological consequences and implications for neurotoxicity. *Eur J Pharmacol* 406:1–13.

Fleckenstein AE, Hanson GR. (2003). Impact of psychostimulants on vesicular monoamine transporter function. *Eur J Pharmacol* 479:283–289.

Fleckenstein AE, Metzger RR, Wilkins DG, et al. (1997b) Rapid and reversible effects of methamphetamine on dopamine transporters. *J Pharmacol Exp Ther* 282:834–838.

Fleckenstein AE, Volz TJ, Riddle EL, et al. (2007). New insights into the mechanism of action of amphetamines. *Annu Rev Pharmacol Toxicol* 47:681–698.

Fleckenstein AE, Wilkins DG, Gibb JW, et al. (1997a). Interaction between hyperthermia and oxygen radical formation in the 5-hydroxytryptaminergic response to a single methamphetamine administration. *J Pharmacol Exp Ther* 283:281–285.

Floor E, Meng L. (1996). Amphetamine releases dopamine from synaptic vesicles by dual mechanisms. *Neurosci Lett* 215:53–56.

Floran B, Floran L, Sierra A, et al. (1997). D_2 receptor-mediated inhibition of

GABA release by endogenous dopamine in the rat globus pallidus. *Neurosci Lett* 237:1–4.

Frankel PS, Hoonakker AJ, Hanson GR, et al. (2005). Differential neurotensin responses to low and high doses of methamphetamine in the terminal regions of striatal efferents. *Eur J Pharmacol* 522:47–54.

Fumagalli F, Gainetdinov RR, Wang YM, et al. (1999). Increased methamphetamine neurotoxicity in heterozygous vesicular monoamine transporter 2 knock-out mice. *J Neurosci* 19:2424–2431.

Galvan A, Wichmann T. (2007). GABA-ergic circuits in the basal ganglia and movement disorders. *Prog Brain Res* 160:287–312.

Garcia-Rates S, Camarasa J, Escubedo E, et al. (2007). Methamphetamine and 3,4-methylenedioxymethamphetamine interact with central nicotinic receptors and induce their up-regulation. *Toxicol Appl Pharmacol* 223(3):195–205.

Gasbarri A, Sulli A, Packard M. (1997). The dopaminergic mesencephalic projections to the hippocampal formation in the rat. *Prog Neuropsychopharmacol Biol Psychiatry* 21:1–22.

Gerfen CR, McGinty JF, Young WS III. (1991). Dopamine differentially regulates dynorphin, substance P, and enkephalin expression in striatal neurons: in situ hybridization histochemical analysis. *J Neurosci* 11:1016–1031.

Gerfen CR. (1984). The neostriatal mosaic: compartmentalization of corticostriatal input and striatonigral output systems. *Nature* 311:461–464.

Gibb JW, Hanson GR, Johnson M. (1994). Neurochemical mechanisms of toxicity. In AK Cho, DS Segal (Eds.), *Amphetamine and its analogs* (pp. 269–295). San Diego: Academic Press.

Gibb JW, Kogan FJ. (1979). Influence of dopamine synthesis on methamphetamine-induced changes in striatal and adrenal tyrosine hydroxylase activity. *Naunyn Schmiedebergs Arch Pharmacol* 310:185–187.

Giovanni A, Liang LP, Hastings TG, et al. (1995). Estimating hydroxyl radical content in rat brain using systemic and intraventricular salicylate: Impact of methamphetamine. *J Neurochem* 64:1819–1825.

Guilarte TR, Nihei MK, McGlothan JL, et al. (2003). Methamphetamine-induced deficits of brain monoaminergic neuronal markers: Distal axotomy or neuronal plasticity. *Neuroscience* 122(2):499–513.

Gygi MP, Gygi SP, Johnson M, et al. (1996). Mechanisms for tolerance to methamphetamine effects. *Neuropharmacology* 35:751–757.

Gygi SP, Gibb JW, Hanson GR. (1994). Differential effects of antipsychotic and psychotomimetic drugs on neurotensin systems of discrete extrapyramidal and limbic regions. *J Pharmacol Exp Ther* 270:192–197.

Gygi SP, Gibb JW, Johnson M, et al. (1993). Blockade of tachykinin NK1 receptors by CP-96345 enhances dopamine release and the striatal dopamine effects of methamphetamine in rats. *Eur J Pharmacol* 250:177–180.

Hamada M, Higashi H, Nairn AC, et al. (2004). Differential regulation of dopamine D_1 and D_2 signaling by nicotine in neostriatal neurons. *J Neurochem* 90(5):1094–1103.

Hanson GR, Bush L, Keefe KA, et al. (2002). Distinct responses of basal ganglia substance P systems to low and high doses of methamphetamine. *J Neurochem* 82:1171–1178.

Hanson GR, Rau KS, Fleckenstein AE. (2004). The methamphetamine experience: A NIDA partnership. *Neuropharmacol* 47(Suppl. 1):92–100.

Hanson GR, Singh N, Bush L, et al. (1991). Response of extrapyramidal and limbic neuropeptides to fenfluramine administration: Comparison with methamphetamine. *J Pharmacol Exp Ther* 259:1197–1202.

Hanson GR, Singh N, Merchant K, et al. (1995). The role of NMDA receptor systems in neuropeptide responses to stimulants of abuse. *Drug Alcohol Depend* 37:107–110.

Harris DS, Reus VI, Wolkowitz O, et al. (2006). Catecholamine response to methamphetamine is related to glucocorticoid levels but not to pleasurable subjective response. *Pharmacopsychiatry* 39:100–108.

Haughey HM, Brown JM, Wilkins DG, et al. (2000b). Differential effects of methamphetamine on Na(+)/Cl(–)-dependent transporters. *Brain Res* 863:59–65.

Haughey HM, Fleckenstein AE, Hanson GR. (1999). Differential regional effects of methamphetamine on the activities of tryptophan and tyrosine hydroxlase. *J Neurochem* 72:661–668.

Haughey HM, Fleckenstein AE, Metzger RR, et al. (2000a). The effects of methamphetamine on serotonin transporter activity: Role of dopamine and hyperthermia. *J Neurochem* 75:1608–1617.

Hogan KA, Staal RG, Sonsalla PK. (2000). Analysis of VMAT2 binding after methamphetamine or MPTP treatment: Disparity between homogenates and vesicle preparations. *J Neurochem* 74:2217–2220.

Horner KA, Keefe KA. (2006). Regulation of psychostimulant-induced preprodynorphin, c-fos and zif/268 messenger RNA expression in the rat dorsal striatum by mu opioid receptor blockade. *Eur J Pharmacol* 532:61–73.

Hotchkiss A, Morgan ME, Gibb JW. (1979). The long-term effects of multiple doses of methamphetamine on neostriatal tryptophan hydroxlase, tyrosine hydroxylase, choline acetyltransferase and glutamate decarboxylase activities. *Life Sci* 25:1373–1378.

Hutson PH, Suman-Chauhan N. (1990). Activation of postsynaptic striatal dopamine receptors, monitored by efflux of cAMP *in vivo*. *Neuropharmacology* 29:1011–1016.

Ikarashi Y, Takahashi A, Ishimaru H, et al. (1997). Regulation of dopamine D_1 and D_2 receptors on striatal acetylcholine release in rats. *Brain Res Bull* 43(1):107–115.

Ikemoto K, Satoh K, Maeda T, et al. (1995). Neurochemical heterogeneity of the primate nucleus accumbens. *Exp Brain Res* 104(2):177–190.

Imam SZ, Newport GD, Itzhak Y, et al. (2001). Peroxynitrite plays a role in methamphetamine-induced dopaminergic neurotoxicity: Evidence from mice lacking neuronal nitric oxide synthase gene or overexpressing copperzinc superoxide dismutase. *J Neurochem* 76:745–749.

In SW, Son EW, Rhee DK, et al. (2005). Methamphetamine administration produces immunomodulation in mice. *J Toxicol Environ Health A* 68:2133–2145.

Ishikawa A, Kadota T, Kadota K, et al. (2005). Essential role of D_1 but not D_2 receptors in methamphetamine-induced impairment of long-term potentiation in hippocampal–prefrontal cortex pathway. *Eur J Neurosci* 22:1713–1719.

Itzhak Y, Ali SF. (1996). The neuronal nitric oxide synthase inhibitor, 7-nitroindazole, protects against methamphetamine-induced neurotoxicity *in vivo*. *J Neurochem* 67:1770–1773.

Jedynak JP, Uslaner JM, Esteban JA, et al. (2007). Methamphetamine-induced structural plasticity in the dorsal striatum. *Eur J Neurosci* 25:847–853.

John CE, Jones SR. (2007). Voltammetric characterization of the effect of monoamine uptake inhibitors and releasers on dopamine and serotonin uptake in mouse caudate-putamen and substantia nigra slices. *Neuropharmacology* 52:1596–1605.

Johnson RA, Eshleman AJ, Meyers T, et al. (1998). [$_3$H]substrate- and cell-specific effects of uptake inhibitors on human dopamine and serotonin transporter-mediated efflux. *Synapse* 30:97–106.

Johnson RG. (1988). Accumulation of biological amines into chromaffin granules: A model for hormone and neurotransmitter transport. *Physiol Rev* 68:232–307.

Johnson-Davis KL, Fleckenstein AE, Wilkins DG. (2003). The role of hyperthermia and metabolism as mechanisms of tolerance to methamphetamine neurotoxicity. *Eur J Pharmacol* 482:151–154.

Johnson-Davis KL, Truong JG, Fleckenstein AE, et al. (2004). Alterations in vesicular dopamine uptake contribute to tolerance to the neurotoxic effects of methamphetamine. *J Pharmacol Exp Ther* 309:578–586.

Kahlig KM, Binda F, Khoshbouei H, et al. (2005). Amphetamine induces dopamine efflux through a dopamine transporter channel. *Proc Natl Acad Sci USA* 102:3495–3500.

Kalivas PW. (2007). Neurobiology of cocaine addiction: implications for new pharmacotherapy. *Am J Addict* 16:71–78.

Kaye S, McKetin R, Duflou J, et al. (2007). Methamphetamine and cardiovascular pathology: A review of the evidence. *Addiction* 102:1204–1211.

Kazahaya Y, Akimoto K, Otsuki S. (1989). Subchronic methamphetamine treatment enhances methamphetamine- or cocaine-induced dopamine efflux *in vivo*. *Biol Psychiatry* 25:903—912.

Kish SJ, Kalasinsky KS, Furukawa Y, et al. (1999). Brain choline acetyltransferase activity in chronic human users of cocaine, methamphetamine, and heroin. *Mol Psychiatry* 4:26–32.

Kitanaka N, Kitanaka J, Takemura M. (2003). Behavioral sensitization and alteration in monoamine metabolism in mice after single versus repeated methamphetamine administration. *Eur J Pharmacol* 474:63–70.

Koda LY, Gibb JW. (1973). Adrenal and striatal tyrosine hydroxylase activity after methamphetamine. *J Pharmacol Exp Ther* 185:42–48.

Kogan FJ, Nichols WK, Gibb JW. (1976). Influence of methamphetamine on nigral and striatal tyrosine hydroxylase activity and on striatal dopamine levels. *Eur J Pharmacol* 36:363–371.

Kokoshka JM, Fleckenstein AE, Wilkins DG, et al. (2000). Age-dependent dif-

ferential responses of monoaminergic systems to high doses of methamphetamine. *J Neurochem* 75:2095–2102.

Kokoshka JM, Vaughan RA, Hanson GR, et al. (1998a). Nature of methamphetamine-induced rapid and reversible changes in dopamine transporters.
Eur J Pharmacol 361:269–275.

Kokoshka JM, Metzger RR, Wilkins DG, et al. (1998b). Methamphetamine
treatment rapidly inhibits serotonin, but not glutamate, transporters in rat
brain. *Brain Res* 799:78–83.

Kuczenski R, Segal DS, Cho AK, et al. (1995). Hippocampus norepinephrine,
caudate dopamine and serotonin, and behavioral responses to the stereoisomers of amphetamine and methamphetamine. *J Neurosci* 15:1308–1317.

Larsen KE, Fon EA, Hastings TG, et al. (2002). Methamphetamine-induced
degeneration of dopaminergic neurons involves autophagy and upregula-
tion of dopamine synthesis. *J Neurosci* 22:8951–8960.

LaVoie MJ, Hastings TG. (1999). Dopamine quinone formation and protein
modification associated with the striatal neurotoxicity of methamphetamine: evidence against a role for extracellular dopamine. *J Neurosci*
19:1484–1491.

Li Y, Kolb B, Robinson TE. (2003). The location of persistent amphetamine-
induced changes in the density of dendritic spines on medium spiny neurons in the nucleus accumbens and caudate-putamen. *Neuropsychopharmacology* 28:1082–1085.

Liang NY, Rutledge CO. (1982). Comparison of the release of [$_3$H]dopamine
from isolated corpus striatum by amphetamine, fenfluramine, and unla-
belled dopamine. *Biochem Pharmacol* 31:983–992.

Ligeiro-Oliveira AP, Fialho de Araujo AM, Lazzarini R, et al. (2004). Effects
of amphetamine on immune-mediated lung inflammatory response in rats.
Neuroimmunomodulation 11(3):181–190.

Liu XY, Chu XP, Mao LM, et al. (2006). Modulation of D2R–NR2B interactions in response to cocaine. *Neuron* 52:897–909.

Marek GJ, Vosmer G, Seiden LS. (1990). Dopamine uptake inhibitors block
long-term neurotoxic effects of methamphetamine upon dopaminergic
neurons. *Brain Res* 513:274–279.

Mark KA, Quinton MS, Russek SJ, et al. (2007). Dynamic changes in vesicular
glutamate transporter 1 function and expression related to methamphetamine-induced glutamate release. *J Neurosci* 27:6823–6831.

Mark KA, Soghomonian JJ, Yamamoto BK. (2004). High-dose methamphetamine acutely activates the striatonigral pathway to increase striatal glutamate and mediate long-term dopamine toxicity. *J Neurosci* 24:11449–
11456.

Marshall JF, Belcher AM, Feinstein EM, et al. (2007). Methamphetamine-
induced neural and cognitive changes in rodents. *Addiction* 102(Suppl.
1):61–69.

Martorana A, Fusco FR, D'Angelo V, et al. (2003). Enkephalin, neurotensin, and
substance P immunoreactivite neurones of the rat GP following 6-hydroxy-
dopamine lesion of the substantia nigra. *Exp Neurol* 183:311–319.

Melega WP, Williams AE, Schmitz DA, et al. (1995). Pharmacokinetic and pharmacodynamic analysis of the actions of D-amphetamine and D-metham-phetamine on the dopamine terminal. *J Pharmacol Exp Ther* 274:90–96.

Merchant KM, Hanson GR, Dorsa DM. (1994). Induction of neurotensin and c-fos mRNA in distinct subregions of rat neostriatum after acute metham-phetamine: Comparison with acute haloperidol effects. *J Pharmacol Exp Ther* 269:806–812.

Metzger RR, Haughey HM, Wilkins DG, et al. (2000). Methamphetamine-induced rapid decrease in dopamine transporter function: Role of dop-amine and hyperthermia. *J Pharmacol Exp Ther* 295:1077–1085.

Miyamoto Y, Yamada K, Nagai T, et al. (2004). Behavioural adaptations to addictive drugs in mice lacking the NMDA receptor epsilon1 subunit. *Eur J Neurosci* 19:151–158.

Morgan ME, Gibb JW. (1980). Short-term and long-term effects of metham-phetamine on biogenic amine metabolism in extra-striatal dopaminergic nuclei. *Neuropharmacology* 9:989–995.

Moriguchi S, Watanabe S, Kita H, et al. (2002). Enhancement of N-methyl-D-aspartate receptor-mediated excitatory postsynaptic potentials in the neo-striatum after methamphetamine sensitization: An *in vitro* slice study. *Exp Brain Res* 144:238–246.

Nishikawa T, Mataga N, Takashima M, et al. (1983). Behavioral sensitiza-tion and relative hyperresponsiveness of striatal and limbic dopaminergic neurons after repeated methamphetamine treatment. *Eur J Pharmacol* 88:195–203.

O'Dell SJ, Weihmuller FB, Marshall JF. (1993). Methamphetamine-induced dopamine overflow and injury to striatal dopamine terminals: attenuation by dopamine D_1 or D_2 antagonists. *J Neurochem* 60:1792–1799.

O'Neil ML, Kuczenski R, Segal DS, et al. (2006). Escalating dose pretreatment induces pharmacodynamic and not pharmacokinetic tolerance to a subse-quent high-dose methamphetamine binge. *Synapse* 60:465–473.

Peat MA, Warren PF, Bakhit C, et al. (1985). The acute effects of metham-phetamine, amphetamine, and p-chloroamphetamine on the cortical sero-tonergic system of the rat brain: Evidence for differences in the effects of methamphetamine and amphetamine. *Eur J Pharmacol* 116:11–16.

Pereira FC, Lourenco E, Milhazes N, et al. (2006). Methamphetamine, mor-phine, and their combination: Acute changes in striatal dopaminergic transmission evaluated by microdialysis in awake rats. *Ann N Y Acad Sci* 1074:160–173.

Pu C, Vorhees CV. (1993). Developmental dissociation of methamphetamine-induced depletion of dopaminergic terminals and astrocyte reaction in rat striatum. *Brain Res Dev Brain Res* 72:325–328.

Pu C, Vorhees CV. (1995). Protective effects of MK-801 on methamphetamine-induced depletion of dopaminergic and serotonergic terminals and striatal astrocytic response: An immunohistochemical study. *Synapse* 19:97–104.

Raiteri M, Cerrito F, Cervoni AM, et al. (1979). Dopamine can be released by two mechanisms differentially affected by the dopamine transport inhibi-tor nomifensine. *J Pharmacol Exp Ther* 208:195–202.

Raudensky J, Yamamoto BK. (2007). Effects of chronic unpredictable stress and methamphetamine on hippocampal glutamate function. *Brain Res* 1135:129–135.

Reid MS, Herrera-Marschitz M, Hokfelt T, et al. (1990). Striatonigral GABA, dynorphin, substance P, and neurokinin A modulation of nigrostriatal dopamine release: Evidence for direct regulatory mechanisms. *Exp Brain Res* 82:293–303.

Ricaurte GA, Schuster CR, Seiden LS. (1980). Long-term effects of repeated methylamphetamine administration on dopamine and serotonin neurons in the rat brain: A regional study. *Brain Res* 193:153–163.

Richfield EK, Penney JB, Young AB. (1989). Anatomical and affinity state comparisons between dopamine D_1 and D_2 receptors in the rat central nervous system. *Neuroscience* 30:767–777.

Riddle EL, Hanson GR, Fleckenstein AE. (2007). Therapeutic doses of amphetamine and methylphenidate selectively redistribute the vesicular monoamine transporter-2. *Eur J Pharmacol* 571:25–28.

Riddle EL, Topham MK, Haycock JW, et al. (2002). Differential trafficking of the vesicular monoamine transporter-2 by methamphetamine and cocaine. *Eur J Pharmacol* 449:71–74.

Robinson TE, Kolb B. (1997). Persistent structural modifications in nucleus accumbens and prefrontal cortex neurons produced by previous experience with amphetamine. *J Neurosci* 17:8491–8497.

Rotllant D, Nadal R, Armario A. (2007) Differential effects of stress and amphetamine administration on Fos-like protein expression in corticotropin releasing factor-neurons of the rat brain. *Dev Neurobiol* 67:702–714.

Sandoval V, Riddle EL, Hanson GR, et al. (2003). Methylphenidate alters vesicular monoamine transport and prevents methamphetamine-induced dopaminergic deficits. *J Pharmacol Exp Ther* 304:1181–1187.

Sandoval V, Riddle EL, Ugarte YV, et al. (2001). Methamphetamine-induced rapid and reversible changes in dopamine transporter function: An *in vitro* model. *J Neurosci* 21:1413–1419.

Saunders C, Ferrer JV, Shi L, et al. (2000). Amphetamine-induced loss of human dopamine transporter activity: An internalization-dependent and cocaine-sensitive mechanism. *Proc Natl Acad Sci USA* 97:6850–6855.

Schmidt CJ, Gehlert DR, Peat MA, et al. (1985a). Studies on the mechanism of tolerance to methamphetamine. *Brain Res* 343:305–313.

Schmidt CJ, Ritter JK, Sonsalla PK, et al. (1985b). Role of dopamine in the neurotoxic effects of methamphetamine. *J Pharmacol Exp Ther* 233:539–544.

Schwartz JW, Novarino G, Piston DW, et al. (2005). Substrate binding stoichiometry and kinetics of the norepinephrine transporter. *J Biol Chem* 280:19177–19184.

Scott JC, Woods SP, Matt GE, et al. (2007). Neurocognitive effects of methamphetamine: A critical review and meta-analysis. *Neuropsychol Rev* 17(3):275–297.

Selden N, Geula C, Hersh L, et al. (1994). Human striatum: Chemoarchitecture of the caudate nucleus, putamen, and ventral striatum in health and Alzheimer's disease. *Neuroscience* 60:621–636.

Segal DS, Kuczenski R. (2006). Human methamphetamine pharmacokinetics simulated in the rat: Single daily intravenous administration reveals elements of sensitization and tolerance. *Neuropsychopharmacology* 31:941–955.

Sekine Y, Iyo M, Ouchi Y, et al. (2001). Methamphetamine-related psychiatric symptoms and reduced brain dopamine transporters studied with PET. *Am J Psych* 158:1206–1214.

Sharma HS, Sjoquist PO, Ali SF. (2007). Drugs of abuse–induced hyperthermia, blood–brain barrier dysfunction, and neurotoxicity: Neuroprotective effects of a new antioxidant compound H-290/51. *Curr Pharm Des* 13:1903–1923.

Singh NA, Bush LG, Gibb JW, et al. (1992). Role of N-methyl-D-aspartate receptors in dopamine D1-, but not D2-mediated changes in striatal and accumbens neurotensin systems. *Brain Res* 571:260–264.

Sitte HH, Huck S, Reither H, et al. (1998). Carrier-mediated release, transport rates, and charge transfer induced by amphetamine, tyramine, and dopamine in mammalian cells transfected with the human dopamine transporter. *J Neurochem* 71:1289–1297.

Smith AJ, McGinty JF. (1994). Acute amphetamine or methamphetamine alters opioid peptide mRNA expression in rat striatum. *Brain Res Mol Brain Res* 21:359–362.

Smith SM, Vaughan JM, Donaldson CJ, et al. (2004). Cocaine- and amphetamine-regulated transcript activates the hypothalamic-pituitary-adrenal axis through a corticotropin-releasing factor receptor-dependent mechanism. *Endocrinology* 145:5202–5209.

Sonders MS, Zhu SJ, Zahniser NR, et al. (1997). Multiple ionic conductances of the human dopamine transporter: The actions of dopamine and psychostimulants. *J Neurosci* 17:960–974.

Sonsalla PK, Gibb JW, Hanson GR. (1986). Roles of D_1 and D_2 dopamine receptor subtypes in mediating the methamphetamine-induced changes in monoamine systems. *J Pharmacol Exp Ther* 238:932–937.

Sonsalla PK, Nicklas WJ, Heikkila RE. (1989). Role for excitatory amino acids in methamphetamine-induced nigrostriatal dopaminergic toxicity. *Science* 243:398–400.

Sorkina T, Doolan S, Galperin E, et al. (2003). Oligomerization of dopamine transporters visualized in living cells by fluorescent resonance energy transfer microscopy. *J Biol Chem* 278:28274–28283.

Stephans S, Yamamoto B. (1996). Methamphetamines pretreatment and the vulnerability of the striatum to methamphetamine neurotoxicity. *Neuroscience* 72:593–600.

Stephans SE, Whittingham TS, Douglas AJ, et al. (1998). Substrates of energy metabolism attenuate methamphetamine-induced neurotoxicity in striatum. *J Neurochem* 71:613–621.

Stephans SE, Yamamoto BK. (1994). Methamphetamine-induced neurotoxicity: Roles for glutamate and dopamine efflux. *Synapse* 17:203–209.

Stone DM, Hanson GR, Gibb JW. (1989b). *In vitro* reactivation of rat cortical tryptophan hydroxylase following *in vivo* inactivation by methylenedioxymethamphetamine. *J Neurochem* 53:572–581.

Stone DM, Johnson M, Hanson GR, et al. (1989a). Acute inactivation of trypto-phan hydroxylase by amphetamine analogs involves the oxidation of sulf-hydryl sites. *Eur J Pharmacol* 172:93–97.

Sulzer D, Chen T-K, Lau YY, et al. (1995). Amphetamine redistributes dop-amine from synaptic vesicles to the cytosol and promotes reverse transport. *J Neurosci* 15:4102–4106.

Sulzer D, Maidment NT, Rayport S. (1993). Amphetamine and other weak bases act to promote reverse transport of dopamine in ventral midbrain neurons. *J Neurochem* 60:527–535.

Sulzer D, Rayport S. (1990). Amphetamine and other psychostimulants reduce pH gradients in midbrain dopaminergic neurons and chromaffin granules: A mechanism of action. *Neuron* 6:797–808.

Sulzer D, Sonders MS, Poulsen NW, et al. (2005). Mechanisms of neurotrans-mitter release by amphetamines: A review. *Prog Neurobiol* 75:406–433.

Surmeier DJ, Ding J, Day M, et al. (2007). D_1 and D_2 dopamine-receptor modu-lation of striatal glutamatergic signaling in striatal medium spiny neurons. *Trends Neurosci* 30:228–235.

Suzuki O, Hattori H, Asano M, et al. (1980). Inhibition of monoamine oxidase by *d*-methamphetamine. *Biochem Pharmacol* 29:2071–2073.

Suzuki T, Mizuo K, Nakazawa H, et al. (2003). Prenatal and neonatal exposure to bisphenol-A enhances the central dopamine D_1 receptor-mediated action in mice: Enhancement of the methamphetamine-induced abuse state. *Neu-roscience* 117:639–644.

Taguchi K, Atobe J, Kato M, et al. (1998). The effect of methamphetamine on the release of acetylcholine in the rat striatum. *Eur J Pharmacol* 360:131–137.

Tata DA, Yamamoto BK. (2007). Interactions between methamphetamine and environmental stress: Role of oxidative stress, glutamate, and mitochon-drial dysfunction. *Addiction* 102(Suppl. 1):49–60.

Tekes K, Magyar K. (2000). Effect of MAO inhibitors on the high-affinity reuptake of biogenic amines in rat subcortical regions. *Neurobiology* (Bp) 8(3–4):257–264.

Thiriet N, Deng X, Solinas M, et al. (2005). Neuropeptide Y protects against methamphetamine-induced neuronal apoptosis in the mouse striatum. *J Neurosci* 25:5273–5279.

Thomas DM, Walker PD, Benjamins JA, et al. (2004). Methamphetamine neu-rotoxicity in dopamine nerve endings of the striatum is associated with microglial activation. *J Pharmacol Exp Ther* 311:1–7.

Tisch S, Silberstein P, Limousin-Dowsey P, et al. (2004). The basal ganglia: Anatomy, physiology, and pharmacology. *Psychiatr Clin North Am* 27:757–799.

Truong JG, Wilkins DG, Baudys J, et al. (2005). Age-dependent methamphet-amine-induced alterations in vesicular monoamine transporter-2 function: Implications for neurotoxicity. *J Pharmacol Exp Ther* 314:1087–1092.

Ujike H, Takaki M, Kodama M, et al. (2002). Gene expression related to syn-aptogenesis, neuritogenesis, and MAP kinase in behavioral sensitization to psychostimulants. *Ann NY Acad Sci* 965:55–67.

Varner KJ, Ogden BA, Delcarpio J, et al. (2002). Cardiovascular responses elicited by the "binge" administration of methamphetamine. *J Pharmacol Exp Ther* 301:152–159.

Viggiano D, Vallone D, Ruocco LA, et al. (2003). Behavioural, pharmacological, morpho-functional molecular studies reveal a hyperfunctioning mesocortical dopamine system in an animal model of attention deficit and hyperactivity disorder. *Neurosci Biobehav Rev* 27:683–689.

Volkow ND, Chang L, Wang GJ, et al. (2001a). Loss of dopamine transporters in methamphetamine abusers recovers with protracted abstinence. *J Neurosci* 21:9414–9418.

Volkow ND, Chang L, Wang GJ, et al. (2001b). Association of dopamine transporter reduction with psychomotor impairment in methamphetamine abusers. *Am J Psychiatry* 158:377–382.

Völlm BA, de Araujo IE, Cowen PJ, et al. (2004). Methamphetamine activates reward circuitry in drug naive human subjects. *Neuropsychopharmacology* 29:1715–1722.

Volz TJ, Hanson GR, Fleckenstein AE. (2007). The role of the plasmalemmal dopamine and vesicular monoamine transporters in methamphetamine-induced dopaminergic deficits. *J Neurochem* 101:883–888.

Wagner GC, Carelli RM, Jarvis MF. (1985). Pretreatment with ascorbic acid attenuates the neurotoxic effects of methamphetamine in rats. *Res Commun Chem Pathol Pharmacol* 47:221–228.

Wagner GC, Lucot JB, Schuster CR, et al. (1983). Alpha-methyltyrosine attenuates and reserpine increases methamphetamine-induced neuronal changes. *Brain Res* 270:285–288.

Wagner GC, Ricaurte GA, Seiden LS, et al. (1980). Long-lasting depletions of striatal dopamine and loss of dopamine uptake sites following repeated administration of methamphetamine. *Brain Res* 181:151–160.

Wagstaff JD, Bush LG, Gibb JW, et al. (1994). Endogenous neurotensin antagonizes methamphetamine-enhanced dopaminergic activity. *Brain Res* 665:237–244.

Wagstaff JD, Gibb JW, Hanson GR. (1996). Microdialysis assessment of methamphetamine-induced changes in extracellular neurotensin in the striatum and nucleus accumbens. *J Pharmacol Exp Ther* 278:547–554.

Wan FJ, Lin HC, Kang BH, et al. (1999). D-amphetamine-induced depletion of energy and dopamine in the rat striatum is attenuated by nicotinamide pretreatment. *Brain Res Bull* 50:167–171.

Wang GJ, Volkow ND, Chang L, et al. (2004). Partial recovery of brain metabolism in methamphetamine abusers after protracted abstinence. *Am J Psychiatry* 161:242–248.

Wang R, Boules M, Tiner W, et al. (2004). Effects of repeated injections of the neurotensin analog NT69L on dopamine release and uptake in rat striatum *in vitro*. *Brain Res* 1025:21–28.

Westfall T, Westfall D. (2006). Adrenergic agonists and antagonists. In L Brunton, J Lazo, K Parker (Eds.), *The pharmacological basis of therapeutics* (11th ed., pp. 237–295). New York: McGraw-Hill.

Wilson JM, Kalasinsky KS, Levey AI, et al. (1996). Striatal dopamine nerve terminal markers in human, chronic methamphetamine users. *Nat Med* 2:699–703.

Woolverton WL, Ricaurte GA, Forno L, et al. (1989). Long-term effects of chronic methamphetamine administration in rhesus monkeys. *Brain Res* 486:73–78.

Xie T, McCann UD, Kim S, et al. (2000). Effect of temperature on dopamine transporter function and intracellular accumulation of methamphetamine: Implications for methamphetamine-induced dopaminergic neurotoxicity. *J Neurosci* 20:7838–7845.

Xu W, Zhu JP, Angulo JA. (2005). Induction of striatal pre- and postsynaptic damage by methamphetamine requires the dopamine receptors. *Synapse* 58:110–121.

Yamamoto BK, Bankson MG. (2005). Amphetamine neurotoxicity: Cause and consequence of oxidative stress. *Crit Rev Neurobiol* 17:87–117.

Yamamoto BK, Zhu W. (1998). The effects of methamphetamine on the production of free radicals and oxidative stress. *J Pharmacol Exp Ther* 287:107–114.

Yamamoto H, Kitamura N, Lin XH, et al. (1999). Differential changes in glutamatergic transmission via N-methyl-D-aspartate receptors in the hippocampus and striatum of rats behaviourally sensitized to methamphetamine. *Int J Neuropsychopharmacology* 2:155–163.

Yui K, Goto K, Ikemoto S. (2004). The role of noradrenergic and dopaminergic hyperactivity in the development of spontaneous recurrence of methamphetamine psychosis and susceptibility to episode recurrence. *Ann NY Acad Sci* 1025:296–306.

Zaczek R, Culp S, De Souza EB. (1991). Interactions of [³H]amphetamine with rat brain synaptosomes. II. Active transport. *J Pharmacol Exp Ther* 257:830–835.

Zahm DS, Williams E, Wohltmann C. (1996). Ventral striatopallidothalamic projection: IV. Relative involvements of neurochemically distinct subterritories in the ventral pallidum and adjacent parts of the rostroventral forebrain. *J Comp Neurol* 364:340–362.

Zhang X, Lee TH, Xiong X, et al. (2006). Methamphetamine induces long-term changes in GABAA receptor alpha2 subunit and GAD67 expression. *Biochem Biophys Res Commun* 351(1):300–305.

Zhu JP, Xu W, Angulo JA. (2006a). Distinct mechanisms mediating methamphetamine-induced neuronal apoptosis and dopamine terminal damage share the neuropeptide substance p in the striatum of mice. *Ann NY Acad Sci* 1074:135–148.

Zhu JP, Xu W, Angulo JA. (2006b). Methamphetamine-induced cell death: Selective vulnerability in neuronal subpopulations of the striatum in mice. *Neuroscience* 140:607–622.

Chapter 4

Methamphetamine and the Brain
Findings from Brain Imaging Studies

Doris Payer and Edythe D. London

Noninvasive neuroimaging techniques have proven essential for clarifying the effects of methamphetamine (MA) on the human brain by linking MA-related behavioral and cognitive abnormalities to neural circuits. The techniques include positron emission tomography (PET), single photon emission computed tomography (SPECT), functional and structural magnetic resonance imaging (MRI), magnetic resonance spectroscopy (MRS), and electroencephalography (EEG). Their application to the study of MA abuse and dependence has helped form a more complete picture of the disorder and its underlying neural substrates. This review covers the body of neuroimaging findings related to acute MA intoxication, MA psychosis, and consequences of long-term MA abuse through investigations of early and prolonged abstinence.

Acute Intoxication

Few studies have assessed the acute effects of MA on human brain function, and only a handful of behavioral investigations have confirmed that MA administration is perceived as rewarding, reinforcing, and pleasurable, through self-report measures or self-administration procedures in healthy (Hart et al., 2001) and MA-experienced individuals (Harris et al., 2003; Newton et al., 2005, 2006). Although these studies suggested that activation of reward- and affect-related neural circuitry was the basis for the positive subjective responses, reports on the precise neu-

61

ral underpinnings remain sparse. As predicted, however, the small body of work on acute MA intoxication converges on a set of brain regions linked to reward and approach behaviors.

Kleinschmidt et al. (1999) noted MRI signal increases in frontotemporal grey matter, subcortical regions, and cerebellum after MA administration, while Gouzoulis-Mayfrank et al. (1999) reported decreases (relative to the global metabolic rate) in cortical glucose metabolism and increases in cerebellar glucose metabolism when studied with [^{18}F] fluorodeoxyglucose (FDG) and PET. Both studies speculated on the relationship between the observed changes in brain activity and subjective effects, so that a heightened sense of wellness was linked to greater subcortical (i.e., striatal) than cortical signal change (Kleinschmidt et al., 1999), and anxiety, intensity of the drug experience, and unpleasant feelings were linked to increased glucose metabolism in the cerebellum and decreased glucose metabolism in frontal and parietal cortex (Gouzoulis-Mayfrank et al., 1999). Völlm et al. (2004) directly addressed hypotheses about MA and reward circuitry by administering MA to psychostimulant-naïve volunteers and performing functional MRI while the subjects rated their experience of "mind racing" (a measure that correlates with overall psychostimulant effect and "buzz"). Constraining analyses to reward-related regions of interest—orbitofrontal cortex (OFC), anterior cingulate cortex (ACC), and ventral striatum—they found MA-induced activation in medial OFC, rostral ACC, and right caudate nucleus, as well as correlations between subjective effects ("mind racing") and activation in caudate nucleus and rostral ACC. Following removal of phasic motor-related activity, medial OFC remained the only region with robust MA-induced increases, suggesting that OFC is among the regions underlying the rewarding effects of MA and associated subjective states. Together the studies show predictable activity in regions related to reward and approach following MA administration, confirming the neural basis for the acute subjective effects.

MA administration also results in a number of acute effects that are not obviously linked to reward, ranging from enhanced alertness and vigilance (Kleinschmidt et al., 1999; Wiegmann et al., 1996), improved performance on cognitive tasks (Mohs et al., 1978, 1980; Gouzoulis-Mayfrank et al., 1999), and "jittery" or "stimulated" states (Hart et al., 2001), to aggressive violence (Szuster, 1990) and risky sexual behavior (Semple et al., 2006). The neural circuitry that mediates these effects has not been investigated, but given the similarity of MA to *d*-amphetamine (both in terms of structure/pharmacology and mechanism of action/ subjective effects), we can glean some information about relevant neural correlates from neuroimaging research involving *d*-amphetamine administration.

Paralleling the effects of acute MA administration, d-amphetamine induces dopamine release in the ventral subdivisions of the striatum (Martinez et al., 2003; Drevets et al., 2001; Leyton et al., 2002); this effect is accompanied by proportional increases in euphoria, "drug-wanting," alertness, and restlessness (Laruelle et al., 1995; Drevets et al., 2001; Leyton, 2002), and its magnitude correlates with the trait of novelty-seeking (Leyton et al., 2002). In addition, assays of cerebral glucose metabolism revealed amphetamine-induced increases in relative activity of subcortical, limbic, and frontal regions (scaled to global activity) (Ernst et al., 1997), and increases in absolute metabolic rate for glucose in the caudate nucleus, putamen, cingulate cortex, and thalamus (Vollenweider et al., 1998). Ernst et al. (1997) also found a relative increase in cerebellar and relative decrease in temporal cortical glucose metabolism. Metabolic changes in the frontal cortex, caudate nucleus, and putamen correlated with mania-like symptoms (Vollenweider et al., 1998) and increases in good mood (Ernst et al., 1997; but see Wolkin et al., 1987, for reports of amphetamine-induced decrease in glucose metabolism). This parallel in subjective effects and implicated neural circuitry encourages further comparisons between acute effects of d-amphetamine and MA.

As with MA, administration of d-amphetamine has been associated with improved speed and performance on cognitive tasks when compared with placebo, and these improvements have been linked to region-specific changes in the circuits underlying task performance. For example, d-amphetamine administration enhanced perfusion of the prefrontal cortex during the Wisconsin Card Sorting Test (WCST; a test of set shifting) and of the hippocampus during the Ravens Progressive Matrices (a visuospatial reasoning test) (Mattay et al., 1996). In addition, d-amphetamine induced prefrontal activation during a working memory task (Mattay et al., 2000), activation of auditory cortex during an auditory attention task, and activation of sensory cortex during a motor task (Uftring et al., 2001). Although one study somewhat paradoxically demonstrated signal *reductions* and fewer active pixels in cingulate and parietal regions during a word-generation task; insula and dorsolateral prefrontal cortex during a working-memory task; and lingual gyrus, occipital cortex, and precuneus during a spatial attention task (Willson et al., 2004), the d-amphetamine-induced changes in neural activity were nonetheless region specific according to task, and the general consensus appears to be that d-amphetamine "focuses" neural activity to highlight the circuits necessary for task performance (Mattay et al., 1996). Finally, d-amphetamine administration (compared with placebo) has also been shown to enhance amygdala responsivity to threatening facial expressions (Hariri et al., 2002), providing a possible link to the emotion-enhancing and anxiogenic properties of the drug.

In addition to providing clues on possible neural mechanisms for the acute effects of MA, research with *d*-amphetamine also highlights another important issue: the impact of individual differences on these effects and on the subsequent risk for progression to drug abuse and dependence. Studies with healthy individuals under *d*-amphetamine challenge have shown that sex, genotype (e.g., polymorphisms for catechol-O-methyltransferase [COMT], dopamine, serotonin, and norepinephrine transporters [DAT, SERT, NET], and brain-derived neurotrophic factor [BDNF]), personality factors (e.g., reward sensitivity, fearlessness, novelty seeking, experience seeking, disinhibition, and boredom susceptibility), and environmental experiences (e.g., life stress), all can predict or modulate striatal dopamine release, cortical activation during task performance, or subjective response to the drug (Lott et al., 2005, 2006; Munro et al., 2006; Mattay et al., 2003; Flanagin et al., 2006; Dlugos et al., 2007; White et al., 2006; Hutchison et al., 1999; Leyton et al., 2002; Oswald et al., 2007). Given the parallels between the acute subjective effects of *d*-amphetamine and MA, and possibly between the neural underpinnings of these effects, it is likely that individual variation is equally important in modulating the acute effects of MA. Knowledge of factors that modulate individual responses to acute intoxication can help understand progression from MA use to abuse and dependence.

Another potential contributing factor to this progression is the loss of reinforcing properties with repeated administration. A study testing the subjective effects of repeated MA administration to healthy individuals in a laboratory setting found that by the third day of MA administration (5 or 10 mg delivered orally twice a day), positive effects, such as "good drug effect" and "high," diminished, while the negative subjective effects, such as dizziness and "flu-like symptoms," increased over time (Comer et al., 2001). This pattern is consistent with the rapid development of tolerance following repeated administration of MA and possible sensitization in the systems underlying the negative effects. Such a pattern is commonly thought to underlie dose escalation in an effort to regain positive and avoid negative effects, potentially resulting in repeated high-level administration that can ultimately result in MA psychosis and dependence.

MA Psychosis

In some cases, repeated high-level MA administration can induce MA psychosis, a state of paranoia, delusion, hallucination, and aggressiveness thought to resemble paranoid schizophrenia. Although neuroimaging research has focused on individuals who have suffered MA psychosis in the past but are in remission at the time of study, some consistent patterns have emerged that can hint at the acute neurobiological changes that occur during this state.

First neuroimaging studies (primarily using PET and SPECT) have shown that monoamine neurotransmitter systems are dysregulated in individuals who have previously experienced MA psychosis. Iyo et al. (1993) found a lower ratio of striatal D_2 dopamine receptor binding availability to prefrontal 5-HT$_2$ serotonin receptor availability in MA-abusing individuals compared with healthy individuals and suggested that this may represent a susceptibility factor for MA psychosis. Subsequent studies also found that residual psychiatric symptoms in MA-abusing subjects correlated negatively with DAT binding potential in the caudate/putamen and nucleus accumbens (Iyo et al., 2004), and that flashbacks to MA-induced psychotic episodes were linked to norepinephrine hyper-reactivity and increased dopamine release in response to stressful events (Yui et al., 2004). Furthermore, certain genetic variants were found to be more common in individuals who experienced MA psychosis and spontaneous relapse to a psychotic state, such as the polymorphism of the gene for COMT that results in greater synaptic dopamine concentration (*met* allele), and certain polymorphisms of the PICK1 gene, which is involved in DAT targeting and clustering (Suzuki et al., 2006; Matsuzawa et al., 2007). These studies suggest that dysregulation in monoamine neurotransmitter systems, in combination with some potential susceptibility factors, can be linked to a persistent or recurring psychotic state following high-dose MA abuse.

MA psychosis has also been investigated using event-related potentials (ERP), a time-locked variant of EEG. In these studies, individuals with a history of MA psychosis and normal control subjects differed in the amplitude and latency of the P300, a component associated with prefrontal functions such as attention, novelty detection, context updating, and effort (Iwanami et al., 1993, 1998). The P300 is also thought to reflect phasic noradrenergic function (Iwanami et al., 1998), corroborating the notion of monoaminergic dysregulation described above. Together the ERP studies suggest that MA psychosis is related to excessive monoamine transmission, which could negatively influence prefrontal executive functions.

Finally, a structural MRI study showed that in a group of individuals with MA psychosis, D_2 dopamine receptor genotype influenced grey matter concentration in the temporal lobe and insula such that individuals homozygous for the A2 allele had narrower temporal lobes than individuals with A1/A2 genotypes (Harano et al., 2004). Interestingly, the A1 allele has been associated with delayed onset of psychosis and better treatment response, suggesting that a genetic basis exists for localized structural deficits that could influence severity and outcome of the psychotic state. A SPECT study on a group of MA-abusing individuals with psychotic symptoms also found focal perfusion deficits in frontal, parietal, and temporal regions, reminiscent of patterns seen in violent and aggressive individuals (Buffenstein et al., 1999); however, the behavioral implications of these studies remain uncertain.

Long-Term MA Abuse

To study the consequences of prolonged high-level administration, we must turn to individuals who have been self-administering MA regularly for substantial amounts of time; however, in order to dissociate the effects of interest from the effects of acute or residual MA intoxication, an abstinence period must be imposed. These factors make some of the literature on the subject difficult to disentangle, as MA-dependent research participants are often studied in varying stages of abstinence, ranging from 2 weeks to several years, and the symptoms and neural correlates noted depend on the stage of abstinence. Nonetheless, evidence converges on a set of differences from healthy individuals in mood/emotion and cognition, and these differences appear linked to dysregulated subcortical systems and a loss of prefrontal control over these systems.

Early Abstinence (<1 Month)

Early abstinence is associated with a syndrome that consists of depressive and anhedonic states, anxiety, craving for the drug, and cognitive difficulties (e.g., poor concentration) (Newton et al., 2004a; McGregor et al., 2005). These symptoms tend to resolve within the first week of abstinence, after which they remain at low levels comparable to those of healthy individuals (McGregor et al., 2005).

A number of neuroimaging methods have been applied to study the early abstinence syndrome. Using EEG to measure electrical activity across the head, 11 MA-dependent individuals after 4 days of abstinence were found to exhibit greater EEG power (during the eyes-closed resting state) in the delta and theta frequency bands than were 11 healthy individuals, a pattern that is consistent with a range of cognitive and psychiatric abnormalities (Newton et al., 2003). Furthermore, in a sample of nine MA-dependent individuals, theta power correlated positively with reaction time and negatively with performance on a working memory task (Newton et al. 2004b), suggesting that high theta power reflects frontoparietal dysfunction. Within 5 to 14 days of abstinence, a sample of 27 MA-dependent individuals also performed more poorly than 18 healthy comparison individuals on a number of measures associated with prefrontal cortical function, including attention and psychomotor speed, verbal learning and memory, and executive measures (Kalechstein et al., 2003), and within the first 5 to 7 days of abstinence, 11 MA-dependent individuals performed more poorly than comparison individuals on the stop-signal task (SST) (Monterosso et al., 2005), which measures executive control and relies on the integrity of prefrontal cortical/basal ganglia pathways (Aron et al., 2007).

While the EEG measures and neuropsychological impairments suggest frontoparietal and frontolimbic dysfunction, other imaging methods can provide insight into more specific regional deficits. London et al. (2005) studied regional cerebral glucose metabolism, using FDG and PET, in 17 MA-dependent individuals during the first 4 to 7 days of abstinence, and showed poorer performance (more errors) in the MA-dependent group than the healthy comparison group on a vigilance task testing sustained attention. Performance correlated negatively with metabolic activity in the anterior and middle cingulate gyrus and the insula, suggesting that prefrontal and insular dysregulation in the early abstinence period could underlie some of the cognitive deficits. Furthermore, a subset of 10 of the MA-dependent individuals, retested after 4 weeks of abstinence, showed greater variance in task accuracy and reaction times, accompanied by a global increase in cerebral glucose metabolism that was largely localized to bilateral parietal cortex, but also included OFC, supragenual cingulate cortex, insula, and thalamus (Figure 4.1); none of these changes were apparent in the healthy comparison group (Berman et al., 2008). These findings suggest either that cortical abnormalities (indexed by an increase in cerebral glucose metabolism) evolve after the first week of abstinence, or that a chronic elevation in glucose metabolism resulting from prolonged MA use is still masked by residual MA effects during days 4–7 of abstinence.

To study more complex behavioral patterns, functional MRI was used to investigate the discounting of delayed rewards in 12 recently abstinent MA-abusing subjects (Monterosso et al., 2007a). The study uncovered MA-related deficits in prefrontal cortical efficiency during difficult ("less money now" vs. "more money later") compared with easy ("more money now" vs. "less money later") decisions, accompanied by steeper discounting functions in the MA-dependent group (i.e., MA-dependent subjects tended to find rewards less valuable after a delay), suggesting that prefrontal cortical deficits also accompany impulsive decision making during early abstinence (Monterosso et al., 2007a).

Finally, a recent SPECT study found that while striatal DAT levels were lower in seven MA-dependent subjects than in seven healthy comparison subjects at baseline (immediately following the last episode of

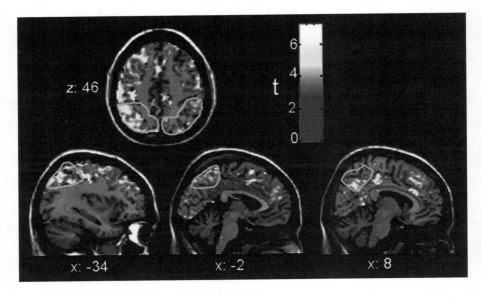

FIGURE 4.1. Cerebral glucose metabolism increase, measured with FDG and PET, from 4–7 days of abstinence to 4 weeks of abstinence. Global glucose metabolism increased more in nine MA-abusing subjects than seven comparison subjects. The parietal lobe region of interest (ROI) is outlined in light grey. Lighter shades indicate greater increases in glucose metabolic rate from initial PET session to 4 weeks later.

MA intoxication), levels partially recovered after 2 weeks of abstinence to a level that was still lower than, but no longer significantly different from, levels in the healthy group; this recovery showed a borderline correlation with improvement on WCST performance (Chou et al., 2007), consistent with prefrontal functional recovery as the abstinence syndrome resolves. Together the neuroimaging findings parallel the time course of recovery suggested by McGregor et al. (2005) and provide increasingly specific neural correlates for the cognitive deficits exhibited in early abstinence.

To investigate the neural substrates associated with symptoms of dysregulated mood and emotion, which are also prominent during acute abstinence, neuroimaging techniques have been applied in conjunction with specific probe tasks or subjective reports. Regional cerebral glucose metabolism (scaled to the global mean) during a vigilance task was measured using PET in a group of 17 MA-dependent individuals abstinent 4 to 7 days and a group of 18 healthy subjects, and was related to self-reported measures of mood states (depression measured via the

Beck Depression Inventory [BDI]; anxiety measured by the State–Trait Anxiety Inventory [STAI; London et al., 2004]). In the MA-dependent group, depressive symptoms correlated positively with relative glucose metabolism in limbic regions (perigenual ACC and amygdala), and anxiety scores correlated positively with amygdala activity and negatively with activity in OFC. This relative hypoactivity in prefrontal cortex and hyperactivity in limbic regions points to a loss of control over limbic circuitry in the MA-dependent individuals, potentially underlying the heightened emotional states during early abstinence. After 4 weeks of abstinence, BDI scores in a subsample of 10 of the MA-dependent subjects still correlated positively with relative glucose metabolism in right parietal cortex, right amygdala, and bilateral striatum, and negatively with relative glucose metabolism in right infragenual cingulate cortex, right supragenual cingulate cortex, and right insula (Berman et al., 2008), suggesting that some loss of cortical control over subcortical regions persists.

Extending the research on emotional dysregulation during early abstinence, a recent fMRI study found higher task-related activation in dorsal ACC of 12 MA-dependent individuals (abstinent 5–16 days) than 12 healthy individuals, and lower task-related activation in ventrolateral prefrontal cortex during a task that required processing of emotional facial expressions (Payer et al., 2008). Higher activation in ACC correlated with self-reports of hostility and interpersonal sensitivity in the MA-abusing group, and lower prefrontal activation (as well as less activation in temporal/parietal regions associated with social cognition; Figure 4.2) could point to a failure to inhibit impulsive actions triggered by the ACC response. Together the findings suggest that limbic hyperreactivity, along with depressive symptoms, anxiety, and social hypersensitivity could contribute to some of the abnormal mood states and social behaviors (violence, aggression) exhibited during early abstinence.

In summary, the imaging literature suggests that the defining aspects of the MA early-abstinence syndrome—that is, cognitive deficits and transient increases in negative mood and antisocial behaviors—are associated with lower function of prefrontal and anterior cingulate cortices, resulting in disrupted control over emotion- and reward-related regions of the brain (e.g., limbic system, basal ganglia), which in turn can lead to impulsive choices and disinhibition (for additional reviews, see Goldstein & Volkow, 2002; Kalivas & Volkow, 2005). Cognitive functions that are subserved by prefrontal systems, such as working memory and executive function, are also affected during early abstinence, which in turn can lead to poor decision making and a lack of foresight in behavior. As negative mood states are stressful and diminished cognitive capacity can promote impulsive choices, the early-abstinence period is particu-

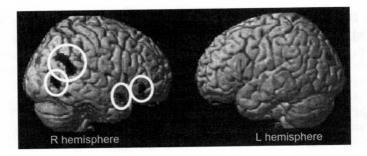

FIGURE 4.2. Healthy > MA contrast from a functional MRI study of facial affect processing. Twelve healthy participants showed greater task-related activity than 12 MA-dependent participants during Emotion Match (relative to Shape Match) trials in a set of cortical regions consisting of right ventrolateral prefrontal cortex, anterior and posterior lateral temporal cortex, and temporoparietal junction (circled), as well as fusiform gyrus and left cuneus.

larly sensitive to the risk of relapse (Huber et al., 1997), and continued exploration of the neural systems affected during this stage can help identify novel targets for intervention and relapse prevention.

Prolonged Abstinence (>1 Month)

Even after the acute abstinence syndrome resolves, cognitive, affective, and regional brain deficits persist. These deficits are more likely to reflect the long-lasting effects of chronic MA abuse than the manifestations of withdrawal during acute abstinence. Behaviorally, the impact of chronic MA use is apparent in cognitive function, in particular in executive functions that rely on frontal/basal ganglia systems (e.g., Woods et al., 2005). Specifically, MA-abusing individuals show deficits in strategic learning and retrieval, psychomotor speed, attention, and interference resolution (Woods et al., 2005; Gonzalez et al., 2004; Simon et al., 2000, 2002). In one study, performance on the Stroop task, which tests selective attention and the ability to suppress task-irrelevant information, was selectively impaired in a group of eight previously MA-dependent men abstinent 2–4 months (Salo et al., 2002). Similarly, a group of 36 subjects abstinent for up to 5 years committed more errors on the Stroop task than a group of 16 healthy control subjects (Salo et al., 2005), suggesting that deficits in executive capabilities can persist for long periods of time following initiation of abstinence. Steep discounting of delayed rewards also persists beyond the immediate abstinence phase (see Monterosso et al., 2005), as 41 MA-abusing subjects, abstinent 2–24 weeks, still discounted delayed rewards more (i.e., found delayed rewards less valuable) than 41 of their healthy counterparts, and this tendency was correlated with the degree of verbal memory impairment (Hoffman et al., 2006). The same group of subjects also showed more psychiatric symptoms than the healthy control subjects did, replicating earlier findings (see section on MA psychosis, p. 64).

As executive cognitive function is thought to rely on frontostriatal systems and the integrity of dopaminergic systems (Goldstein & Volkow, 2002; Kalivas & Volkow, 2005; Nordahl et al., 2003), and psychiatric and affective symptoms on frontolimbic systems and the integrity of the serotonergic system (Baicy & London, 2007), neuroimaging has been applied to elucidate the neural underpinnings of these persistent deficits after prolonged abstinence. The first study to investigate the issue of long-lasting effects of MA on neural systems was a postmortem study (Wilson et al., 1996) that found reduced markers for dopamine nerve terminals (dopamine itself, as well as tyrosine hydroxylase and DAT) in striatum and reduced markers for serotonergic terminals in ventrome- dial prefrontal cortex (Brodmann areas 11 and 12) of 12 MA-abusing individuals. However, the study found normal levels of the vesicular monoamine transporter and DOPA decarboxylase in striatum, suggest- ing that instead of MA-induced neuronal degeneration, terminals adapt to chronic dopamine stimulation by downregulating presynaptic mark- ers. A later study by the same group (Moszczynska et al., 2004) showed the same pattern of dopamine reduction in the striatum in an expanded sample of 20 MA-abusing individuals, but added that the reduction was greater in the caudate nucleus than the putamen. Since the caudate nucleus subserves cognitive functions and putamen motor functions, this finding helped explain why individuals who abuse MA show no signs of Parkinson's disease (as patients with Parkinson's disease show the oppo- site pattern, with greater DA depletion in putamen than in caudate), but instead show more cognitive deficits.

Subsequent neuroimaging studies corroborated these findings by showing similar reductions in dopaminergic and serotonergic mark- ers *in vivo*. PET studies have demonstrated significant reductions in DAT binding in the striatum (Volkow et al., 2001a; Sekine et al., 2001; Johanson et al., 2006; McCann et al., 1998), orbitofrontal and dorsolat- eral prefrontal cortex (Sekine et al., 2001, 2003), and amygdala (Sekine et al., 2003) of MA-abusing individuals (sample sizes ranging from 6 to 15 MA-dependent subjects; abstinence duration ranging from 7 days to several years). Volkow et al. (2001b) added evidence of the postsynaptic impact of prolonged MA abuse by showing reduced dopamine D_2 recep- tor availability in the striatum that correlated with orbitofrontal glucose metabolism in a group of 15 formerly MA-abusing subjects (abstinent

2 weeks to 5 months). The studies provide evidence that the striato–thalamo–orbitofrontal relationships involved in drive and perseverative behaviors are disrupted in MA-dependent individuals, even after months of abstinence. Another postmortem study of 12 MA-abusing individuals also found a reduction of D_2 dopamine markers at trend levels, but surprisingly, a marked elevation of D_1 dopamine receptor protein (Worsley et al., 2000), indicating that striatal dopamine dysregulation is not limited to D_2 dopamine receptors, and that the changes accompanying chronic MA administration are complex. Behaviorally, striatal DAT reduction was correlated with psychomotor impairment (Volkow et al., 2001a), although in some cases, performance fell within a normal range (Johanson et al., 2006; McCann et al., 1998). Striatal (Sekine et al., 2001) and prefrontal (Sekine et al., 2003) DAT reduction also related to severity and duration of residual psychiatric symptoms, and although no functional correlate was found for the decrease in amygdalar DAT binding, it is conceivable that low DAT availability contributes to the mood disturbances and psychiatric symptoms displayed even after prolonged abstinence (e.g., Hoffman et al., 2006), and/or drug craving (Baicy & London, 2007).

Because MA also affects non-dopaminergic systems (Wilson et al., 1996; also see section on acute effects, p. 61), neuroimaging studies have also investigated deficits in other systems. Using PET, serotonin transporter (SERT) density was found to be lower in 12 formerly MA-abusing subjects, abstinent 1.6 ± 1.3 years, than a healthy control group, in widespread regions encompassing midbrain, thalamus, caudate, putamen, cerebral cortex, and cerebellum, and SERT density in orbitofrontal, temporal, and anterior cingulate areas correlated with aggressive symptoms in the formerly MA-abusing group (Sekine et al., 2006). A postmortem study also found elevated vesicular acetylcholine transporter levels in the caudate nucleus of 20 MA-abusing subjects, compared with 16 control subjects (Siegal et al., 2004), further suggesting dysregulation of multiple transmitter systems in frontrostriatal circuits. Finally, an FDG PET study showed lower relative glucose metabolism in 15 MA-abusing subjects (abstinent 2 weeks–35 months) than in 20 control subjects in subcortical regions that have known dopaminergic innervation (thalamus, caudate, putamen), consistent with the notion of disrupted dopaminergic function, but also showed elevated relative metabolism in parietal cortex, a region with no known dopaminergic innervation (Volkow et al., 2001c). More recently, another FDG PET study replicated the finding of elevated cortical glucose metabolism by demonstrating an increase in parietal metabolism from the first to the fourth week of abstinence in a sample of 10 MA-dependent individuals (Berman et al., 2008). In both studies, parietal metabolism in the MA group correlated with task performance (grooved pegboard task [Volkow et al., 2001c] or continuous performance task [Berman et al., 2008]), suggesting that this dysregulation of both dopaminergic and nondopaminergic systems contributes to the cognitive, motor, and mood deficits observed with longtime MA abuse.

Another approach to assessing the functional deficits associated with long-term MA abuse is measuring whole-brain integrity through perfusion and glucose metabolism. Twenty formerly MA-abusing subjects, abstinent 8 ± 2 months, were found to have lower relative perfusion than control subjects in putamen/insular cortex and lateral parietal cortex, potentially reflecting neuronal injury, and higher relative perfusion than control subjects in temporoparietal white matter and occipital and parietal regions, potentially reflecting gliosis and/or dopamine- and serotonin-related changes in microvasculature (Chang et al., 2002). Although these subjects performed in the normal range on neuropsychological tests, they performed some tasks more slowly than did control subjects, especially those that require working memory, suggesting that the differences in blood flow reflect some disruption in the necessary networks. Perfusion deficits, potentially reflecting vascular changes, were also seen in frontal and temporal cortices in six of nine subjects using SPECT, even after protracted abstinence (>3 years); however, no relationship was found between duration of MA use or abstinence and perfusion (Iyo et al., 1997). Cerebral glucose metabolism also remains abnormal throughout protracted abstinence. As discussed above, Volkow et al. (2001c) showed higher relative parietal and lower relative subcortical glucose metabolism (after scaling to global metabolism) in a group of formerly MA-dependent individuals compared with healthy individuals, accompanying poorer performance on a visuospatial motor task, which suggests that adaptive processes such as reactive proliferation of glial cells (which have a higher metabolic demand than neurons) take place in response to damage in cortical (especially parietal) regions (also see Berman et al., 2008, for elevated parietal glucose metabolism during early abstinence). In addition, a group of 28 formerly MA-abusing men, abstinent 19.14 ± 27.2 months, were found to have lower glucose metabolism in prefrontal white matter than 15 healthy control subjects had, and the severity of this deficit correlated with impairment on the WCST, which relies on prefrontal integrity (Kim et al., 2005). Finally, glucose metabolism in OFC was higher than that of healthy subjects at rest, and activity correlated positively with personality measures of harm avoidance and constraint in MA-abusing subjects (Goldstein et al., 2002), suggesting a relationship between orbitofrontal function and stable personality traits exhibited by many MA-abusing individuals even after protracted abstinence.

As elevated glucose metabolism at rest has been interpreted as a sign of reactive gliosis resulting from neurotoxic insult (Volkow et al., 2001c; Chang et al., 2007), MR spectroscopy has been applied to measure levels of brain metabolites related to neuronal viability, degeneration, and glial proliferation in abstinent MA-dependent individuals. These studies measure regional concentrations of N-acetylaspartate (NAA), which is a marker of neuronal integrity, choline (CHO), which is a measure of neuronal death, myo-inositol (MI), indicating glial proliferation, and creatine (CR), which is often used as a standard by which to standardize the other metabolite measures. These studies have found deficits in the same regions as the PET and postmortem studies, including low NAA in striatum and frontal white matter, suggesting low local neuronal density, and high levels of CHO in frontal white and grey matter and MI in frontal grey matter, suggesting inflammation or glial proliferation (Chang et al., 2005b; Ernst et al., 2000; Sung et al., 2007), as well as low NAA–CR ratios in anterior cingulate grey matter (Nordahl et al., 2002) in samples ranging from 9 to 36 MA-abusing individuals abstinent 4 weeks to several years. These metabolite deficits have been interpreted as indices of neuronal damage and have been associated with behavioral deficits, where reduced striatal CR–CHO ratio was found to correlate with severity of residual psychiatric symptoms in 13 MA-abusing subjects, abstinent 1.5 ± 1.2 years (Sekine et al., 2002), and levels of NAA in the anterior cingulate of 36 MA-abusing subjects, abstinent 19.87 ± 5.37 months correlated with performance on a task of attentional control (Salo et al., 2007). Possible interpretations of this body of research therefore include MA-induced regional neuron loss or dysfunction, disturbances in energetic expenditure, and/or adaptive changes in glial function, accompanied by functional deficits that persist well into protracted periods of abstinence.

Although MRI cannot distinguish between neurotransmitter systems, functional MRI (fMRI) represents the most direct measure of the relationship between brain and behavioral deficits. Studies using fMRI during decision making (choosing between two equally likely responses, given feedback from the previous trial) showed strategy differences between 10 MA-abusing subjects, abstinent 6–46 days, and 10 healthy control subjects, accompanied by deficits in task-related dorsolateral and ventromedial prefrontal activations in the MA group (Paulus et al., 2002), and later, task-related deficits in a cortical network consisting of orbitofrontal and dorsolateral prefrontal cortex, anterior cingulate, and parietal cortex in 14 MA-dependent subjects abstinent 6–46 days (Paulus et al., 2003). Another study (Leland et al., 2008) showed greater responsivity of the ACC in 19 MA-abusing subjects, abstinent 25–50 days, when primed with valid cues than when primed with invalid cues on a go/no-go task (a test of inhibitory function), suggesting that MA-abusing individuals rely more heavily than healthy individuals do on the presence of cues to resolve conflict. Monterosso et al. (2007a) also found evidence of cortical inefficiency in recently abstinent MA-dependent subjects during decision making in a delay-discounting setting by asking them to resolve easy (large reward now vs. small reward later) compared with difficult (small reward now vs. large reward later) discounting operations. Together the evidence collected using fMRI suggests that task-related cortical dysfunction can be detected in all phases of abstinence.

Finally, structural differences are evident even after prolonged abstinence, as 22 MA-abusing individuals exhibited deficits in grey matter concentration (measured during their first week of abstinence), in particular in the cingulate–limbic cortex (a region also found to have metabolic abnormalities [London et al., 2004]) and the ventrolateral prefrontal cortex (Figure 4.3), but also in the hippocampus, where the structural measure was associated with deficits in a word recall task (Thompson et al., 2004). In addition, preliminary evidence using voxel-based morphometry (a measure of grey matter volume) suggests that a region of inferior frontal gyrus contains less grey matter in eight abstinent MA-dependent subjects than control subjects, and that this deficit correlates with performance on the stop-signal task, which tests inhibitory control (Monterosso et al., 2007b). Somewhat paradoxically, other structural studies show abnormally *high* grey matter volumes, such as greater basal ganglia volumes in 50 MA users abstinent 4 ± 6.2 months, and greater parietal cortical volumes in 21 MA-abusing subjects abstinent approximately 3 months (Chang et al., 2005a; Jernigan et al., 2005).

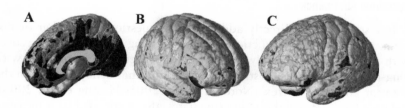

FIGURE 4.3. Grey matter deficits on medial and lateral cortical surfaces, measured with MRI. Maps of group differences on the left medial (A), right (B), and left lateral (C) surfaces represent mean percentage differences in grey matter volumes between the control group average and the MA group average. The cingulate gyrus (A), as well as ventrolateral prefrontal cortex (B and C), showed significant grey matter deficits (dark shades), whereas other brain regions were comparatively spared.

However, these studies differ in the regions investigated, as well as in the period of abstinence in which they were conducted (early vs. prolonged abstinence); the proposed mechanism of initial neuronal injury followed by reactive gliosis and axonal arborization (Volkow et al., 2001c; Berman et al., 2008) could account for this pattern. Notably, Thompson et al. (2004) also showed white matter hypertrophy in temporal and occipital regions, which could be a further indication of gliosis. Finally, there is evidence for shape changes in the corpus callosum of MA-abusing subjects (Oh et al., 2005), where the curvature of the genu was greater in 27 MA users, abstinent 20.5 ± 35.4 months, than in 18 healthy control subjects, and the width of posterior midbody/isthmus was smaller. Because the genu contains fibers connecting prefrontal cortex of the two hemispheres and the midbody contains fibers connecting parietal regions, this finding suggests that fewer fibers pass between these cortical regions in abstinent MA-abusing individuals.

Taken together, the neuroimaging evidence points to frontostriatal deficits, in particular in relation with the dopaminergic system, as underlying the cognitive deficits, compulsive behaviors, and poor decision making often exhibited long after initiating abstinence from MA. Similarly, frontolimbic circuitry and the serotonin system remain impaired throughout prolonged abstinence and can underlie some of the dysregulated affective responses, such as aggression and residual psychotic symptoms. Like the cognitive deficits, many of the affective symptoms could also stem from inhibitory deficits and a loss of executive control, and the two domains are probably intertwined; the interaction between the two is likely to give a more thorough account of the reasons for relapse after prolonged abstinence.

Sustained Abstinence

A few studies have directly addressed the question of whether or not cognitive function and function in the underlying neural systems recover with time. Studies directly comparing short-term (< 6 months) with long-term (> 6 months) abstinence have found that deficits persist in the anterior cingulate cortex (Nordahl et al., 2005; Hwang et al., 2006). Relative levels of metabolic intermediates also were used as a measure of damage and recovery in 16 recently abstinent (2.95 ± .4 months) and eight long-time abstinent (37.5 ± 5.87 months) individuals who had abused MA, and revealed low NAA/CR levels in the anterior cingulate in the MA-dependent group compared to 16 healthy control subjects, regardless of duration of abstinence; however, recently abstinent MA-abusing subjects had much higher levels of CHO/NAA in the ACC than MA-abusing individuals abstinent more than 1 year, who had similar levels to healthy control subjects, suggesting that ACC neurochemistry normalizes with time (Nordahl et al., 2005). Similarly, although a sample of 40 MA-abusing individuals had lower blood flow than 23 healthy control subjects in the ACC, those abstinent >6 months (27 individuals) had greater blood flow in the region than those abstinent <6 months (13 individuals) (Hwang et al., 2006). Grey matter density in right middle frontal cortex also appeared to recover (Kim et al., 2006), as long-term abstinence (18 individuals) was associated with less grey matter deficit than short-term abstinence (11 individuals), although as a group, MA-dependent subjects still had lower grey matter density than control subjects. In addition, MA-dependent subjects performed more poorly on the WCST than control subjects did, suggesting prefrontal dysfunction, but longer duration of abstinence was associated with better performance. This suggests that, with time, prefrontal neurochemistry, structure, and function recover, although not to the level of healthy comparison subjects.

Basal ganglia function has also been investigated in the context of short-term versus long-term abstinence. DAT levels measured in the same five MA-dependent individuals after short-term (<6 months) and long-term (12–17 months) abstinence increased significantly, no longer showing a significant difference from control levels after protracted abstinence, and although performance on a neuropsychological evaluation containing memory and motor tasks did not recover completely, the DAT recovery points to reversible adaptations of dopamine terminals (although it could also represent an increase in arborization of surviving neurons; Volkow et al., 2001d). Glucose metabolism of five MA-abusing subjects, while recovering to control levels in thalamus after 12–17 months, did not recover in striatum (in particular caudate and nucleus accumbens). However, the duration-dependent thalamic increases in glucose metabolism were associated with improved performance on motor and verbal memory tasks (Wang et al., 2004). In summary, although the evidence is still sparse, there are some indications of recovery or compensation after significant amounts of time without MA use.

Current Controversies

Controversy at this time revolves around the issue of whether or not the MA-related deficits in neural circuitry signify permanent neurotoxic damage, or a manifestation of adaptive, reversible changes. In other words, it is unclear whether brain structure and function recover to levels predating MA abuse after sufficient time has passed in abstinence. Some of the preclinical literature points toward neurotoxic damage, as chronic high-dose administration of MA leads to neuronal death in rodents and nonhuman primates (e.g., Chang et al., 2007; but see Harvey et al., 2000, for evidence of DAT recovery with time and failure to detect cell loss in vervet monkeys). This pattern cannot be ascertained in humans, however, as studies using human *in vivo* techniques rely on cross-sectional samples rather than longitudinal data, and dose, frequency, and route of administration cannot be systematically controlled in human studies. Spectroscopy and structural MRI data suggest a picture of neuronal damage in frontostriatal and paralimbic circuits (Nordahl et al., 2003; Thompson et al., 2004; see Figure 4.3), by showing lower levels of markers for neuronal integrity and lower grey matter concentration (interpreted as neuronal loss), higher markers for reactive gliosis (interpreted as an adaptive response to neuronal injury), and long-lasting cognitive deficits and psychiatric symptoms (interpreted as functional consequences to the substrate loss). These neurochemical and structural deficits appear to be paralleled by decreases in available dopamine and serotonin binding sites (Volkow et al., 2001a; McCann et al., 1998; Sekine et al., 2002, 2006). Given that these deficits can be detected after up to 35 months of abstinence (Volkow et al., 2001a), they have been interpreted as irreversible damage in the relevant neural circuitry. On the other hand, postmortem studies in humans that have found similar evidence for decreases in striatal dopamine and DAT levels also found normal levels of vesicular monoamine transporter (VMAT) suggesting that the terminals in fact survived, but DAT proteins expressed on the surface may have been downregulated or internalized into the cell membrane, accounting for the inability of PET tracers to bind (Wilson et al., 1996; Moszczynska et al., 2004). However, a recent PET study found slight decreases in VMAT binding (Johanson et al., 2006), highlighting the importance of replicating this finding in larger samples and with multiple techniques. Arguing for the reversibility of deficits, recovery was observed in regional DAT binding and normalization of glucose metabolism after sustained abstinence (Volkow et al., 2001d; Wang et al., 2004), suggesting that the measured deficits in early abstinence represent reversible changes that renormalize with time. This "normalization" in binding potential or metabolism could also reflect compensatory axonal arborization from the surviving neurons (Jernigan et al., 2005) and/or inflammation/gliosis (Volkow et al., 2001d); furthermore, failure to recover in all regions investigated or failure to recover to levels comparable to those of healthy control subjects could still point to region-specific sustained deficits indicative of neuronal death. Resolution of this debate will require detailed longitudinal studies with sufficient statistical power and sensitivity to detect regional changes over time. In the end, however, it is of little consequence whether permanent damage occurs with chronic MA administration, as a wealth of imaging evidence points to functional and structural deficits during early abstinence; understanding those deficits, regardless of their underlying neurochemistry or trajectory, will help identify treatment targets and improve intervention and relapse prevention.

The notion of "incomplete recovery" noted above also highlights another point of controversy, namely that it is unclear from human *in vivo* studies whether premorbid levels of transporter protein, metabolites, or cortical structure/function of individuals who become MA-dependent were ever comparable to those of the control subjects. Using neuroimaging techniques, we can only observe correlations between MA abuse and these neuronal measures, but not causation; lower levels of brain-integrity markers could also reflect a condition that predates and perhaps even predisposes to MA addiction. Across the population, many markers of brain structure and function exist on a range of levels that are determined by genetic and environmental factors, and a particular combination of predisposing factors could impart greater risk of becoming MA-dependent. A number of genetic polymorphisms in the DA system are highly common in MA-abusing populations (see Barr et al., 2006, for review), suggesting that genetic mechanisms modulate the reinforcing effects of MA by influencing function (and conceivably structure) of relevant systems in the brain, and that those individuals who become MA dependent could be those who try to compensate for an intrinsically hyporesponsive dopamine system. Similarly, susceptibility to MA psychosis has been linked to genetic factors (Suzuki et al., 2006; Matsuzawa et al., 2007), and imaging studies detecting differences between MA-dependent and healthy populations cannot discern between factors that precipitated MA abuse/psychosis and those that are a consequence. As a striking example, recent PET research in rodents has shown that those rats who exhibited impulsive behavioral traits had lower striatal $D_{2/3}$ receptor availability, and were also more likely to self-administer cocaine (Dalley et al., 2007). Although the link to MA-abusing humans is not clear, the study shows that genetic variability can underlie behavioral choices as well as PET findings, irrespective of putative neurotoxic effects of the drug. Because MA acutely improves cognitive function (see section on acute effects, p. 61), individuals with cognitive deficits might also be more likely to use MA to improve cognitive function, and individuals with mood or social disorders may use MA to attain a less emotionally disruptive or aversive state. Measurements comparing groups, then, would detect differences that do not necessarily arise as a consequence of MA abuse, but rather arise as a result of biased cross-sectional sampling. Environmental factors such as stress also lead to both greater likelihood of drug abuse and lower markers of brain structure and function (e.g., Radley & Morrison, 2005; Eluvathingal et al., 2006), creating the appearance of MA-induced deficits when it is also plausible that MA abuse and deficits have an underlying but unrelated common environmental cause. One argument against this line of reasoning is that cognitive and brain deficits correlate with duration of use before initiating abstinence, amount used, and duration of abstinence. Abstinent individuals with a longer history of MA abuse had less prefrontal white matter NAA and lower DAT and SERT binding (Ernst et al., 2000; Sekine et al., 2006; Volkow et al., 2001a), and individuals with greater cumulative amounts used had smaller basal ganglia volumes and performed more poorly on a task of motor inhibition (Monterosso et al., 2005; Chang et al., 2005a; but see Simon et al., 2000, for a failure to find such correlations). Again, however, those individuals with the greatest premorbid neurochemical deficits may be those who initiate MA abuse the earliest, or escalate to greater doses the fastest. Resolution of this debate will require thorough characterization of premorbid factors that potentially influence results, and matching MA-abusing and healthy individuals on those factors. In the end, as before, what matters most is an understanding of the nature of these group differences, regardless of whether they reflect vulnerability to, or consequences, of MA abuse, as this will lead to more sensitive and effective strategies for intervention.

Relation to Treatment

Ultimately, much of the research on MA abuse and associated neural deficits is conducted in an effort to design effective treatments. Although treatment development has been the motivation for a number of the imaging studies reviewed here, only one study, to our knowledge, has addressed this topic directly. Paulus et al. (2005) used fMRI to test MA-dependent subjects during early abstinence while they performed a decision-making task. Regional activity during task performance correctly predicted relapse in 20 of 22 subjects who had relapsed at follow-up, and correctly predicted sustained abstinence in 17 of 18 subjects who had not relapsed at follow-up, demonstrating that cognitive function during early abstinence can predict treatment success. Since the most successful current treatments for MA addiction are behavioral therapies, the study also underscores the importance of understanding which cognitive functions are affected in MA abuse, and which of those are amenable to improvement. Many of the studies testing cognitive function in MA-abusing individuals in conjunction with neuroimaging have made strides toward answering that question.

One area of cognitive function that has received particular attention with respect to treatment is inhibitory control, as imparted by prefrontal cortical regions over striatal, thalamic, and limbic targets (for review, see Goldstein & Volkow, 2002; Kalivas & Volkow, 2005; Baicy & London, 2007). Inhibitory control has been operationalized as the ability to ignore task-irrelevant information via the Stroop task (e.g., Salo et al., 2002, 2005), and as the ability to inhibit motor responses that are already under way via the stop-signal task (Monterosso et al., 2005, 2007b). In both cases, performance was poorer in MA-dependent than in healthy subjects, and accompanied structural and functional deficits in relevant brain regions. As treatment adherence relies in large part on the ability of the patient to exercise executive inhibitory control in responding to cues that trigger impulses for drug-seeking during everyday circumstances, behavioral therapies might benefit from interventions that specifically improve inhibitory function. This idea is currently being tested using several promising compounds, and if results show improvement in brain function and task performance, this strategy could be applied to treatment populations to test its utility in predicting and improving treatment retention.

Similarly, emotional self-control is a part of successful behavioral treatment, in that cognitive strategies can be employed to alleviate stressful affective states such as depression, anxiety, and craving, which are in turn associated with risk for relapse (e.g., Vocci et al., 2005). Neuroimaging research can help identify potential targets for improvement in emotion control, as studies have shown some of the neural abnormalities associated with negative or maladaptive affective states during abstinence from MA (London et al., 2004; Payer et al., 2007; Sekine et al., 2006). As described earlier, pharmacological interventions could target the affected circuitry, improving the capacity of MA-abusing individuals to control or alleviate negative affect, which might further improve treatment success.

Finally, studies of delay discounting may be valuable for the improvement of contingency-management-based treatments, as this approach relies on rewarding patients for sustained abstinence, and as such is vulnerable to the tendency of MA-abusing individuals to discount delayed rewards, as demonstrated by a lower capacity for awaiting large rewards in favor of "cashing in" small, immediate rewards (e.g., Monterosso et al., 2007a; Hoffman et al., 2006). Functional MRI suggests that cortical deficits are associated with decision making in this type of delay-discounting setting (Monterosso et al., 2007a). Continued pursuit of this line of research, along with the neural circuitry of impulsive decision-making, could help establish optimal reward size and delay length during contingency management; if discounting functions can be established for each patient and rewards tailored accordingly, patients may be less likely to choose immediate rewards (i.e., MA). Combined with improved inhibitory and other cognitive functions, patients may then be able to improve their ability for awaiting delayed rewards, and thus be more capable of benefiting from the behavioral treatments.

Unanswered Questions

Despite ongoing efforts to elucidate the nature and extent of neural and behavioral deficits associated with MA abuse, a number of unanswered questions remain, making research often difficult to interpret. For example, unless studies directly relate their findings to treatment outcome (e.g., Paulus et al., 2005), it is difficult to determine the meaning, or ecological validity, of group differences in some marker of brain structure or function, or in behavior. Not only are findings from *in vivo* imaging studies only inferential, meaning we do not know the underlying neurochemical deficit or generator of signal difference, but the finding could also be unrelated to MA addiction (as discussed earlier, it could predate the addiction or represent a marker of a population that also happens to be more susceptible to drug addiction), or even if it is MA-related, it could be meaningless in terms of functional significance or predictive power, meaning the deficit could have no implications for treatment. We do not currently have reliable predictors for relapse risk or treatment success, and as such, no way to assess who is likely to respond to treatment. To answer this question, more studies will have to be conducted that directly link some experimental manipulation and technique to real-world outcomes such as treatment retention and sustained abstinence.

Another unanswered question revolves around brain connectivity. Although imaging research has found a number of regional differences and deficits in MA-abusing individuals, it is unclear whether the deficits are truly localized or represent a deficit in connectivity between regions that could conceivably be functioning properly. Although some evidence, such as white matter hyperintensities and callosal shape changes, point to white matter dysfunction (Bae et al., 2006; Oh et al., 2005), methodologies such as diffusion tensor imaging are needed to determine whether brain deficits are indeed regional, a manifestation of a breakdown in the connections between regions, or both.

Yet another confounding factor that is currently poorly understood is that of comorbidity, as individuals who abuse only MA, and MA-abusing individuals who only have a single diagnosis of substance dependence are rare. Individuals who abuse MA tend to abuse stimulants in general, including cocaine, and tend to use marijuana and tobacco. Abuse of each of these substances is associated with its own set of neural and behavioral dysfunctions, partially overlapping those of MA abuse, and how to disentangle potential deleterious effects of these substances from those of MA alone is a difficult issue in many neuroimaging studies. Furthermore, individuals who abuse MA often have comorbid diagnoses of ADHD, depression, anxiety, personality disorders, or HIV, and may be undergoing pharmacotherapy for some of these disorders. How these factors affect neuroimaging results, especially when they are not always detected or disclosed and thus not taken into consideration in the interpretation of results, remains unanswered.

Finally, although some promising targets have been identified, little is known about the individual differences that may affect risk for abuse, treatment success, and/or neuroimaging results. In terms of effect on imaging results, a growing number of studies are detecting differences in brain structure and function that are determined by genetic polymorphisms even in healthy individuals, in particular in systems that are implicated in drug abuse (e.g., Hariri & Weinberger, 2003; Meyer-Lindenberg et al., 2005; Eisenberger et al., 2007). Whether failure to take these factors into consideration in imaging studies can bias or obscure results, whether and how many of such differences remain undiscovered, and how they influence interpretation of imaging results also remains a set of unanswered questions.

Conclusion

Despite the controversies and unanswered questions described here, neuroimaging research has substantially contributed to uncovering and describing many of the neurochemical, structural, and functional deficits associated with the abuse of MA. The continued use of emerging technologies in neuroimaging promises to offer great help in providing information that can eventually be used to inform treatment for MA dependence.

Acknowledgments

Research was supported by NIH grants P20 DA022539, R01 DA020726, and F31 DA025422.

References

Aron A, Behrens T, Smith S, et al. (2007). Triangulating a cognitive control network using diffusion-weighted magnetic resonance imaging (MRI) and functional MRI. *J Neurosci* 27:3743–3752.

Bae S, Lyoo I, Sung Y, et al. (2006). Increased white matter hyperintensities in male methamphetamine abusers. *Drug Alcohol Depend* 81:83–88.

Baicy K, London E. (2007). Corticolimbic dysregulation and chronic methamphetamine abuse. *Addiction* 102(Suppl. 1):5–15.

Barr A, Panenka W, MacEwan G, et al. (2006). The need for speed: An update on methamphetamine addiction. *J Psychiatry Neurosci* 31:301.

Berman S, Voytek B, Mandelkern M, et al. (2008). Changes in cerebral glucose metabolism during early abstinence from chronic methamphetamine abuse. *Mol Psychiatry* 13(9):897–908.

Buffenstein A, Heaster J, Ko P. (1999). Chronic psychotic illness from methamphetamine. *Am J Psychiatry* 156:662.

Chang L, Alicata D, Ernst T, et al. (2007). Structural and metabolic brain changes in the striatum associated with methamphetamine abuse. *Addiction* 102:16–32.

Chang L, Cloak C, Patterson K, et al. (2005a). Enlarged striatum in abstinent methamphetamine abusers: A possible compensatory response. *Biol Psychiatry* 57:967–974.

Chang L, Ernst T, Speck O, et al. (2005b). Additive effects of HIV and chronic methamphetamine use on brain metabolite abnormalities. *Am J Psychiatry* 162:361–369.

Chang L, Ernst T, Speck O, et al. (2002). Perfusion MRI and computerized cognitive test abnormalities in abstinent methamphetamine users. *Psychiatry Res* 114:65–79.

Chou Y, Huang W, Su T, et al. (2007). Dopamine transporters and cognitive function in methamphetamine abusers after a short abstinence: A SPECT study. *Eur Neuropsychopharmacol* 17:46–52.

Comer S, Hart C, Ward A, et al. (2001). Effects of repeated oral methamphetamine administration in humans. *Psychopharmacology* 155:397–404.

Dalley J, Fryer T, Brichard L, et al. (2007). Nucleus accumbens D2/3 receptors predict trait impulsivity and cocaine reinforcement. *Science* 315:1267–1270.

Dlugos A, Freitag C, Hohoff C, et al. (2007). Norephinephrine transporter gene variation modulates acute response to d-amphetamine. *Biol Psychiatry* 61:1296–1305.

Drevets W, Gautier C, Price J, et al. (2001). Amphetamine-induced dopamine release in human ventral striatum correlates with euphoria. *Biol Psychiatry* 49:81–96.

Eisenberger N, Way B, Taylor S, et al. (2007). Understanding genetic risk for aggression: Clues from the brain's response to social exclusion. *Biol Psychiatry* 61:1100–1108.

Eluvathingal T, Chugani H, Behen M, et al. (2006). Abnormal brain connectivity in children after early severe socioemotional deprivation: A diffusion tensor imaging study. *Pediatrics* 117:2093–2100.

Ernst M, Zametkin A, Matochik J, et al. (1997). Intravenous dextroamphetamine and brain glucose metabolism. *Neuropsychopharmacology* 17:391–401.

Ernst T, Chang L, Leonido-Yee M, et al. (2000). Evidence for long-term neurotoxicity associated with methamphetamine abuse: A 1H MRS study. *Neurology* 54:1344–1349.

Flanagin B, Cook E, de Wit H. (2006). An association study of the brain-derived neurotrophic factor Val66Met polymorphism and amphetamine response. *Am J Med Genet B Neuropsychiatr Genet* 141:576–583.

Goldstein R, Volkow N. (2002). Drug addiction and its underlying neurobiological basis: Neuroimaging evidence for the involvement of the frontal cortex. *Am J Psychiatry* 159:1642–1652.

Goldstein R, Volkow N, Chang L, et al. (2002). The orbitofrontal cortex in methamphetamine addiction: Involvement in fear. *Neuroreport* 13:2253–2257.

Gonzalez R, Rippeth J, Carey C, et al. (2004). Neurocognitive performance of methamphetamine users discordant for history of marijuana exposure. *Drug Alcohol Depend* 76:181–190.

Gouzoulis-Mayfrank E, Schreckenberger M, Sabri O, et al. (1999). Neurometabolic effects of psilocybin, 3,4-methylenedioxyethylamphetamine (MDE) and d-methamphetamine in healthy volunteers: A double-blind, placebo-controlled PET study with [18F]FDG. *Neuropsychopharmacology* 20:565–581.

Harano M, Uchimura N, Abe H, et al. (2004). A polymorphism of DRD2 gene and brain atrophy in methamphetamine psychosis. *Ann NY Acad Sci* 1025:307–315.

Hariri A, Mattay V, Tessitore A, et al. (2002). Dextroamphetamine modulates the response of the human amygdala. *Neuropsychopharmacology* 27:1036–1040.

Hariri A, Weinberger D. (2003). Functional neuroimaging of genetic variation in serotonergic neurotransmission. *Genes Brain Behav* 2:341–349.

Harris D, Reus V, Wolkowitz O, et al. (2003). Altering cortisol level does not change the pleasurable effects of methamphetamine in humans. *Neuropsychopharmacology* 28:1677–1684.

Hart C, Ward A, Haney M, et al. (2001). Methamphetamine self-administration by humans. *Psychopharmacology* 157:75–81.

Harvey D, Lacan G, Tanious S, et al. (2000). Recovery from methamphetamine induced long-term nigrostriatal dopaminergic deficits without substantia nigra cell loss. *Brain Res* 871:259–270.

Hoffman W, Moore M, Templin R, et al. (2006). Neuropsychological function and delay discounting in methamphetamine-dependent individuals. *Psychopharmacology* 188:162–170.

Huber A, Ling W, Shoptaw S, et al. (1997). Integrating treatments for methamphetamine abuse: A psychosocial perspective. *J Addict Dis* 16:41–50.

Hutchison K, Wood M, Swift R. (1999). Personality factors moderate subjective and psychophysiological responses to d-amphetamine in humans. *Exp Clin Psychopharmacol* 7:493–501.

Hwang J, Lyoo I, Kim S, et al. (2006). Decreased cerebral blood flow of the right anterior cingulate cortex in long-term and short-term abstinent methamphetamine users. *Drug Alcohol Depend* 82:177–181.

Iwanami A, Kuroki N, Iritani S, et al. (1998). P3a of event-related potential in chronic methamphetamine dependence. *J Nerv Ment Dis* 186:746–751.

Iwanami A, Suga I, Kato N, et al. (1993). Event-related potentials in methamphetamine psychosis during an auditory discrimination task: A preliminary report. *Eur Arch Psychiatry Clin Neurosci* 242:203–208.

Iyo M, Namba H, Yanagisawa M, et al. (1997). Abnormal cerebral perfusion in chronic methamphetamine abusers: a study using 99MTc-HMPAO and SPECT. *Prog Neuropsychopharmacol Biol Psychiatry* 21:789–796.

Iyo M, Nishio M, Itoh T, et al. (1993). Dopamine D_2 and serotonin S_2 receptors in susceptibility to methamphetamine psychosis detected by positron emission tomography. *Psychiatry Res* 50:217–231.

Iyo M, Sekine Y, Mori N. (2004). Neuromechanism of developing methamphetamine psychosis: A neuroimaging study. *Ann NY Acad Sci* 1025:288–295.

Jernigan T, Gamst A, Archibald S, et al. (2005). Effects of methamphetamine dependence and HIV infection on cerebral morphology. *Am J Psychiatry* 162:1461–1472.

Johanson C, Frey K, Lundahl L, et al. (2006). Cognitive function and nigrostriatal markers in abstinent methamphetamine abusers. *Psychopharmacology* 185:327–338.

Kalechstein A, Newton T, Green M. (2003). Methamphetamine dependence is associated with neurocognitive impairment in the initial phases of abstinence. *J Neuropsychiatry Clin Neurosci* 15:215–220.

Kalivas P, Volkow N. (2005). The neural basis of addiction: A pathology of motivation and choice. *Am J Psychiatry* 162:1403–1413.

Kim S, Lyoo I, Hwang D, et al. (2005). Frontal glucose hypometabolism in abstinent methamphetamine users. *Neuropsychopharmacology* 30:1383–1391.

Kim S, Lyoo I, Hwang J, et al. (2006). Prefrontal grey-matter changes in short-term and long-term abstinent methamphetamine abusers. *Int J Neuropsychopharmacol* 9:221–228.

Kleinschmidt A, Bruhn H, Kruger G, et al. (1999). Effects of sedation, stimulation, and placebo on cerebral blood oxygenation: A magnetic resonance neuroimaging study of psychotropic drug action. *NMR Biomed* 12:286–292.

Leland D, Arce E, Miller D, et al. (2008) Anterior cingulate cortex and benefit of predictive cueing on response inhibition in stimulant dependent Individuals. *Biol Psychiatry* 63(2):184–190.

Leyton M, Boileau I, Benkeifat C, et al. (2002). Amphetamine-induced increases in extracellular dopamine, drug wanting, and novelty seeking: A PET/[11C] raclopride study in healthy men. *Neuropsychopharmacology* 27:1027–1035.

London E, Berman S, Voytek B, et al. (2005). Cerebral metabolic dysfunction and impaired vigilance in recently abstinent methamphetamine abusers. *Biol Psychiatry* 58:770–778.

London E, Simon S, Berman S, et al. (2004). Mood disturbances and regional cerebral metabolic abnormalities in recently abstinent methamphetamine abusers. *Arch Gen Psychiatry* 61:73–84.

Lott D, Kim S, Cook E, et al. (2005). Dopamine transporter gene associated with diminished subjective response to amphetamine. *Neuropsychopharmacology* 30:602–609.

Lott D, Kim S, Cook E, et al. (2006). Serotonin transporter genotype and acute subjective response to amphetamine. *Am J Addict* 15:327–335.

Martinez D, Slifstein M, Broft A, et al. (2003). Imaging human mesolimbic dopamine transmission with positron emission tomography. Part II: Amphetamine-induced dopamine release in the functional subdivisions of the striatum. *J Cereb Blood Flow Metab* 23:285–300.

Matsuzawa D, Hashimoto K, Miyatake R, et al. (2007). Identification of functional polymorphisms in the promoter region of the human PICK1 gene and their association with methamphetamine psychosis. *Am J Psychiatry* 164(7):999–1001.

Mattay V, Berman K, Ostrem J, et al. (1996). Dextroamphetamine enhances "neural network-specific" physiological signals: A positron-emission tomography rCBF study. *J Neurosci* 16:4816–4822.

Mattay V, Callicott J, Bertolino A, et al. (2000). Effects of dextroamphetamine on cognitive performance and cortical activation. *Neuroimage* 12:268–275.

Mattay V, Goldberg T, Fera F, et al. (2003). Catechol O-methyltransferase val158-met genotype and individual variation in the brain response to amphetamine. *Proc Natl Acad Sci USA* 100:6186–6191.

McCann U, Wong D, Yokoi F, et al. (1998). Reduced striatal dopamine transporter density in abstinent methamphetamine and methcathinone users: Evidence from positron emission tomography studies with [^{11}C]WIN-35,428. *J Neurosci* 18:8417–8422.

McGregor C, Srisurapanont M, Jittiwutikarn J, et al. (2005). The nature, time course, and severity of methamphetamine withdrawal. *Addiction* 100:1320–1329.

Meyer-Lindenberg A, Kohn P, Kolachana B, et al. (2005). Midbrain dopamine and prefrontal function in humans: Interaction and modulation by COMT genotype. *Nat Neurosci* 8:594–596.

Mohs R, Tinklenberg J, Roth W, et al. (1978). Methamphetamine and diphenhydramine effects on the rate of cognitive processing. *Psychopharmacology* 59:13–19.

Mohs R, Tinklenberg J, Roth W, et al. (1980). Sensitivity of some human cognitive functions to effects of methamphetamine and secobarbital. *Drug Alcohol Depend* 5:145–150.

Monterosso J, Ainslie G, Xu J, et al. (2007a). Frontoparietal cortical activity of methamphetamine-dependent and comparison subjects performing a delay discounting task. *Hum Brain Mapp* 28:383–393.

Monterosso J, Aron A, Cordova X, et al. (2005). Deficits in response inhibition associated with chronic methamphetamine abuse. *Drug Alcohol Depend* 79:273–277.

Monterosso J, Tabibnia G, Chakrapani S, et al. (2007b, November). *Does higher grey matter density in right inferior frontal gyrus predict better stop signal reaction time? Voxel-based morphometry in methamphetamine-dependent and healthy comparison subjects.* Paper presented at the 37th annual meeting of the Society for Neuroscience, San Diego.

Moszczynska A, Fitzmaurice P, Ang L, et al. (2004). Why is parkinsonism not a feature of human methamphetamine users? *Brain* 127:363–370.

Munro C, McCaul M, Wong D, et al. (2006). Sex differences in striatal dopamine release in healthy adults. *Biol Psychiatry* 59:966–974.

Newton T, Cook I, Kalechstein A, et al. (2003). Quantitative EEG abnormalities in recently abstinent methamphetamine dependent individuals. *Clin Neurophysiol* 114:410–415.

Newton T, De La Garza R, Kalechstein A, et al. (2005). Cocaine and methamphetamine produce different patterns of subjective and cardiovascular effects. *Pharmacol Biochem Behav* 82:90–97.

Newton T, Kalechstein A, Duran S, et al. (2004a). Methamphetamine abstinence syndrome: Preliminary findings. *Am J Addict* 13:248–255.

Newton T, Kalechstein A, Hardy D, et al. (2004b). Association between quantitative EEG and neurocognition in methamphetamine-dependent volunteers. *Clin Neurophysiol* 115:194–198.

Newton T, Roache J, De La Garza R, et al. (2006). Bupropion reduces methamphetamine-induced subjective effects and cue-induced craving. *Neuropsychopharmacology* 31:1537–1544.

Nordahl T, Salo R, Leamon M. (2003). Neuropsychological effects of chronic methamphetamine use on neurotransmitters and cognition: A review. *J Neuropsychiatry Clin Neurosci* 15:317–325.

Nordahl T, Salo R, Natsuaki Y, et al. (2005). Methamphetamine users in sustained abstinence: A proton magnetic resonance spectroscopy study. *Arch Gen Psychiatry* 62:444–452.

Nordahl T, Salo R, Possin K, et al. (2002). Low N-acetyl-aspartate and high choline in the anterior cingulum of recently abstinent methamphetamine-dependent subjects: A preliminary proton MRS study. *Psychiatry Res* 116:43–52.

Oh J, Lyoo I, Sung Y, et al. (2005). Shape changes of the corpus callosum in abstinent methamphetamine users. *Neurosci Lett* 384:76–81.

Oswald L, Wong D, Zhou Y, et al. (2007). Impulsivity and chronic stress are associated with amphetamine-induced striatal dopamine release. *Neuroimage* 36:153–166.

Paulus M, Hozack N, Frank L, et al. (2003). Decision making by methamphetamine-dependent subjects is associated with error-rate-independent decrease in prefrontal and parietal activation. *Biol Psychiatry* 53:65–74.

Paulus M, Hozack N, Zauscher B, et al. (2002). Behavioral and functional neuroimaging evidence for prefrontal dysfunction in methamphetamine-dependent subjects. *Neuropsychopharmacology* 26:53–63.

Paulus M, Tapert S, Schuckit M. (2005). Neural activation patterns of methamphetamine-dependent subjects during decision making predict relapse. *Arch Gen Psychiatry* 62:761–768.

Payer DE, Lieberman MD, Monterosso JR, et al. (2008). Differences in cortical activity between methamphetamine-dependent and healthy individuals performing a facial affect matching task. *Drug Alcohol Depend* 93(1–2):93–102.

Payer DE, Lieberman MD, Rowny S, et al. (2007, November) *Amygdala down-regulation via affect labeling is disrupted in methamphetamine-dependent individuals*. Paper presented at the 37th annual meeting of the Society for Neuroscience, San Diego.

Radley J, Morrison J. (2005). Repeated stress and structural plasticity in the brain. *Ageing Res Rev* 4:271–287.

Salo R, Nordahl T, Moore C, et al. (2005). A dissociation in attentional control: Evidence from methamphetamine dependence. *Biol Psychiatry* 57:310–313.

Salo R, Nordahl T, Natsuaki Y, et al. (2007). Attentional control and brain metabolite levels in methamphetamine abusers. *Biol Psychiatry* 61:1272–1280.

Salo R, Nordahl T, Possin K, et al. (2002). Preliminary evidence of reduced cognitive inhibition in methamphetamine-dependent individuals. *Psychiatry Res* 111:65–74.

Sekine Y, Iyo M, Ouchi Y, et al. (2001). Methamphetamine-related psychiatric symptoms and reduced brain dopamine transporters studied with PET. *Am J Psychiatry* 158:1206–1214.

Sekine Y, Minabe Y, Kawai M, et al. (2002). Metabolite alterations in basal ganglia associated with methamphetamine-related psychiatric symptoms: A proton MRS study. *Neuropsychopharmacology* 27:453–461.

Sekine Y, Minabe Y, Ouchi Y, et al. (2003). Association of dopamine transporter loss in the orbitofrontal and dorsolateral prefrontal cortices with methamphetamine-related psychiatric symptoms. *Am J Psychiatry* 160:1699–1701.

Sekine Y, Ouchi Y, Takei N, et al. (2006). Brain serotonin transporter density and aggression in abstinent methamphetamine abusers. *Arch Gen Psychiatry* 63:90–100.

Semple S, Zians J, Grant I, et al. (2006). Methamphetamine use, impulsivity, and sexual risk behavior among HIV-positive men who have sex with men. *J Addict Dis* 25:105–114.

Siegal D, Erickson J, Varogui H, et al. (2004). Brain vesicular acetylcholine transporter in human users of drugs of abuse. *Synapse* 52:223–232.

Simon S, Domier C, Carnell J, et al. (2000). Cognitive impairment in individuals currently using methamphetamine. *Am J Addict* 9:222–231.

Simon S, Domier C, Sim T, et al. (2002). Cognitive performance of current methamphetamine and cocaine abusers. *J Addict Dis* 21:61–74.

Sung Y, Cho S, Hwang J, et al. (2007). Relationship between *N*-acetyl-aspartate in grey and white matter of abstinent methamphetamine abusers and their history of drug abuse: A proton magnetic resonance spectroscopy study. *Drug Alcohol Depend* 88:28–35.

Suzuki A, Nakamura K, Sekine Y, et al. (2006). An association study between catechol-O-methyl transferase gene polymorphism and methamphetamine psychotic disorder. *Psychiatr Genet* 16:133–138.

Szuster R. (1990). Methamphetamine in psychiatric emergencies. *Hawaii Med J* 49:389–391.

Thompson P, Hayashi K, Simon S, et al. (2004). Structural abnormalities in the brains of subjects who use methamphetamine. *J Neurosci* 24:6028–6036.

Uftring S, Wachtel S, Chu D, et al. (2001). An fMRI study of the effect of amphetamine on brain activity. *Neuropsychopharmacology* 25:925–935.

Vocci F, Acri J, Elkashef A. (2005). Medication development for addictive disorders: The state of the science. *Am J Psychiatry* 162:1432–1440.

Volkow N, Chang L, Wang G, et al. (2001a). Low level of brain dopamine D_2 receptors in methamphetamine abusers: Association with metabolism in the orbitofrontal cortex. *Am J Psychiatry* 158:2015–2021.

Volkow N, Chang L, Wang G, et al. (2001b). Higher cortical and lower subortical metabolism in detoxified methamphetamine abusers. *Am J Psychiatry* 158:383–389.

Volkow N, Chang L, Wang G, et al. (2001c). Loss of dopamine transporters in methamphetamine abusers recovers with protracted abstinence. *J Neurosci* 21:9414–9418.

Volkow N, Chang L, Wang G, et al. (2001d). Association of dopamine transporter reduction with psychomotor impairment in methamphetamine abusers. *Am J Psychiatry* 158:377–382.

Vollenweider F, Maguire R, Leenders K, et al. (1998). Effects of high amphetamine dose on mood and cerebral glucose metabolism in normal volunteers using positron emission tomography (PET). *Psychiatry Res* 83:149–162.

Völlm B, de Araujo I, Cowen P, et al. (2004). Methamphetamine activates reward circuitry in drug naïve human subjects. *Neuropsychopharmacology* 29:1715–1722.

Wang G, Volkow N, Chang L, et al. (2004). Partial recovery of brain metabolism in methamphetamine abusers after protracted abstinence. *Am J Psychiatry* 161:242–248.

White T, Lott D, de Wit H. (2006). Personality and the subjective effects of acute amphetamine in healthy volunteers. *Neuropsychopharmacology* 31:1064–1074.

Wiegmann D, Stanny R, McKay D, et al. (1996). Methamphetamine effects on cognitive processing during extended wakefulness. *Int J Aviat Psychol* 6:379–397.

Willson M, Wilman A, Bell E, et al. (2004). Dextroamphetamine causes a change in regional brain activity in vivo during cognitive tasks: A functional magnetic resonance imaging study of blood oxygen level-dependent response. *Biol Psychiatry* 56:284–291.

Wolkin A, Angrist B, Wolf A, et al. (1987). Effects of amphetamine on local cerebral metabolism in normal and schizophrenic subjects as determined by positron emission tomography. *Psychopharmacology* 92:241–246.

Woods S, Rippeth J, Conover E, et al. (2005). Deficient strategic control of verbal encoding and retrieval in individuals with methamphetamine dependence. *Neuropsychology* 19:35–43.

Worsley J, Moszczynska A, Falardeau P, et al. (2000). Dopamine D$_1$ receptor protein is elevated in nucleus accumbens of human, chronic methamphetamine users. *Mol Psychiatry* 5:664–672.

Yui K, Goto K, Ikemoto S. (2004). The role of noradrenergic and dopaminergic hyperactivity in the development of spontaneous recurrence of methamphetamine psychosis and susceptibility to episode recurrence. *Ann NY Acad Sci* 1025:296–306.

Chapter 5

Behavioral Pharmacology and Psychiatric Consequences of Methamphetamine

Craig R. Rush, William W. Stoops, and Walter Ling

Methamphetamine (MA) abuse and dependence is a significant public health concern (Drug and Alcohol Services Information System [DASIS] Report, 2004). The number of Americans who reported MA use increased 250% between 1996 and 2002 (4.8 million in 1996, 12 million in 2002; Substance Abuse and Mental Health Services Administration [SAMHSA], 2003). The number of individuals reporting recent use of MA has remained relatively stable over the past 4 years with approximately 731,000 Americans reporting past-month use in 2005 (SAMHSA, 2007). Rates of primary treatment admissions for MA increased nearly 200% between 2000 and 2004 (National Drug Intelligence Center [NDIC], 2006). By contrast, treatment admissions for cocaine decreased 24% between 1992 and 2002 (DASIS, 2005). This decrease may be attributable to some cocaine users' switching to MA because it is cheaper and produces longer-lasting effects (Community Epidemiology Work Group [CEWG], 2004). MA is a public health concern similar in magnitude to, or perhaps greater than, that of cocaine.

Alarmingly, the dependence process may proceed more rapidly for MA than cocaine (Castro et al., 2000). In this study, 39 regular users of MA, but not cocaine, were compared to 90 regular users of cocaine, but not MA. The period of time from initial to regular use, as well as entry into treatment, was significantly shorter for the MA users. These clinical findings, along with the epidemiological data reviewed above, underscore the need for effective treatments for MA dependence.

MA use is associated with a number of health problems, including cardiovascular complications, risky sexual behavior resulting in sexually transmitted disease, and burns (Chin et al., 2006; Danks et al., 2004; Halkitis et al., 2005; Yen et al., 1994). Considerable attention has been given to the impact of MA use on mental health (Meredith et al., 2005; Scott et al., 2007). The purpose of this chapter is to provide an overview of the behavioral pharmacology and psychiatric consequences of MA.

Human Behavioral Pharmacology of MA

The abuse-related effects of MA can be assessed using drug self-administration or discrimination procedures. These behavioral procedures were developed using nonhuman laboratory animals, but have been adapted for use with human research participants. In a drug self-administration study, the delivery of a drug or vehicle is contingent on the emission of a behavior. Drugs that maintain behavior at levels greater than vehicle are considered to function as reinforcing stimuli. An alternative method for assessing the reinforcing effects of drugs involves a choice procedure wherein volunteers sample the drug or a placebo under double-blind conditions on separate days and are then given the opportunity to choose which drug they wish to take on subsequent days. The reliable selection of the drug-containing capsules demonstrates that the drug is a reinforcer (Johanson & Uhlenhuth, 1980a, 1980b). Drug self-administration studies have successfully identified the factors that influence the reinforcing effects of abused drugs. The availability of an alternative reinforcer, for example, decreases the reinforcing efficacy of abused drugs (e.g., Higgins et al., 1994). As another example, behavioral demands following drug ingestion systematically influence the reinforcing effects of drugs (Stoops et al., 2005a, 2005b).

In a drug-discrimination experiment, a behavior (e.g., lever pressing) is differentially reinforced, contingent on the presence or absence of a specific drug stimulus. Under this arrangement, abused drugs control the behavior (Glennon et al., 1991). This procedure is pharmacologically specific in that the discriminative-stimulus effects of drugs are mediated via receptor mechanisms. Typically, drugs from the same class as the training drug increase drug-appropriate responding in a dose-dependent manner, while drugs from different classes generally produce placebo-appropriate responding (Glennon et al., 1991). The discriminative effects of abused drugs may be involved in relapse to drug-taking behavior in that an initial dose (i.e., a lapse) may function as a discriminative stimulus signaling the availability of more drug (Bickel & Kelly, 1988; DeGrandpre & Bickel, 1993).

With human research participants the behavioral pharmacological effects of abused drugs are most often assessed using subjective-effects questionnaires. A range of acute doses are administered, and volunteers complete a battery of subjective drug-effect questionnaires before drug administration and periodically afterward for several hours. These questionnaires ask the volunteers to rate their affective state or perception of a drug effect. Standardized mood questionnaires like the Addiction Research Center Inventory (ARCI) or Profile of Mood States (POMS) are often employed along with investigator-constructed instruments. The investigator-constructed instruments usually consist of several items (e.g., good effects, like drug, stimulated, willing to take drug again) that are rated using a 5-point ordinal scale (i.e., 0 = Not at All, 4 = Extremely) or a 100-mm visual-analog line (e.g., leftmost extreme labeled "Not at All" and rightmost extreme label "An Awful Lot"). Most abused drugs produce a constellation of positive subjective ratings (e.g., good effects or like drug).

Below we provide an overview of the behavioral pharmacological effects of MA in humans, which will demonstrate that there is a dearth of such studies. By contrast, there is a plethora of studies that characterize the behavioral pharmacological effects of d-amphetamine and cocaine in humans. These studies provide valuable information that can be used to better understand the behavioral effects of MA that contribute to its abuse.

Reinforcing Effects of MA

The reinforcing effects of MA may be the single most important behavioral processes involved in its abuse. We know of three published studies in which the reinforcing effects of MA were explicitly assessed in humans (Hart et al., 2001; Johnson et al., 2005, 2007). In the first study, the reinforcing effects of oral MA (0, 5, and 10 mg) were assessed in eight stimulant users using a choice procedure (Hart et al., 2001). Participants sampled each dose condition and then were given eight opportunities to choose between the drug dose and a one-dollar voucher. Both active MA doses were chosen significantly more than placebo, although they did not differ from each other. Future studies should test a wide range of doses to determine whether the reinforcing effects of MA are dose dependent.

In the other two studies the reinforcing effects of MA were assessed as part of larger trials designed to determine the efficacy of isradipine and topiramate as putative pharmacotherapies for MA dependence (Johnson et al., 2005, 2007). During these trials participants were maintained on placebo, and the reinforcing effects of MA were established using a multiple-choice procedure that provided a contingency-based assessment of the monetary value of several drug conditions and was developed as an efficient method for assessing drug reinforcement in humans (Griffiths et al., 1993, 1996). In this procedure, participants receive a drug dose and after a predetermined amount of time (e.g., 24 hours) and complete a drug versus money multiple-choice form. The multiple-choice form typically consists of several drug versus money choices (e.g., yesterday's drug vs. $0.25; yesterday's drug vs. $0.50; yesterday's drug vs. $1; yesterday's drug vs. $2; yesterday's drug vs. $4; yesterday's drug vs. $8; yesterday's drug vs. $16; yesterday's drug vs. $32; yesterday's drug vs. $64). Each of these choices is labeled numerically (i.e., 1–9). An identical form is completed after each of the test doses, except that the drug versus money choices are assigned different numerical labels (e.g., 10–18 for the second dose condition; 19–27 for the third dose condition). A "reinforcement session" is then conducted after the participants have been exposed to all of the experimental dose conditions. During the reinforcement session, participants draw one number from a container holding several numbered chips. Based on the above example, the chips would be labeled from 1 to 27, and the choice corresponding to that randomly selected number is reinforced. If, for example, the participant chooses drug, then that specific dose of drug is re-administered. If the participant chooses money, then the indicated amount of money is added to his/her study earnings. The outcome measure for the multiple-choice form is the maximum dollar value at which participants choose the drug dose over money. This dollar value is defined as the "crossover point." The reinforcing effects of intravenous MA (0, 15, and 30 mg) were assessed in both studies that used the multiple-choice procedure (Johnson et al., 2005, 2007). In the first study, 18 MA-dependent individuals participated. In the second study, 10 MA-dependent individuals participated. In both studies the active doses of intravenous MA increased the "crossover point" above levels observed with placebo.

The results of these experiments suggest that MA, like other commonly abused stimulants, reliably functions as a reinforcer in humans. Altering the reinforcing effects of MA, as well as other abused stimulants, may be essential for initiating abstinence (Higgins et al., 2004). Contingency management procedures, for example, are effective for initiating abstinence (Lussier et al., 2006, Prendergast et al., 2006). Briefly, contingency management procedures attenuate the reinforcing effects of drugs by providing an alternative reinforcer contingent upon drug abstinence. The alternative reinforcer is usually a voucher that is redeemable for material items. Drug abstinence is verified via a biological sample provided several times weekly, and the alternative reinforcer is withheld if the biological sample indicates recent drug use. The results of clinical trials and laboratory studies suggest that contingency management procedures are effective for initiating abstinence from MA (Roll, 2007; Roll et al., 2006). However, contingency management procedures are costly and may not be feasible in community-based treatment facilities. Pharmacotherapies that attenuate the reinforcing effects of MA or enhance the effects of contingency management may also be useful for initiating abstinence.

Discriminative-Stimulus Effects of MA

The discriminative effects of MA may be involved in relapse to drug-taking behavior in that an initial dose (i.e., a lapse) may function as a discriminative stimulus signaling the availability of more drug (Bickel & Kelly, 1988; DeGrandpre & Bickel, 1993). We know of only two studies in which MA was explicitly established as a discriminative stimulus in humans (Hart et al., 2002; Sevak et al., 2008). The results of these studies are consistent in that the MA discrimination was readily acquired, its discriminative effects were an orderly function of dose, and the discriminative effects overlapped extensively with those of other stimulants, but not drugs from other pharmacological classes. In the first study, the discriminative-stimulus effects of a range of doses of MA (5–20 mg) and memantine (0 and 40) were examined, alone and in combination, in six volunteers who had learned to discriminate between oral MA (10 mg) and placebo (Hart et al., 2002). Memantine is an NMDA antagonist. During two experimental sessions, participants received 10 mg MA and placebo to familiarize them with the drug effects. MA and placebo were identified by letter code (e.g., Drug A is 10 mg MA; Drug B is placebo). During a training phase, participants received Drug A or Drug B at least twice but were not informed of the letter code. Participants were asked to identify which drug they had received using a point-distribution task. The criterion for having acquired the discrimination was   80% correct responding on four consecutive sessions. Participants met the discrimination criterion in four to nine sessions. During a test phase, a range of doses of MA (0, 5, 10, and 20 mg) and memantine (0 and 40 mg) were tested to determine whether they shared discriminative-stimulus effects with the training dose. During this phase participants could respond on a novel option if the drug did not feel like either Drug A or Drug B. MA, but not memantine, increased drug-appropriate responding substantially above levels observed with placebo. In the second study the discriminative-stimulus effects of MA (2.5–15 mg), d-amphetamine (2.5–15 mg), methylphenidate (5–30 mg), triazolam (0.0625–0.375 mg), and placebo were examined in seven volunteers with histories of illicit stimulant use who had learned to discriminate 10 mg oral MA (Sevak et al., 2008). Triazolam is a triazolobenzodiazepine hypnotic. During two experimental sessions, participants received 10 mg MA to familiarize them with the drug effects. MA was identified by letter code (i.e., Drug A). During a test-of-acquisition phase, participants received 10 mg MA or placebo at least twice. Participants were instructed to respond on the Drug A option of a point-distribution task if the drug they received that day felt like Drug A. Participants were further instructed to respond on the Not Drug A option of a point-distribution task if they did not feel any drug effect or if the drug effect felt different than Drug A. The criterion for having acquired the discrimination was $\geq 80\%$ correct responding on four consecutive sessions. Participants met the discrimination criterion (i.e., $\geq 80\%$ correct responding during four consecutive sessions) in 4–12 sessions (mean = 6). MA, d-amphetamine, and methylphenidate dose-dependently increased MA-appropriate responding, while triazolam produced low levels of drug-appropriate responding.

There are also two published studies that determined the discriminative-stimulus effects of MA in participants who had learned to discriminate cocaine or d-amphetamine (Johanson et al., 2006b; Lamb & Henningfield, 1994). In the earlier study the discriminative-stimulus effects of a range of doses of d-amphetamine (3.75–45 mg), MA (5–30 mg), and hydromorphone (an opiate analgesic) (1–12) were examined in five volunteers who had learned to discriminate oral d-amphetamine (30 mg) (Lamb & Henningfield, 1994). d-Amphetamine and MA generally dose-dependently increased drug-appropriate responding (see Figure 5.1). Hydromorphone on average occasioned low levels of drug-appropriate responding. In the other study, 10 cocaine-dependent participants attempted to learn to discriminate between intravenous saline and 20 mg/70 kg cocaine (Johanson et al., 2006b). During a sampling session, participants received injections of saline or cocaine to familiarize them with the drug effects. These injections were identified by letter codes (e.g., Injection A is 20 mg/70 kg cocaine; Injection B is saline). During the next three sessions 12 trials were conducted, with cocaine and saline each administered six times in quasi-random order. Thirty minutes after each injection, participants were asked to identify the injection by letter code. Seven of the 10 acquired the discrimination (i.e., ≥ 10 trials correct). A range of doses of cocaine (10, 20, and 40 mg/70 kg), MA (5 and 10 mg/70 kg), pentobarbital (a barbituate hypnotic) (50 and 100 mg/70 kg), and placebo were then tested to determine whether they engendered cocaine-like discriminative-stimulus effect. Cocaine dose dependently increased the number of participants who identified the injection as cocaine. The highest dose of MA and pentobarbital also increased the

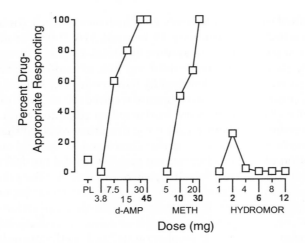

FIGURE 5.1. Dose effects for *d*-amphetamine (d-AMP), methamphetamine (METH), and hydromorphone (HYDROMOR) for percent drug-appropriate responding. *x*-axes: dose in mg. Data points above PL indicate placebo values. Data from Lamb and Henningfield (1994).

number of participants who identified the injection as cocaine above levels observed with placebo.

The results of these studies suggest that MA, like other commonly abused stimulants including *d*-amphetamine, cocaine, and methylphenidate, readily functions as a discriminative stimulus. This discrimination is pharmacologically specific in that in participants who have learned to discriminate MA, other stimulants engender significant levels of drug-appropriate responding, whereas drugs from other pharmacological classes do not. MA also engenders significant levels of drug-appropriate responding in participants who had learned to discriminate other commonly abused stimulants, including *d*-amphetamine and cocaine.

Subjective Effects of MA

MA produces a constellation of positive subjective effects (e.g., increased ratings of good effects and like drug; Martin et al., 1971; Mayfield, 1973; Perez-Reyes et al., 1991). Measurable positive subjective effects are observed when MA is ingested orally, insufflated (i.e., inhaled), injected, or smoked. In the study that administered the experimental drug orally, eight participants sampled MA (0, 5, and 10 mg) as part of the larger drug self-administration study described earlier (Hart et al.,

2001). In the study that administered the experimental drug intranasally, 11 participants received MA (0, 12, 25, and 50 mg) (Hart et al., 2007a). In another study eight participants smoked 40 mg MA (Harris et al., 2003). In the study that administered experimental drug intravenously, 12 participants received MA (0, 17.5, and 35 mg/70 kg) (Mendelson et al., 2006). In each of these studies the subjective effects of MA were measured using a 100 mm visual analog scale. MA increased subject ratings of "Good Effects" that were dose and time dependent, regardless of route of administration. Consistent with the pharmacokinetics of these routes of administration, peak drug effects were observed sooner with smoked and inhaled MA. Larger effects were also observed with smoked and inhaled MA relative to oral or intravenous drug. These differences may, however, be due to testing relatively higher doses of smoked and inhaled MA. The similarity of the drug effects across these experiments suggest that laboratory findings could have implications for understanding MA abuse, regardless of the route of administration.

The behavioral effects of MA are qualitatively and quantifiably similar to those observed with cocaine. In one study, for example, 14 non-treatment-seeking cocaine-dependent participants received an injection of placebo or 40 mg cocaine, while 11 non-treatment-seeking MA-dependent participants received an injection of placebo or 30 mg MA (Newton et al., 2005). Drug effects were assessed with subjective-effects questionnaires. Although the time to peak effect was quicker with cocaine relative to MA, the magnitude of drug effects was similar. The similarity of effects across these drugs suggests that laboratory findings with cocaine could have implications for understanding the behavioral pharmacology of MA.

Subjective-Effects Questionnaires, Drug Self-Administration, and Drug Discrimination as Instruments to Screen Pharmacotherapies for MA Dependence

The studies reviewed here provide important information concerning the basic human behavioral pharmacology of MA. MA functions as a reinforcer and discriminative stimulus, and it produces a constellation of positive subjective effects. These behavioral assays are commonly used to determine the initial efficacy of putative pharmacotherapies for stimulant dependence. Identifying an effective pharmacotherapy for substance-use disorders in general, and stimulant-use disorders in particular, is an arduous process that requires a multitude of controlled studies. Human behavioral pharmacology studies are integral in this process so that the initial safety and tolerability of a putative pharmacotherapy in combination with MA can be determined. These studies also include outcome measures to determine whether the putative pharmaco-therapy alters the behavioral effects of MA. A putative pharmacotherapy that is well tolerated and alters at least some of the behavioral effects of the MA should then be tested in a clinical trial. Double-blind, placebo-controlled, randomized trials are, of course, the gold standard of clinical research. Clinical trials, however, are costly, time consuming, and labor intensive. Double-blind, placebo-controlled, randomized trials should be reserved for only the most promising medications (i.e., compounds that are well tolerated and alter at least some of the behavioral effects under controlled laboratory conditions).

Subjective-effects questionnaires are perhaps the most widely used behavioral assay in human laboratory experiments designed to screen putative pharmacotherapies for stimulant dependence. The premise is that the positive subjective effects of MA contribute significantly to its abuse. Identifying medications that attenuate the subjective effects of MA would be predicted to be effective clinically because drug taking would cease when the patient no longer experiences these desired effects. However, the predictive validity of human laboratory studies that use subjective-effects questionnaires as the primary outcome measure is unclear.

We know of only a single compound, bupropion, that has been tested as a putative pharmacotherapy for MA in a laboratory-based study and a double-blind, placebo-controlled clinical trial (Elkashef et al., 2006; Newton et al., 2006). In the laboratory-based study, the subjective effects of intravenous MA (0, 15, and 30 mg) were determined in volunteers maintained on 150 mg bupropion (n = 10; twice daily for 6 days) or placebo (n = 10) (Newton et al., 2006). Both doses of MA increased subjective ratings of any effect and feeling high in placebo- and bupropion-maintained volunteers. However, these increases were significantly lower in the buproprion-maintained volunteers when compared with those of the placebo-maintained volunteers. A similar trend was noted for subjective ratings of stimulated. Bupropion also attenuated cue-induced increases in subjective ratings of craving. In the clinical trial, MA-dependent patients were randomly assigned to receive placebo (n = 72) or sustained-release bupropion (150 mg twice daily) (n = 79) (Elkashef et al., 2006). Drug urine tests were conducted thrice weekly and were the primary outcome measure. The bupropion- and placebo-treated patients did not differ significantly in terms of amphetamine-negative urine samples (p = .09). The discordance between these laboratory and clinical findings suggest subjective-effects questionnaires may produce false-positive results and not accurately predict the efficacy of putative pharmacotherapies for MA dependence.

There is a voluminous literature involving the administration of cocaine to humans as well as studies that attempted to identify a pharmacotherapy that might attenuate the subjective effects of cocaine. A widely effective pharmacotherapy has not yet been identified. Identifying an effective pharmacotherapy for cocaine dependence has been limited, in part, by uncertainty regarding the predictive validity of laboratory methods used to screen novel medications. The successes and failures encountered while attempting to identify a pharmacotherapy for cocaine dependence provide valuable information that can be used to guide the development of a medication for MA dependence.

We know of at least 19 compounds that were tested under controlled laboratory conditions and in double-blind, placebo-controlled clinical trials to determine their efficacy as putative pharmacotherapies for cocaine dependence. Bupropion (Oliveto et al., 2001; Poling et al., 2006), desipramine (Campbell et al., 2003; Fischman et al., 1990), fluoxetine (Covi et al., 1995; Grabowski et al., 1995; Walsh et al., 1994), naltrexone (Schmitz et al., 2004; Sofuoglu et al., 2003), pergolide (Focchi et al., 2005; Haney et al., 1998; Malcolm et al., 2000), risperidone (Grabowski et al., 2000, 2004; Newton et al., 2001), and venlafaxine (Ciraulo et al., 2005; Foltin et al., 2003) attenuated some of the subjective effects of experimentally administered cocaine but failed to reduce drug use in clinical trials. Like the studies described above that tested bupropion as a pharmacotherapy for MA dependence, the results of these studies suggest the use of subjective-effects questionnaires often resulted in false-positive outcomes when testing medications as putative pharmacotherapies for cocaine dependence.

Baclofen (Haney et al., 2006; Lile et al., 2003; Shoptaw et al., 2003), disulfiram (Carroll et al., 2004; McCance-Katz et al., 1998), methylphenidate (Collins et al., 2006; Levin et al., 2007; Rush et al., 2007; Winhusen et al., 2006; cf. Grabowski et al., 1997), phenytoin (Crosby et al., 1996; Sofuoglu et al., 1999), and tiagabine (Gonzalez et al., 2003, 2007; Lile et al., 2004; Winhusen et al., 2005), by contrast, did not attenuate the subjective effects of cocaine, but reduced drug use in clinical trials. The discordance between these laboratory and clinical findings suggest subjective-effects questionnaires also produced false-negative results and did not accurately predict the efficacy of putative pharmacotherapies for cocaine dependence.

Amantadine (Collins et al., 2003; Shoptaw et al., 2002), bromocriptine (Handelsman et al., 1997; Preston et al., 1992), carbamazepine (Cornish et al., 1995; Hatsukami et al., 1991; Kranzler et al., 1995; Montoya et al., 1995), gabapentin (Bisaga et al., 2006; Gonzalez et al., 2007; Hart et al., 2007b, 2007c), and mazindol (Margolin et al., 1995; Preston et al., 1993; Stine et al., 1995) did not attenuate the subjective effects of cocaine, nor did they reduce drug use in clinical trials. While the results of these last studies suggest data from subjective-effects questionnaires predict clinical results, they must be viewed cautiously because both out-comes are negative.

We know of only two instances in which the results of studies that used subjective-effects questionnaires accurately predicted clinical suc-cess. Buprenorphine (Foltin & Fischman, 1996; Montoya et al., 2004) and modafinil (Dackis et al., 2003, 2005; Hart et al., 2007d; Malcolm et al., 2006) attenuated the subjective effects of cocaine and reduced drug use in clinical trials. Worth noting is that two of these laboratory-based studies also included a direct measure of drug reinforcement (Foltin & Fischman, 1996; Hart et al., 2007d). Overall, then, the concordance between human laboratory studies and clinical trials is low when the former employed only subjective-effects questionnaires as the outcome measure. In other words, human laboratory studies that employ subjec-tive-effects questionnaires as the behavioral outcome measure do not accurately predict the clinical success of candidate medications.

The results of human laboratory studies and clinical trials suggest that drug self-administration procedures may more accurately predict the eventual efficacy of putative pharmacotherapies in clinical trials. The premise of these studies is that the reinforcing effects of cocaine are cen-tral to its abuse (Fischman & Foltin, 1998). Medications that attenuate the reinforcing effects of cocaine would be predicted to be effective clini-cally because drug taking would cease.

We know of 10 compounds that were tested under controlled labo-ratory conditions to determine whether they attenuate the reinforcing effects of cocaine. These compounds have also been tested in double-blind, placebo-controlled clinical trials to determine their efficacy in the management of cocaine dependence. Baclofen (Haney et al., 2006; Shoptaw et al., 2003), buprenorphine (Foltin & Fischman, 1996; Mon-toya et al., 2004), methylphenidate (Collins et al., 2006; Levin et al., 2007; cf. Grabowski et al., 1997), and modafinil (Dackis et al., 2005; Hart et al., 2007c) significantly attenuated the reinforcing effects of cocaine under controlled laboratory conditions and reduced cocaine-taking behavior in double-blind, placebo-controlled clinical trials. Amantadine (Collins et al., 2003; Shoptaw et al., 2002), desipramine (Campbell et al., 2003; Fischman et al., 1990), gabapentin (Bisaga et al., 2006; Gonzalez et al., 2007; Hart et al., 2007b, 2007c), pergolide (Focchi et al., 2005; Haney et al., 1998; Malcolm et al., 2000), and venlafaxine (Ciraulo et al., 2005; Foltin et al., 2003) did not attenuate the reinforcing effects of cocaine, nor did they reduce drug use in dou-ble-blind, placebo-controlled clinical trials. We know of only a single instance in which the results of a human drug self-administration study are discordant with those from the double-blind, placebo-controlled trial. Phenytoin did not attenuate the reinforcing effects of cocaine, but reduced drug use in a clinical trial (Crosby et al., 1996; Sofuoglu et al., 1999). Thus there is good concordance between the results of human laboratory studies that used drug self-administration procedures to assess the initial efficacy of medication for cocaine dependence and clinical trials. This high degree of concordance, although not absolute, suggests that human drug self-administration procedures may be well suited for determining the initial efficacy of putative pharmacotherapies for stimulant dependence.

Finally, we know of only one compound, gabapentin, that was tested to determine whether it attenuates the discriminative effects of cocaine (Haney et al., 2005). The premise of this approach is that the discriminative-stimulus effects of an abused drug (e.g., cocaine) may be involved in relapse to drug-taking behavior in that an initial dose (i.e., a lapse) may function as a discriminative stimulus signaling the availability of more drug. Pharmacotherapies that attenuate the discriminative-stimulus effects of stimulants may be developed further as "anti-relapse" medications. Gabapentin has also been tested as a putative pharmacotherapy in double-blind, placebo-controlled clinical trials (Bisaga et al., 2006; Gonzalez et al., 2007). In the discrimination study, volunteers learned to discriminate 25 mg smoked cocaine. After acquiring the discrimination, a range of cocaine doses (0, 6, 12, 25, and 50 mg) was tested to determine if they engendered cocaine-appropriate responding during three gabapentin maintenance conditions (0, 600, and 1,200 mg/day). Cocaine dose-dependently increased cocaine responding regardless of the gabapentin maintenance condition. These findings are concordant with the results of clinical trials that suggest gabapentin does not prevent relapse to drug taking (Bisaga et al., 2006; Gonzalez et al., 2007). Although the results of these studies suggest drug discrimination procedures may predict clinical outcome, they too must be viewed cautiously because both outcomes are negative. More research is needed to determine the extent to which human drug discrimination procedures might be used to screen pharmacotherapies for stimulant dependence. Specifically, drug-discrimination procedures should be used with a putative pharmacotherapy with demonstrated clinical efficacy.

Summary

In summary, MA, like other abused stimulants, functions as reinforcer and discriminative stimulus and produces a constellation of positive subjective effects in humans. Recent efforts have been devoted to determining whether putative pharmacotherapies may attenuate these behavioral effects of MA. A pharmacotherapy that attenuates the reinforcing, discriminative, or subjective effects of MA may be effective as a pharmacotherapy for the management of MA dependence. Because it has emerged as a public health concern somewhat recently, the development of a pharmacotherapy for MA dependence is in its infancy. The development of an effective pharmacotherapy may be expedited if appropriate human laboratory procedures are used to screen candidate medications. Identifying an effective pharmacotherapy for cocaine dependence has been limited, in part, by uncertainty regarding the predictive validity of laboratory methods used to screen novel medications. The extensive literature involving the administration of cocaine to humans in studies aimed at identifying a pharmacotherapy suggests that sophisticated behavioral procedures like self-administration and drug discrimination may more accurately predict the clinical success of candidate medications than subjective-effects questionnaires.

Psychiatric Consequences of MA Use

MA use has been correlated with a number of health problems, including cardiovascular complications, risky sexual behavior resulting in sexually transmitted disease, and burns (Chin et al., 2006; Danks et al., 2004; Halkitis et al., 2005; Yen et al., 1994). In addition to physical health problems, much attention has been given to the impact of MA use on mental health (Meredith et al., 2005; Scott et al., 2007). MA has been associated with both acute problems like psychosis during heavy use and neurocognitive deficits following long-term use, even during abstinence. Below we review representative literature on both the acute and long-term effects of MA use.

Acute Effects of MA Use

As described earlier, experimental administration of MA to humans produces prototypical stimulant-like effects (e.g., increased heart rate and blood pressure, increased ratings of high and euphoric). Early studies also demonstrated that experimental administration of high amphetamine doses resulted in schizotypal psychotic episodes (Angrist & Gershon, 1970; Bell, 1973; Griffith et al., 1972). In those studies repeated dosing of either MA or d-amphetamine to volunteers with histories of stimulant abuse resulted in psychotic symptoms including paranoia or irrational, violent behavior. Importantly, the development of symptoms varied across volunteers in terms of dose and time of onset, indicating that individual differences play a role in amphetamine-induced psychosis. The development of psychotic symptoms following administration of MA has been associated with increased catecholamine, particularly dopamine, release (Lieberman et al., 1990; Snyder, 1972).

Because of ethical concerns associated with chronic high-dose administration of MA to humans, more recent research has surveyed the prevalence and correlates of psychotic symptoms in MA users that present for treatment or are hospitalized on inpatient psychiatric units (Batki & Harris, 2004; Chen et al., 2003; McKetin et al., 2006; Pasic et al., 2007; Srisurapanont et al., 2003).

The results of the studies that examined the prevalence of psychosis or psychotic symptoms in MA users are concordant with those of early laboratory findings indicating that MA produces these symptoms (Chen et al., 2003; McKetin et al., 2006; Pasic et al., 2007). In the first study 435 MA users recruited from a psychiatric hospital or detention center completed a series of screens that included assessments for premorbid diagnoses (via interviews with parents), as well as current comorbid diagnoses (Chen et al., 2003). Of these 435 subjects, 40% had experienced MA-induced psychosis, well above the prevalence levels for the general population in Taiwan, where the survey was conducted. These individuals were more likely to be diagnosed with current major depression, alcohol dependence, and antisocial personality disorder relative to those who had not experienced MA-induced psychosis. In addition, individuals who experienced psychosis were more likely to have premorbid schizoid/schizotypal traits.

In the second study, 309 MA-using individuals were interviewed (McKetin et al., 2006). Although these individuals did not necessarily have heavy MA use histories (i.e., the inclusion criterion was monthly MA use over the past year), 13% had experienced MA-induced psychosis and 23% experienced psychotic symptoms. These numbers are much higher than those for the general population in Australia, where the survey was conducted. The likelihood of MA psychosis was increased in MA-dependent individuals. In the most recent study, which used a case-control design, 60 MA-using patients were compared with 60 non-using patients from the same unit on a range of variables (Pasic et al., 2007). While MA-using patients were less likely to have reported a psychiatric history, they were more likely to be admitted to the unit for psychosis and dysphoria than were the case controls. In addition, MA users were more likely to be referred to the unit by police and had a longer duration of stay on the unit. While the populations surveyed in the studies described earlier varied (e.g., use rates differed across studies and populations were drawn from different pools), the findings demonstrate the high prevalence of psychosis or psychotic symptoms in MA-using individuals. It is also apparent that certain factors like MA dependence or preexisting schizoid/schizotypal traits result in a predisposition to develop MA-induced psychosis.

Other research has demonstrated correlations between MA use and specific psychosis symptoms (Batki & Harris, 2004; Harris & Batki, 2000; Srisurapanont et al., 2003). In the Batki and Harris/Harris and Batki studies, 19 subjects admitted to a psychiatric emergency services unit following presentation to a hospital with psychotic symptoms and admitting stimulant (cocaine or amphetamine) use completed a battery of questionnaires and submitted urine and blood samples that were assayed for quantitative drug levels (Batki & Harris, 2004; Harris & Batki, 2000). Because the focus of this chapter is amphetamine, only results from the amphetamine-using individuals ($n = 14$) will be described here. MA users presented largely with positive psychosis symptoms, although a number of negative symptoms were also observed. MA and amphetamine levels were positively correlated with a number of psychotic symptoms including global hyperkinesia (including stereotypies) and scores on the activation scale, positive scale, and total score of the Positive and Negative Syndrome Scale (PANSS). Srisurapanont and colleagues reviewed charts from 168 patients hospitalized on psychiatric units in several different countries to determine the structure of psychotic symptoms associated with MA use (Srisurapanont et al., 2003). As with the Batki and Harris/Harris and Batki studies, the majority of symptoms observed were positive-type psychosis symptoms like persecutory delusions and auditory hallucinations, although some negative symptoms were also observed. The results of these studies from hospitalized patients support the notion that MA use is associated with psychotic symptoms, and while these symptoms are mainly positive in nature, negative symptoms also occur, mirroring psychotic symptoms associated with schizophrenia.

Taken together, the findings described above demonstrate that acute MA use is associated with psychosis or psychotic symptoms. It is important to note that MA-associated psychosis is correlated with the development of later psychotic symptoms in the absence of drug use (Flaum & Schultz, 1996; Sato, 1992; Sato et al., 1983).

Long-Term Effects of MA Use

The long-term psychiatric effects of MA during abstinence in humans remain controversial because it has not been definitively determined that the presence of these effects are due to MA use or were present prior to MA use. The primary focus of research in long-term MA users has focused on comorbid psychiatric diagnoses and neurocognitive deficits (Hoffman et al., 2006; Kalechstein et al., 2000; London et al., 2005;

Scott et al., 2007; Sekine et al., 2001; Shoptaw et al., 2003; Simons et al., 2005; Stoops et al., 2005c; Vik, 2007; Zweben et al., 2004).

We review the results of three studies that examined the prevalence of psychiatric disorders in MA users compared to controls (Kalechstein et al., 2000; Sekine et al., 2001; Stoops et al., 2005c). In the first study MA-using prison inmates in California were compared with nonusers (Kalechstein et al., 2000). After controlling for demographic variables and other substance dependence, MA-dependent individuals were still more likely to report current needs of psychiatric assistance, previous suicidal ideation, and presence of depressive symptoms in the past year relative to those that had not used MA.

In the second study abstinent MA users were compared to nonusing controls with PET scanning and the Brief Psychiatric Rating Scale (BPRS) (Sekine et al., 2001). The PET scan revealed decreased dopamine transporter levels in a number of brain areas in MA users relative to controls. Importantly, dopamine transporter density was significantly associated with years of MA use. Moreover, MA use was associated with increased scores on the BPRS positive symptoms scale. In the third study MA-using drug court clients were compared to non-MA-using drug court clients (Stoops et al., 2005c). Although differences in scores on the Brief Symptom Inventory (BSI) were limited, perhaps due to the wide-ranging extent of MA use in the group under study, MA users were more likely to report use of a number of drugs, indicating that use of MA is associated with other drug use, abuse, and dependence.

Although it cannot be determined whether the differences between MA users and control subjects described earlier were a result of MA use or represent some underlying condition, the results of these studies demonstrate that MA use is associated with comorbid psychiatric symptoms, changes in brain neurotransmitter function, and increased substance abuse or dependence.

These associations with psychiatric comorbidity like depression and substance abuse/dependence are supported by findings from other studies, which found high prevalence of a number of psychiatric risk factors or comorbid psychiatric disorders in MA-using subjects (Shoptaw et al., 2003; Simons et al., 2005; Vik, 2007; Zweben et al., 2004). In one study, for example, MA use was associated with increased levels of impulsivity (Simons et al., 2005). In another study, MA use was associated with increased scores relative to population norms on a number of including the Beck Depression Inventory (BDI) and BSI (Zweben et al., 2004).

Neurocognitive deficits associated with MA use have also been explored in a large number of studies (reviewed in Scott et al., 2007). In that review, a meta-analysis was conducted on previously published literature to determine effect sizes for multiple neurocognitive domains

(Scott et al., 2007). Moderate effect sizes were observed across all domains, indicating that MA use was associated with deficits in learning, executive function, memory, information-processing speed, motor coordination, attention, visual construction of objects, reaction time, and verbal ability. Although these findings are provocative, it is important to note that the studies reviewed used varying populations of MA users and use of frequency or abstinence was not always associated with observed neurocognitive deficits (Hoffman et al., 2006; Johanson et al., 2006).

In addition to the demonstrated neurocognitive deficits noted above, other studies have demonstrated increased impulsivity in MA users, although it has yet to be determined whether increased impulsivity is pre- or postmorbid to MA use (Hoffman et al., 2006; Monterosso et al., 2005). Taken together, it is apparent that MA use is associated with, but may not cause, a number of long-term effects. These effects likely interfere with treatment and intervention efforts, particularly because comorbid psychiatric diagnoses, neurocognitive deficits and impulsivity are associated with worse clinical outcomes in drug treatment (Miller, 1991; Patkar et al., 2004).

Conclusion

The results of the representative studies described above demonstrate a clear link between acute MA use and psychosis or psychotic symptoms. These symptoms are similar to those observed with schizophrenia and may be due to the interaction of MA with brain catecholamine systems. MA-induced psychosis has been associated with increased risk for non-drug-induced psychosis. Other possible long-term effects of MA include increased depressive symptomatology and neurocognitive deficits, although it remains to be definitively determined whether these effects are pre- or postmorbid to MA use. Regardless of the temporal nature of these effects, it is apparent that MA use is associated with increased psychiatric comorbidity and cognitive deficits, which must be considered when developing intervention or treatment strategies.

Acknowledgments

National Institute on Drug Abuse Grant Nos. R01 DA010325, R01 DA020429, R01 DA017711, and R01 DA021155 (to Craig R. Rush) supported this research. We would like to thank Rajkumar J. Sevak, PhD, Andrea R. Vansickel, MA, and Megan Poole, BA, for their thoughtful comments. We would also like to thank Derek Roe, BA, for his editorial comments.

References

Angrist BM, Gershon S. (1970). The phenomenology of experimentally induced amphetamine psychosis—preliminary observations. *Biol Psychiatry* 2:95–107.

Batki SL, Harris DS. (2004). Quantitative drug levels in stimulant psychosis: Relationship to symptom severity, catecholamines and hyperkinesia. *Am J Addict* 13:461–470.

Bell DS. (1973). The experimental reproduction of amphetamine psychosis. *Arch Gen Psychiatry* 29:35–40.

Bickel WK, Kelly TH. (1988). The relationship of stimulus control to the treatment of substance abuse. *NIDA Res Monog* 84:122–140.

Bisaga A, Aharonovich E, Garawi F, et al. (2006). A randomized placebo-controlled trial of gabapentin for cocaine dependence. *Drug Alcohol Depend* 81:267–274.

Campbell J, Nickel EJ, Penick EC, et al. (2003). Comparison of desipramine or carbamazepine to placebo for crack cocaine-dependent patients. *Am J Addict* 12:122–136.

Carroll KM, Fenton LR, Ball SA, et al. (2004). Efficacy of disulfiram and cognitive behavior therapy in cocaine-dependent outpatients: A randomized placebo-controlled trial. *Arch Gen Psychiatry* 61:264–272.

Castro GF, Barrington EH, Walton MA, et al. (2000). Cocaine and methamphetamine: Differential addiction rates. *Psychol Addict Behav* 14:390–396.

Chen CK, Lin SK, Sham PC, et al. (2003). Pre-morbid characteristics and co-morbidity of methamphetamine users with and without psychosis. *Psychol Med* 33:1407–1414.

Chin KM, Channick RN, Rubin LJ. (2006). Is methamphetamine use associated with idiopathic pulmonary arterial hypertension? *Chest* 130:1657–1663.

Ciraulo DA, Sarid-Segal O, Knapp CM, et al. (2005). Efficacy screening trials of paroxetine, pentoxifylline, riluzole, pramipexole and venlafaxine in cocaine dependence. *Addiction* 100(Suppl. 1):12–22.

Collins ED, Vosburg SK, Hart CL, et al. (2003). Amantadine does not modulate reinforcing, subjective, or cardiovascular effects of cocaine in humans. *Pharmacol Biochem Behav* 76:401–407.

Collins SL, Levin FR, Foltin RW, et al. (2006). Response to cocaine, alone and in combination with methylphenidate, in cocaine abusers with ADHD. *Drug Alcohol Depend* 82:158–167.

Community Epidemiology Work Group. (2004). *Epidemiological trends in drug abuse.* U.S. Department of Health and Human Services.

Cornish JW, Maany I, Fudala PJ, et al. (1995). Carbamazepine treatment for cocaine dependence. *Drug Alcohol Depend* 38:221–227.

Covi L, Hess JM, Kreiter NA, et al. (1995). Effects of combined fluoxetine and counseling in the outpatient treatment of cocaine abusers. *Am J Drug Alcohol Abuse* 21:327–344.

Crosby RD, Pearson VL, Eller C, et al. (1996). Phenytoin in the treatment of cocaine abuse: A double-blind study. *Clin Pharmacol Therapeutics* 59:458–468.

Dackis CA, Kampman KM, Lynch KG, et al. (2005). A double-blind, placebo-controlled trial of modafinil for cocaine dependence. *Neuropsychopharmacology* 30:205–211.

Dackis CA, Lynch KG, Yu E, et al. (2003). Modafinil and cocaine: A double-blind, placebo-controlled drug interaction study. *Drug Alcohol Depend* 70:29–37.

Danks RR, Wibbenmeyer LA, Faucher LD, et al. (2004). Methamphetamine-associated burn injuries: A retrospective analysis. *J Burn Care Rehab* 25:425–429.

DeGrandpre RJ, Bickel WK. (1993). Stimulus control and drug dependence. *Psychol Record* 43:651–666.

Drug and Alcohol Services Information System [DASIS] Report. (2004). *Primary methamphetamine/amphetamine treatment admissions increase: 1992–2002.* Office of Applied Studies, Substance Abuse and Mental Health Services Administration [SAMHSA]. Retrieved November 15, 2007, from *www.oas.samhsa.gov/2k4/methTX/methTX.cfm.*

Drug and Alcohol Services Information System [DASIS] Report. (2005). *Smoked methamphetamine/amphetamines, 1992–2002.* Office of Applied Studies, Substance Abuse and Mental Health Services Administration [SAMHSA]. Retrieved November 15, 2007, from *www.oas.samhsa.gov/2k4/meth-Smoked/methSmoked.htm.*

Elkashef AM, Rawson RA, Smith E, et al. (2006). *Bupropion for the treatment of methamphetamine dependence.* Paper presented at the Annual Meeting of the College on Problems of Drug Dependence, Scottsdale, AZ.

Fischman MW, Foltin RW. (1998). Cocaine self-administration research: Implications for rational pharmacotherapy. In ST Higgins, JL Katz (Eds.), *Cocaine abuse research: Pharmacology, behavior and clinical applications* (pp. 181–208). San Diego: Academic Press.

Fischman MW, Foltin RW, Nestadt G, et al. (1990). Effects of desipramine maintenance on cocaine self-administration by humans. *J Pharmacol Exp Ther* 253:760–770.

Flaum M, Schultz SK. (1996). When does amphetamine-induced psychosis become schizophrenia? *Am J Psychiatry* 153:812–815.

Focchi GR, Leite MC, Andrade AG, at al. (2005). Use of dopamine agonist pergolide in outpatient treatment of cocaine dependence. *Subst Use Misuse* 40:1169–1177.

Foltin RW, Fischman MW. (1996). Effects of methadone or buprenorphine maintenance on the subjective and reinforcing effects of intravenous cocaine in humans. *J Pharmacol Exp Ther* 278:1153–1164.

Foltin RW, Ward AS, Collins ED, et al. (2003). The effects of venlafaxine on the subjective, reinforcing, and cardiovascular effects of cocaine in opioid-dependent and non-opioid-dependent humans. *J Exp Clin Psychopharmacol* 11:123–130.

Glennon RA, Järbe TUC, Frankenheim J. (1991). Drug discrimination: Applications to drug abuse research. Rockville, MD: National Institute on Drug Abuse.

Gonzalez G, Desai R, Sofuoglu M, et al. (2007). Clinical efficacy of gabapentin versus tiagabine for reducing cocaine use among cocaine-dependent methadone-treated patients. *Drug Alcohol Depend* 87:1–9.

Gonzalez G, Severing K, Sofuoglu M, et al. (2003). Tiagabine increases cocaine-free urines in cocaine-dependent methadone-treated patients: Results of a randomized pilot study. *Addiction* 98:1625–1632.

Grabowski J, Rhoades H, Elk R, et al. (1995). Fluoxetine is ineffective for treatment of cocaine dependence or concurrent opiate and cocaine dependence: Two placebo-controlled double-blind trials. *J Clin Psychopharmacol* 15:163–174.

Grabowski J, Roache JD, Schmitz JM, et al. (1997). Replacement medication for cocaine dependence: Methylphenidate. *J Clin Psychopharmacol* 17:485–488.

Grabowski J, Rhoades H, Silverman P, et al. (2000). Risperidone for the treatment of cocaine dependence: Randomized, double-blind trial. *J Clin Psychopharmacol* 20:305–310.

Grabowski J, Rhoades H, Stotts A, et al. (2004). Agonist-like or antagonist-like treatment for cocaine dependence with methadone for heroin dependence: Two double-blind randomized clinical trials. *Neuropsychopharmacology* 29:969–981.

Griffith JD, Cavanaugh J, Held J, et al. (1972). Dextroamphetamine: Evaluation of psychomimetic properties in man. *Arch Gen Psychiatry* 26:97–100.

Griffiths RR, Rush CR, Puhala KA. (1996). Validation of the multiple-choice procedure for investigating drug reinforcement in humans. *Exp Clin Psychopharmacol* 4:97–106.

Griffiths RR, Troisi JR, Silverman K, et al. (1993). Multiple-choice procedure: An efficient approach for investigating drug reinforcement in humans. *Behav Pharmacol* 4:3–13.

Halkitis PN, Shrem MT, Martin FW. (2005). Sexual behavior patterns of methamphetamine-using gay and bisexual men. *Subst Use Misuse* 40:703–719.

Handelsman L, Rosenblum A, Palij M, et al. (1997). Bromocriptine for cocaine dependence: A controlled clinical trial. *Am J Addict* 6:54–64.

Haney M, Foltin RW, Fischman MW. (1998). Effects of pergolide on intravenous cocaine self-administration in men and women. *Psychopharmacology* 137:15–24.

Haney M, Hart C, Collins ED, et al. (2005). Smoked cocaine discrimination in humans: Effects of gabapentin. *Drug Alcohol Depend* 80:53–61.

Haney M, Hart CL, Foltin RW. (2006). Effects of baclofen on cocaine self-administration: Opioid- and nonopioid-dependent volunteers. *Neuropsychopharmacology* 31:1814–1821.

Harris D, Batki SL. (2000). Stimulant psychosis: Symptom profile and acute clinical course. *Am J Addict* 9:28–37.

Harris DS, Boxenbaum H, Everhart ET, et al. (2003). The bioavailability of intranasal and smoked methamphetamine. *Clin Pharmacol Ther* 74:475–486.

Hart CL, Gunderson EW, Perez A, et al. (2007a). Acute physiological and behavioral effects of intranasal methamphetamine in humans. *Neuropsychopharmacology* 33(8):1847–1855.

Hart CL, Haney M, Collins ED, et al. (2007b). Smoked cocaine self-administration by humans is not reduced by large gabapentin maintenance doses. *Drug Alcohol Depend* 86:274–277.

Hart CL, Haney M, Foltin RW, et al. (2002). Effects of the NMDA antagonist memantine on human methamphetamine discrimination. *Psychopharmacology (Berl)* 164:376–384.

Hart CL, Haney M, Vosburg SK, et al. (2007c). Gabapentin does not reduce smoked cocaine self-administration: Employment of a novel self-administration procedure. *Behav Pharmacol* 18:71–75.

Hart CL, Haney M, Vosburg SK, et al. (2007d). Smoked cocaine self-administration is decreased by modafinil. *Neuropsychopharmacology* 33(4):761–768.

Hart CL, Ward AS, Haney M, et al. (2001). Methamphetamine self-administration by humans. *Psychopharmacology (Berl)* 157:75–81.

Hatsukami D, Keenan R, Halikas J, et al. (1991). Effects of carbamazepine on acute responses to smoked cocaine-base in human cocaine users. *Psychopharmacology* 104:120–124.

Higgins ST, Heil SH, Lussier JP. (2004). Clinical implications of reinforcement as a determinant of substance use disorders. *Ann Rev Psychology* 55:431–461.

Hoffman WF, Moore M, Templin R, et al. (2006). Neuropsychological function and delay discounting in methamphetamine-dependent individuals. *Psychopharmacology* 188:162–170.

Johanson CE, Frey KA, Lundahl L, et al. (2006a). Cognitive function and nigrostriatal markers in abstinent methamphetamine abusers. *Psychopharmacology* 185:327–338.

Johanson CE, Lundahl LH, Lockhart N, et al. (2006b). Intravenous cocaine discrimination in humans. *Exp Clin Psychopharmacol* 14:99–108.

Johanson CE, Uhlenhuth EH. (1980a). Drug preference and mood in humans: *d*-Amphetamine. *Psychopharmacology* 71:275–279.

Johanson CE, Uhlenhuth EH. (1980b). Drug preference and mood in humans: Diazepam. *Psychopharmacology* 71:269–273.

Johnson BA, Roache JD, Ait-Daoud N, et al. (2005). Effects of isradipine, a dihydropyridine-class calcium-channel antagonist, on *d*-methamphetamine's subjective and reinforcing effects. *Int J Neuropsychopharmacology* 8:203–213.

Johnson BA, Roache JD, Ait-Daoud N, et al. (2007). Effects of acute topiramate dosing on methamphetamine-induced subjective mood. *Int J Neuropsychopharmacology* 10:85–98.

Kalechstein AD, Newton TF, Longshore D, et al. (2000). Psychiatric comorbidity of methamphetamine dependence in a forensic sample. *J Neuropsychiatry Clin Neurosci* 12:480–484.

Kranzler HR, Bauer LO, Hersh D, et al. (1995). Carbamazepine treatment of cocaine dependence: A placebo-controlled trial. *Drug Alcohol Depend* 38:203–211.

Lamb RJ, Henningfield JE. (1994). Human *d*-amphetamine drug discrimination: Methamphetamine and hydromorphone. *J Exp Anal Behav* 61:169–180.

Levin FR, Evans SM, Brooks DJ, et al. (2007). Treatment of cocaine-dependent treatment seekers with adult ADHD: Double-blind comparison of methylphenidate and placebo. *Drug Alcohol Depend* 87:20–29.

Lieberman JA, Kinon BJ, Loebel AD. (1990). Dopaminergic mechanisms in idiopathic and drug-induced psychoses. *Schizophrenia Bull* 16:97–110.

Lile JA, Stoops WW, Allen TS, et al. (2003). Baclofen does not alter the reinforcing, subject-rated, or cardiovascular effects of intranasal cocaine in humans. *Psychopharmacology* 171:441–449.

Lile JA, Stoops WW, Glaser PEA, et al. (2004). Tiagabine does not alter the discriminative-stimulus, reinforcing, subject-rated or cardiovascular effects of cocaine in humans. *Drug Alcohol Depend* 76:81–91.

London ED, Berman SM, Voytek B, et al. (2005). Cerebral metabolic dysfunction and impaired vigilance in recently abstinent methamphetamine abusers. *Biol Psychiatry* 58:770–778.

Lussier JP, Heil SH, Mongeon JA, et al. (2006). A meta-analysis of voucher-based reinforcement therapy for substance use disorders. *Addiction* 101:192–203.

Malcolm R, Kajdasz DK, Herron J, et al. (2000). A double-blind, placebo-controlled outpatient trial of pergolide for cocaine dependence. *Drug Alcohol Depend* 60:161–168.

Malcolm R, Swayngim K, Donovan JL, et al. (2006). Modafinil and cocaine interactions. *Am J Drug Alcohol Abuse* 32:577–587.

Margolin A, Avants SK, Kosten TR. (1995). Mazindol for relapse prevention to cocaine abuse in methadone-maintained patients. *Am J Drug Alcohol Abuse* 21:469–481.

Martin WR, Sloan JW, Sapmra JD, et al. (1971). Physiologic, subjective, and behavioral effects of amphetamine, methamphetamine, ephedrine, phenmetrazine, and methylphenidate in man. *Clin Pharmacol Ther* 12:245–258.

Mayfield DG. (1973). The effect of intravenous methamphetamine on mood. *Int J Addict* 8:565–568.

McCance-Katz EF, Kosten TR, Jatlow P. (1998). Disulfiram effects on acute cocaine administration. *Drug Alcohol Depend* 52:27–39.

McKetin R, McLaren J, Lubman DI, et al. (2006). The prevalence of psychotic symptoms among methamphetamine users. *Addiction* 101:1473–1478.

Mendelson J, Uemura N, Harris D, et al. (2006). Human pharmacology of the methamphetamine stereoisomers. *Clin Pharmacol Ther* 80:403–420.

Meredith CW, Jaffe C, Ang-Lee K, et al. (2005). Implications of chronic methamphetamine use: A literature review. *Harvard Rev Psychiatry* 13:141–154.

Miller L. (1991). Predicting relapse and recovery in alcoholism and addiction:

Neuropsychology, personality, and cognitive style. *J Subst Abuse Treat* 8:277–291.

Monterosso JR, Aron AR, Cordova X, et al. (2005). Deficits in response inhibition associated with chronic methamphetamine abuse. *Drug Alcohol Depend* 79:273–277.

Montoya ID, Gorelick DA, Preston KL, et al. (2004). Randomized trial of buprenorphine for treatment of concurrent opiate and cocaine dependence. *Clin Pharmacol Ther* 75:34–48.

Montoya ID, Levin FR, Fudala PJ, et al. (1995). Double-blind comparison of carbamazepine and placebo for treatment of cocaine dependence. *Drug Alcohol Depend* 38:213–219.

National Drug Intelligence Center. (2006). National methamphetamine threat assessment 2007. Washington, DC: U.S. Department of Justice. Retrieved September 5, 2007, from *www.usdoj.gov/ndic/pubs21/21821/ index.htm*.

Newton TF, De La Garza R, 2nd, Kalechstein AD, et al. (2005). Cocaine and methamphetamine produce different patterns of subjective and cardiovascular effects. *Pharmacol Biochem Behav* 82:90–97.

Newton TF, Ling W, Kalechstein AD, et al. (2001). Risperidone pretreatment reduces the euphoric effects of experimentally administered cocaine. *Psychiatry Res* 102:227–233.

Newton TF, Roache JD, De La Garza R, 2nd, et al. (2006). Bupropion reduces methamphetamine-induced subjective effects and cue-induced craving. *Neuropsychopharmacology* 31:1537–1544.

Oliveto A, McCance-Katz FE, Singha A, et al. (2001). Effects of cocaine prior to and during bupropion maintenance in cocaine-abusing volunteers. *Drug Alcohol Depend* 63:155–167.

Pasic J, Russo JE, Ries RK, et al. (2007). Methamphetamine users in the psychiatric emergency services: A case–control study. *Am J Drug Alcohol Abuse* 33:675–686.

Patkar AA, Murray HW, Mannelli P, et al. (2004). Pretreatment measures of impulsivity, aggression, and sensation seeking are associated with treatment outcome for African American cocaine-dependent patients. *J Addict Dis* 23:109–122.

Perez-Reyes M, White WR, McDonald SA, et al. (1991). Clinical effects of methamphetamine vapor inhalation. *Life Sciences* 49:953–959.

Poling J, Oliveto A, Petry N, et al. (2006). Six-month trial of bupropion with contingency management for cocaine dependence in a methadone-maintained population. *Arch Gen Psychiatry* 63:219–228.

Prendergast M, Podus D, Finney J, et al. (2006). Contingency management for treatment of substance use disorders: A meta-analysis. *Addiction* 101:1546–1560.

Preston KL, Liebson IA, Bigelow GE. (1992). Discrimination of agonist–antagonist opioids in humans trained on a two-choice saline–hydromorphone discrimination. *J Pharmacol Exp Ther* 261:62–71.

Preston KL, Sullivan JT, Berger P, et al. (1993). Effects of cocaine alone and in combination with mazindol in human cocaine abusers. *J Pharmacol Exp Ther* 267:296–307.

Roll JM. (2007). Contingency management: An evidence-based component of methamphetamine use disorder treatments. *Addiction* 102(Suppl. 1):114–120.

Roll JM, Petry NM, Stitzer ML, et al. (2006). Contingency management for the treatment of methamphetamine use disorders. *Am J Psychiatry* 163:1993–1999.

Rush CR, Stoops WW, Hays LR. (2009). Cocaine effects during *d*-amphetamine maintenance: A human laboratory analysis of safety, tolerability and efficacy. *Drug Alcohol Depend* 99(1–3):261–271.

Sato M. (1992). A lasting vulnerability to psychosis in patients with previous methamphetamine psychosis. *Ann NY Acad Sci* 654:160–170.

Sato M, Chen CC, Akiyama K, et al. (1983). Acute exacerbation of paranoid psychotic state after long-term abstinence in patients with previous methamphetamine psychosis. *Biol Psychiatry* 18:429–440.

Schmitz JM, Stotts AL, Sayre SL, et al. (2004). Treatment of cocaine–alcohol dependence with naltrexone and relapse prevention therapy. *Am J Addict* 13:333–341.

Scott JC, Woods SP, Matt GE, et al. (2007). Neurocognitive effects of methamphetamine: A critical review and meta-analysis. *Neuropsychol Rev* 17:275–297.

Sekine Y, Iyo M, Ouchi Y, et al. (2001). Methamphetamine-related psychiatric symptoms and reduced brain dopamine transporters studied with PET. *Am J Psychiatry* 158:1206–1214.

Sevak RJ, Stoops WW, Hays LR, et al. (2008). Discriminative-stimulus and subject-rated effects of methamphetamine, d-amphetamine, methylphenidate and triazolam in methamphetamine-trained humans. *Journal of Pharmacology and Experimental Therapeutics*, Dec 22. [Epub ahead of print].

Shoptaw S, Kintaudi PC, Charuvastra C, et al. (2002). A screening trial of amantadine as a medication for cocaine dependence. *Drug Alcohol Depend* 66:217–224.

Shoptaw S, Peck J, Reback CJ, et al. (2003). Psychiatric and substance dependence comorbidities, sexually transmitted diseases, and risk behaviors among methamphetamine-dependent gay and bisexual men seeking outpatient drug abuse treatment. *J Psychoactive Drugs* 35(Suppl. 1):161–168.

Simons JS, Oliver MN, Gaher RM, et al. (2005). Methamphetamine and alcohol abuse and dependence symptoms: Associations with affect lability and impulsivity in a rural treatment population. *Addict Behav* 30:1370–1381.

Snyder SH. (1972). Catecholamines in the brain as mediators of amphetamine psychosis. *Arch Gen Psychiatry* 27:169–179.

Sofuoglu M, Pentel PR, Bliss RL, et al. (1999). Effects of phenytoin on cocaine self-administration in humans. *Drug Alcohol Depend* 53:273–275.

Sofuoglu M, Singha A, Kosten TR, et al. (2003). Effects of naltrexone and isradipine, alone or in combination, on cocaine responses in humans. *Pharmacol Biochem Behav* 75:801–808.

Srisurapanont M, Ali R, Marsden J, et al. (2003). Psychotic symptoms in methamphetamine psychotic in-patients. *Int J Neuropsychopharmacol* 6:347–352.

Stine SM, Krystal JH, Kosten TR, et al. (1995). Mazindol treatment for cocaine dependence. *Drug Alcohol Depend* 39:245–252.

Stoops WW, Lile JA, Fillmore MT, et al. (2005a). Reinforcing effects of methylphenidate: Influence of dose and behavioral demands following drug administration. *Psychopharmacology* 177:349–355.

Stoops WW, Lile JA, Fillmore MT, et al. (2005b). Reinforcing effects of modafinil: Influence of dose and behavioral demands following drug administration. *Psychopharmacology* 182:186–193.

Stoops WW, Tindall MS, Mateyoke-Scrivner A, et al. (2005c). Methamphetamine use in nonurban and urban drug court clients. *Int J Offend Ther Comp Criminology* 49:260–276.

Substance Abuse and Mental Health Services Administration. (2003). *National Household Survey on Drug Abuse and Health (NHSDAH)*. Retrieved March 1, 2008, from *www.samhsa.gov*.

Substance Abuse and Mental Health Services Administration. (2007). *National Household Survey on Drug Abuse and Health (NHSDAH)*. Retrieved March 1, 2008, from *www.samhsa.gov*.

Vik PW. (2007). Methamphetamine use by incarcerated women: Comorbid mood and anxiety problems. *Womens Health Iss* 17:256–263.

Walsh SL, Preston KL, Sullivan JT, et al. (1994). Fluoxetine alters the effects of intravenous cocaine in humans. *J Clin Psychopharmacol* 14:396–407.

Winhusen T, Somoza E, Singal BM, et al. (2006). Methylphenidate and cocaine: A placebo-controlled drug interaction study. *Pharmacol Biochem Behav* 85:29–38.

Winhusen TM, Somoza EC, Harrer JM, et al. (2005). A placebo-controlled screening trial of tiagabine, sertraline, and donepezil as cocaine dependence treatments. *Addiction* 100(Suppl. 1):68–77.

Yen DJ, Wang SJ, Ju TH, et al. (1994). Stroke associated with methamphetamine inhalation. *Euro Neurol* 34:16–22.

Zweben JE, Cohen JB, Christian D, et al. (2004). Psychiatric symptoms in methamphetamine users. *Am J Addict* 13:181–190.

Chapter 6

Medical Effects
of Methamphetamine Use

Larissa Mooney, Suzette Glasner-Edwards,
Richard A. Rawson, and Walter Ling

Methamphetamine (MA) use is known to be associated with acute and chronic medical conditions affecting multiple organ systems. Toxicity from MA may result from a single dose, but serious medical effects are more common when use is prolonged (Karch, 2002; Kaye et al., 2007). Although the majority of fatalities related to MA intoxication involve accidents or violence, life-threatening medical consequences may also occur, including myocardial infarction, aortic dissection, arrhythmias, seizures, and stroke (Logan et al., 1998; Bailey & Shaw, 1989; Lan et al., 1998). MA intoxication is responsible for increasing incidences of hospital visits, and the rate at which MA is cited as a factor in emergency department (ED) presentations across the nation is rising steadily (Substance Abuse and Mental Health Services Administration [SAMSHA], 2004).

As a central and peripheral sympathetic nervous system stimulant, MA facilitates the release of newly synthesized norepinephrine and dopamine from nerve terminals and, to some extent, blocks their synaptic reuptake (King & Everett, 2005). The resulting catecholamine surge mediates many of the acute symptoms and physiological changes associated with MA intoxication, including elevated heart rate (i.e., tachycardia) and blood pressure. Excess circulating norepinephrine may contribute to organ pathology by causing vasoconstriction and ischemia (i.e., inadequate blood supply to tissues). Likewise, the oxidation of accumu-

117

lated intra- and extracellular catecholamines may lead to the formation of reactive oxygen species and subsequent cellular toxicity (Karch, 2002; Kaye et al., 2007).

Apart from its sympathomimetic effects, other putative mechanisms by which MA use may induce medical illness include direct toxicity to tissues and concurrent effects from other chemical and street drug contaminants (Varner et al., 2002; Albertson et al., 1999). When examining physiologic sequelae of MA use, it is often difficult to differentiate direct effects of the drug from general health consequences of drug-using lifestyles. Specifically, needle sharing, malnutrition, and concomitant use of other substances, such as tobacco and alcohol, may accelerate and exacerbate the onset and clinical course of MA-associated medical consequences, respectively. Prior literature demonstrates that toxicity from MA is amplified when taken with ethanol and opioids, for example (Baselt & Cravey, 1995; Mendelson et al., 1995).

Literature on the medical effects of MA is limited in scope relative to that of other drugs of abuse, including stimulants such as cocaine. Current knowledge of MA-induced medical illness has been influenced primarily by case reports, case series, and autopsy studies. Although the physiological effects of MA are presumed to be similar to those of cocaine, present understanding is limited by a lack of prospective studies and large epidemiological surveys evaluating the extent of medical impairment in this population. MA and cocaine share similar but not identical neurobiological mechanisms of action; their pharmacokinetic and pharmacodynamic properties differ sufficiently such that certain substance-specific medical effects would be anticipated. Acutely, both MA and cocaine use result in elevated norepinephrine and dopamine levels; however, MA acts primarily within the nerve cell by interfering with the vesicular storage of monoamines and facilitating their release into the synaptic cleft, whereas the actions of cocaine are predominantly extracellular, involving monoamine reuptake blockade. Additionally, the half-life of MA is prolonged relative to that of cocaine (11–12 hours vs. 90 minutes, respectively), contributing to longer-lasting subjective and physiological effects (Newton et al., 2005).

The rising use of MA in recent decades has been associated with adverse public health consequences and increasing morbidity and mortality. In addition to general health effects, MA-related medical effects and toxicity have been documented in cardiovascular, pulmonary, gastrointestinal, dermatological, genitourinary, and neurological organs (Albertson et al., 1999). As such, the purpose of this chapter is to summarize and review extant literature on medical sequelae of MA use, organized according to organ systems.

General Health and Acute Presentations

The deleterious effects of MA use on general health are widespread, with underlying mechanisms involving alterations across multiple physiological systems, most prominently the autonomic nervous system. In particular, the sympathetic nervous system activation acutely induced by MA use can cause marked hypertension, tachycardia, increased respiration rate (i.e., tachypnea), peripheral hyperthermia, pupillary dilation, increased perspiration (i.e., diaphoresis), and constriction of blood vessels (i.e., vasoconstriction) (see Meredith et al., 2005). By contrast, the positively reinforcing psychological and physiological effects of MA use include intense euphoria, increased energy and alertness, a sense of heightened physical and mental capacity, and initially, decreased anxiety and enhanced libido (Cretzmeyer et al., 2003; Hart et al., 2001). Routes of MA administration include smoking, injecting, snorting, ingesting, or sublingual use, with injection and smoking producing the most immediate euphoric effects. The high from MA typically lasts between 8 and 12 hours, owing largely to the 12-hour half-life of the drug (Cho et al., 2001). Some of the health risks associated with MA use may be mediated by the effects of toxic agents used in the synthesis of the drug; in particular, the occasional use of lead acetate as a reagent has been linked with acute lead poisoning, observed mostly in intravenous users (Centers for Disease Control and Prevention [CDC], 1989; Allcott et al., 1987).

Like other stimulants, MA suppresses appetite and, during intoxication, the observed increases in energy and goal-directed activities are often accompanied by sleeplessness. With prolonged use, corresponding nutritional deficiencies may occur. As the positively reinforcing effects of MA diminish with repeated use, emergent toxic effects may become manifest in the form of heightened anxiety, irrititability, and/or confusion. Long-term use of MA is also associated with elevated rates of infectious diseases including human immunodeficiency virus (HIV), hepatitis B and C, and endocarditis, or infection of the inner lining of the heart muscle and valves (Albertson et al., 1999; Gonzales et al., 2006). Factors accounting for the heightened risk for infectious diseases in MA-using populations include (1) increased risky sexual behaviors occurring in the context of MA intoxication, practices that are particularly prominent among men who have sex with men (MSM) (see Shoptaw & Reback, 2007) and are mediated in part by facilitation of sexual desire resulting from use (Volkow et al., 2007); and (2) injection drug use and associated risk behaviors (e.g., needle sharing) (CDC, 2006). Moreover, repeated injection use of MA can produce severe infections, including abscesses and cellulitis at the injection sites.

In recent years MA-related ED mentions have increased to approach the frequency of heroin-associated visits, with a 54% increase in such visits across the nation reported between 1995 and 2002 (SAMSHA, 2004). Individuals experiencing acute toxic effects of MA may present to the ED with a variety of symptoms. Psychosis, agitation, suicidality, and cardiovascular abnormalities are among the most common signs of MA toxicity (e.g., Richards et al., 1999a). In a recent study of adults who visited the ED for MA-related problems, psychiatric disorders and trauma were the two most common presenting conditions, followed by skin infections and dental problems (Hendrickson et al., 2008).

Although a causal relationship has yet to be demonstrated, MA use is associated with impulsive, violent, and, at times, homicidal behavior; hence, consideration of MA abuse is warranted when a patient presents in an emergency medical setting with violence, loss of self-control, and/or related trauma (e.g., gunshot wounds, stabbings, and assaults). Given the impairment in judgment and fine motor skills that can result from MA use (e.g., Scott et al., 2007), MA-using populations may be predisposed to injury secondary to motor vehicle accidents. Likewise, in a review of ED visits by 461 patients with positive toxicology screens for MA, blunt trauma, occurring in more than one third of the sample, with the majority involving motor vehicle accidents, was found to be the most common presenting complaint, occurring at a significantly higher rate than that observed in a control group of patients whose ED visits were non-drug related. In that same study, the second most common chief complaint involved altered level of consciousness, observed in 23% of the sample. Tonic–clonic seizures were also reported in a small subgroup of patients who tested positive for MA ($n = 16$; 3.4%); of note, the majority of these cases represented first-onset seizures in the absence of plausible etiology unrelated to MA use (e.g., alcohol withdrawal) (Richards et al., 1999a). MA-induced seizures may occur as isolated phenomena but have been reported to occur in association with other events related to toxicity, including hyperthermia, coma, renal failure, and shock (Albertson et al., 1999).

In addition to deaths associated with assaults, suicides, homicides, and accidents, MA-induced mortality can result from overdose and hypersensitivity to acute physiological effects of the drug, such as hypertension (e.g., Delaney & Estes, 1980). An often-cited mechanism underlying lethality, demonstrated in clinical and animal studies, is hyperthermia (Numachi et al., 2007), which may occur as a consequence of MA's modulation of the hypothalamic temperature centers. Alternatively, increases in body temperature may be accounted for by high levels of motor activity during MA intoxication coupled with the inhibition of heat loss secondary to MA's vasoconstricting effects (Karch, 2002).

Other potentially fatal medical complications of overdose include seizures, hypoxic stress, and cardiovascular complications (Davidson et al.,
2001).

Central Nervous System Effects

Central nervous system (CNS) complications of MA intoxication include
a broad range of mental status changes, neurotoxicity, strokes, and other
brain tissue injury. Relative to its parent compound, amphetamine,
MA exhibits greater CNS effects due to elevated CNS penetration and
potency (Albertson et al., 1999). Psychiatric symptoms have been well
documented in individuals experiencing MA intoxication (see Zweben et
al., 2004). These symptoms, which may vary as a function of individual
differences in sensitivity to MA, escalation in quantity and/or frequency
of use, and route of MA administration, include anxiety, insomnia, irritability, paranoia, hallucinations, and even delirium (Harris & Batki,
2000). Injection users and those with familial loading for psychosis are
at heightened risk for the development of MA-related psychotic symptoms (McKetin et al., 2006; Chen et al., 2005). In some individuals MA
intoxication can mimic hypomania or mania, with symptoms including grandiosity, marked psychomotor agitation, and impaired judgment.
Upon cessation of use, an abstinence syndrome comprising predominant
psychiatric features may emerge, which is particularly prominent among
chronic and injection drug users (e.g., McGregor et al., 2005; Newton
et al., 2004). This syndrome is typically characterized by drug cravings
coupled with marked depressive symptoms including ahedonia, dysphoria, irritability, poor concentration, hypersomnia, low energy, and even
suicidality (Meredith et al., 2005). Anxiety, aggression, and psychosis
have also been reported following cessation of use. Although the severity
of psychiatric symptoms typically declines within a week of abstinence
(Newton et al., 2004), a subset of MA users experience prolonged psychiatric symptomatology, even in the absence of a known prior history
of mental illness (Chen et al., 2003; Iwanami et al., 1994).

Despite the fact that epidemiological surveys have focused more
broadly on amphetamine users rather than targeting MA-dependent
individuals per se, a handful of clinical studies strongly suggest that MA
users have elevated rates of psychiatric disorders (e.g., Shoptaw et al.,
2003; Copeland & Sorenson, 2001; Glasner-Edwards et al., 2007), particularly affective and thought disorders. The distinction between MA-
induced and primary mood disorders poses challenges to clinicians and
researchers seeking to understand the relationship between MA use and
affect dysregulation, and little is known about the order of onset and

respective etiologies of MA abuse versus mood disorders in MA-dependent populations. Relatively more studies have been conducted in efforts to delineate prevalence and risk factors for protracted and/or recurrent psychosis, which clinically may appear similar to schizophrenia (Harris & Batki, 2000). Psychosis occurs at least transiently in a significant proportion of MA users, with wide variation in the duration of symptoms (McKetin et al., 2006). Nevertheless, nearly one third of those with psychosis in the context of MA use have reported prolonged psychotic symptoms lasting more than 6 months (Ujike & Sato, 2004). Although the mechanism underlying variation in the duration of psychotic symptoms is unclear, evidence suggests that genetic factors play a key role (Ujike et al., 2003) and may operate in concert with stress reactivity in the genesis of recurrent psychotic episodes (Iyo et al., 2004; Yui et al., 2002).

In addition to psychiatric impairment, use of MA is associated with neurocognitive deficits; according to recent estimates, 40% of individuals with MA dependence display evidence of global neuropsychological impairment (Rippeth et al., 2004). The effects of MA on neuropsychological functioning may vary according to quantity (Monterosso et al., 2005) and frequency (Simon et al., 2000) of use as well as dependence severity, although some studies have failed to find evidence for these associations (see Scott et al., 2007, for review). Single doses are interestingly associated with enhanced performance in multiple neuropsychological domains in normal human subjects (e.g., Soetens et al., 1995). By contrast, according to a recent meta-analysis of the neuropsychological effects of MA abuse and dependence, chronic use is associated with impairment in several domains, including deficits of medium magnitude (i.e., effect size) in processes engaging frontostriatal and limbic circuits such as episodic memory, executive functions, and psychomotor tasks. To a somewhat lesser extent, MA use is associated with detrimental effects on attention, working memory, language, and visuoconstruction (Scott et al., 2007). The severity of neurocognitive deficits may become worse during initial abstinence relative to active users (Simon et al., 2004) and may persist for 9 months or longer following initial abstinence; however, sustained abstinence is correlated with recovery in dopamine terminal function and at least partial recovery of cognitive functioning in MA-dependent populations (Volkow et al., 2001b; Wang et al., 2004).

MA users may exhibit hyperkinetic movements including repetitive or stereotyped behaviors (Mattson & Calvery, 1968; Sperling & Horowitz, 1994), effects that have been demonstrated even more extensively in animal studies (e.g., Wallace et al., 1999; Kuczenski & Segal, 2001). Choreoathetoid movement disorders have also been observed (Lundh & Tunving, 1981; Rhee et al., 1988). In addition, although it has been suggested that dopaminergic deficits resulting from MA use may produce parkinsonian symptoms, clinical research evidence supporting this theory remains limited (Caliguri & Buitenhuys, 2005). Chronic MA use has been shown to cause neurotoxicity as evidenced by reductions in striatal dopamine transporter (DAT) activity, and this may correlate clinically with impairment in cognition and psychomotor slowing (Volkow et al., 2001a). Moreover, it has been purported that decreased dopaminergic neurotransmission associated with chronic use may predispose MA users to parkinsonism and that associated cognitive deficits involving working memory may represent a form of subclinical parkinsonism (Volkow et al., 2001a; Chang et al., 2002).

In ED settings, MA users may present unconscious as a consequence of overdose, possibly in combination with other drugs of abuse. Alternately, unresponsiveness may occur as a result of tonic-clonic seizure activity in association with MA intoxication, including potentially life-threatening status epilepticus. Although uncommon relative to other health effects, seizures may occur in isolation after amphetamine use or as a secondary consequence of other related medical conditions, such as hyperthermia or metabolic disturbances (Albertson et al., 1999; Meredith et al., 2005; Sommers et al., 2006).

Of public health concern is the growing evidence for stimulant use as a significant risk factor for stroke in young adults (Kaku & Lowenstein, 1990; Westover et al., 2007). MA-related cerebrovascular accidents (CVAs) have been widely documented in case reports and case series in association with various routes of administration (e.g., Rothrock et al., 1988; Lessing & Hyman, 1989; Perez et al., 1999; Yen et al., 1994). Data from histological and autopsy investigations of stroke in MA users is limited relative to existing clinical evidence. As observed in cocaine abusers, amphetamine-related strokes typically affect the frontal lobes, and the etiology is usually hemorrhagic or ischemic (Karch, 2002). Embolic stroke has also been documented but is assumed to be rare (Imanishi et al., 1997). Although cerebrovascular lesions in MA abusers are most often intracerebral, subarachnoid hemorrhages following ruptured berry aneurysms have also been reported (Davis & Swalwell, 1994, 1996).

Although a direct causal link between MA use and CVA has been difficult to establish, findings from a recent analysis of clinical data from a statewide hospital database implicated amphetamine as a significant risk factor for hemorrhagic stroke and for associated in-hospital fatalities. Results also demonstrated that the rate of increase in amphetamine-related CVA was greater during the time period of the study (2000–2003) than that for other drugs of abuse (Westover et al., 2007). Commonly cited mechanisms contributing to stroke involve catecholamine-mediated effects, such as vasospasm and hypertension. Other adverse clinical outcomes associated with MA-induced vasospasm include blindness; in one case, transient cortical blindness was reported in an infant exposed to MA (Gospe, 1995). Cerebral vasculitis has also been described in MA users and may be implicated in the pathogenesis of CVA in some instances (e.g., Salanova & Taubner, 1984; Shibata et al., 1991).

Cardiovascular Effects

MA is associated with cardiac toxicity and cardiovascular tissue pathology, most notably after long-term use (Karch, 2002; Kaye et al., 2007). Cardiovascular consequences have been described in numerous case reports as well as animal, *in vitro*, and autopsy investigations, and effects have been demonstrated regardless of route of administration (Haning & Goebert, 2007). Due to MA's sympathomimetic properties resulting in increased catecholamine activity, heart rate and blood pressure elevation are the most common initial cardiovascular manifestations of MA use. Compensatory lowering of heart rate may also occur (Perez-Rayes et al., 1991; Varner et al., 2002).

According to a recent study by Newton and colleagues (2005), the acute cardiovascular effects of MA administration are longer lasting than those of cocaine. When administered intravenously, MA-induced changes in heart rate and blood pressure peak within 10 minutes and remain significantly elevated for at least 30 minutes, as opposed to the acute cardiovascular effects of cocaine, which return to baseline before 30 minutes post-administration. As suggested by Newton et al., these differences may be only partially attributable to unique pharmacokinetic properties of the two drugs, which include the prolonged elimination half-life of MA relative to cocaine. Pharmacodynamic differences, involving mechanisms of synaptic monoamine level elevation and dopaminergic neurotransmission, may contribute to an even greater extent.

In ED settings, common presenting symptoms related to MA intoxication include chest pain, hypertension, shortness of breath, and tachycardia (Derlet et al., 1989; Richards et al., 1999a; Turnipseed et al., 2003). Although seen less frequently, an important life-threatening complication of MA use is the acute coronary syndrome (ACS) in which chest pain resulting from myocardial ischemia (i.e., insufficient blood supply to cardiac tissue) is a predominant symptom. Among those who present with ACS, electrocardiogram (ECG) abnormalities are common, including ST-segment elevation. Individuals may be diagnosed with unstable angina or acute myocardial infarction and are at risk of adverse events including arrhythmias and cardiogenic shock (i.e., inadequate blood flow due to diminished heart function) (Turnipseed et al., 2003; Wijetunga et al., 2004). Turnipseed and colleagues (2003) recently reported a 25% prevalence of ACS in MA users hospitalized for chest pain, and serious cardiac complications emerged in a significant percentage of patients despite the relatively young average age of the sample (i.e., 40 years old).

Peripheral catecholamine excess is cardiotoxic and understood to be the primary mechanism underlying both immediate MA-related cardiac effects and chronic cardiovascular pathology (Karch, 2002). As demonstrated in prior studies of other stimulant drugs, both central and peripheral sympathetic nervous system activation likely share a role in these outcomes (Vongpatanasin et al., 1999). High levels of catecholamines may cause vasospasm, hypertrophy (i.e., increased size) of myocardial cells, and fibrous tissue formation. Consistent with these effects, elevated heart weight, microvascular changes, and accelerated coronary artery disease are observed in autopsy studies of MA abusers relative to controls. In addition, postmortem histological findings include interstitial fibrosis and hypertrophy of cardiac myocytes and arterioles (Matoba et al., 1986; Karch et al., 1999; Karch, 2002).

Microvascular pathology and fibrous tissue formation are predisposing factors for cardiac arrhythmias (Karch, 2002). In MA users, sudden death due to arrhythmias has been well documented, and evidence suggests that risk is amplified in individuals with preexisting structural abnormalities, including myocardial hypertrophy (Matoba et al., 1984, 1986; Derlet & Horowitz, 1995; Albertson et al., 1999; Kaye et al., 2007). Additional risk of potentially fatal ventricular arrhythmias is conferred by QTc prolongation, an ECG abnormality recently found at elevated and clinically significant rates in two populations of MA-dependent adults (Haning & Goebert, 2007; Mooney et al., in press). Importantly, arrhythmias and sudden death may occur even after low doses of MA (Kaye et al., 2007).

Another infrequent but often lethal complication of MA use is aortic dissection, which involves tearing of the inner layer of the aorta and likely eventual rupture of the aortic wall (Davis & Swalwell, 1994; Swalwell & Davis, 1999; Karch et al., 1999). One cited putative mechanism underlying aortic dissection is untreated MA-induced hypertension, which may contribute to weakening, tearing, and eventual rupture of the aorta. Formation of reactive oxygen species due to excess circulating catecholamines, causing vascular cell death, may also play a role in this rare complication (Karch, 2002; Kaye et al., 2007).

Evidence for amphetamine-related cardiomyopathy has been documented in prior clinical and experimental literature, including case reports and a recent retrospective study (Hong et al., 1991; Smith et al., 1976; Wijetunga et al., 2003; He et al., 1996). Individuals with cardiomyopathy exhibit left ventricular enlargement, signs and symptoms of heart failure, and a variable clinical course. Cardiomyopathy is most commonly observed after chronic MA use, but acute and reversible cases have also been reported (Call et al., 1982; O'Neill et al., 1983; Jacobs, 1989). Although the etiology of cardiomyopathy in MA users has not been fully elucidated, one proposed mechanism involves catecholamine-mediated vasospasm and myocardial cell death (Karch, 2002; Kaye et al., 2007). Recent cellular and animal studies also suggest possible direct toxicity of MA to cardiac tissues (Welder, 1992; He, 1995; Maeno et al., 2000a, 2000b).

Acute myocardial infarction (AMI) has been reported in association with MA use, although less frequently than with cocaine; one cited explanation for this disparity is that MA intoxication causes elevated body temperature and subsequent production of cardiac heat-shock proteins, which may protect the myocardium from ischemic damage (Karch, 2002; Maulik et al., 1995). Nevertheless, to date, there have been multiple reports in the literature of amphetamine-related myocardial infarction (e.g., Farnsworth et al., 1997; Furst et al., 1990; Packe et al., 1990). Of particular concern, an association between amphetamine use and AMI in young individuals has been suggested by a recent case report (Chen, 2007) and a population-based study (Westover et al., 2008). Mechanisms implicated in the pathogenesis of AMI in MA users include coronary vasospasm, platelet aggregation, atherosclerotic plaque rupture, and subsequent thrombus formation (Kaye et al., 2007). AMI secondary to coronary artery aneurysm rupture has also been reported after amphetamine use (Brennan et al., 2004).

Although many of the above-mentioned cardiac complications in MA users are relatively uncommon, autopsy studies demonstrate a strong association between coronary artery disease (CAD) and MA. Postmortem evidence has shown rapid progression of multivessel CAD at relatively young ages in MA users relative to controls (Karch, 2002). In one large autopsy review, Karch and colleagues (1999) found a CAD prevalence rate of nearly 20% in MA users compared with only 5% of controls. Purported etiologies of CAD in this population include catecholamine-induced vasoconstriction and hypertension, platelet aggregation, and vascular injury from free-radical generation (Karch, 2002; Turnipseed et al., 2003).

In conclusion, the relatively small but expanding body of clinical and experimental literature describing the cardiovascular sequelae of MA use supports the link between potentially life-threatening cardiac complications and MA exposure. Cardiovascular consequences are more likely to be observed in long-term users with preexisting cardiac disease; intravenous use may also confer elevated risk as a function of higher and more frequent dosing relative to other routes of administration (Kaye et al., 2007). The primary meditational mechanism of MA-related myocardial pathology is catecholamine excess, although direct toxicity to myocardial cells may also occur (Varner et al., 2002). Although the cardiovascular complications of MA use are serious and wide-ranging, existing case reports and animal studies provide a basis for the assumption that cardiac lesions related to MA use may be potentially reversible upon discontinuation of use of the drug (Jacobs, 1989; Islam et al., 1995). Thus it is imperative to educate both users and treatment providers about these and other potentially devastating medical risks of MA.

Pulmonary Effects

The incidence of respiratory symptoms and pulmonary pathology in MA users is unknown, and the relative contribution of route of administration to frequency and severity of stimulant-related pulmonary toxicity has not been established. Surprisingly limited data regarding pulmonary effects of MA use have been published relative to cocaine, for which an extensive body of evidence exists supporting its link with respiratory symptoms and pathology. It is unknown whether differences in mechanisms of action, frequency of use, or methods of administration between these stimulants may contribute to this discrepancy (Albertson et al., 1995).

MA use can stimulate respiratory system activity, as manifested by acute respiratory symptomatology. Dyspnea, or shortness of breath, has been commonly reported in ED settings and may be secondary to cardiovascular complications related to MA use (Albertson et al., 1995, 1999). Despite clinical observations of dyspnea, due to the bronchodilating properties of MA, wheezing is not directly associated with MA use (Cruz et al., 1998); in fact, amphetamine was once used as an ingredient in inhalers for asthma and nasal allergies in the 1930s (Albertson et al., 1995).

In addition to the respiratory effects of using MA, involvement in MA manufacture poses unique pulmonary risks; in particular, individuals who make MA are subject to inhalation injuries from toxic fumes. The process of MA synthesis involves combining potentially volatile chemicals, causing the release of toxic and corrosive gases, such as phospine. Inhalation of smoke from fires associated with chemical explosions may also contribute to and exacerbate pulmonary injury (Burgess, 2001; Willers-Russo, 1999; Santos et al., 2005). In a recent study of burn victims, mechanical ventilation requirements were significantly greater in subjects with MA-related injury relative to those with burns unrelated to MA production or use (Santos et al., 2005).

Respiratory complications associated with MA use include pulmonary edema and pulmonary hypertension. A case of acute noncardiogenic pulmonary edema, an illness involving fluid accumulation in the lungs, has been reported in a MA smoker (Nestor et al., 1989). Pulmonary edema was also found in more than 70% of MA-related deaths in a large autopsy study conducted by Karch and colleagues (1999). Idiopathic pulmonary arterial hypertension (IPAH) in MA users has been reported, albeit infrequently (Robertson et al., 1976; Schaiberger et al., 1993; Nishida et al., 2003) and a recent retrospective study demonstrated a significant association between MA use and IPAH (Chin et al., 2003).

In their autopsy investigation, Karch and colleagues (1999) noted pneumonia and emphysema in 8% and 5% of MA users, respectively. Birefringent crystals in the pulmonary vasculature were evident in 11% of subjects, suggesting possible intravenous use of crushed tablets containing fillers such as cellulose or cornstarch; when oral pills are administered intravenously, these insoluble particles may occlude small pulmonary vessels and appear as birefringent crystals. Over the long term, intravenous injection may lead to increased pulmonary vascular resistance and, in some individuals, development of pulmonary hypertension and granulomas (i.e., areas of inflammation) (Karch, 2002). In parallel with these observations, injection of the stimulant methylphenidate, which often contains the filler talc, has been linked with the development of talc granulomas and panacinar emphysema (e.g., Schmidt et al., 1991; Stern et al., 1994; Karch, 2002).

Although precise mechanisms underlying the pathogenesis of pulmonary disease such as IPAH in MA users have not been ascertained, they are likely multifactorial. Catecholamine-mediated vasoconstriction and endothelial injury have been proposed in the literature and may play a significant role (Chin et al., 2006), and one small prior study showed increased pulmonary arterial pressure in persons receiving intravenous MA (Kneehans et al., 1975). A direct toxic effect of the drug on pulmonary cells is also plausible, but research evaluating this and other effects of MA on pulmonary cellular functioning is largely lacking. In evaluating the etiology of lung pathology in MA users, it is also important to consider possible toxic effects of drug contaminants as well as the concomitant use of other substances known to compromise pulmonary function, such as marijuana and tobacco (Albertson et al., 1995).

Gastrointestinal Effects

Gastrointestinal complications have not been widely examined in MA users. Acute abdominal pain has been described as a presenting symptom in MA-intoxicated individuals in ED settings (Derlet et al., 1989). In addition, chronic MA use is known to be associated with hepatic toxicity; in a large autopsy investigation of MA-related deaths, fatty liver was the most commonly reported medical abnormality, found in approximately 16% of subjects. Cirrhosis was observed in 9% of subjects, and, to a lesser yet notable extent, infiltration of major hepatic vessels (e.g., portal triad infiltration) and hepatitis were also reported (Karch et al., 1999).

It is difficult to establish a direct causal relationship between MA and liver pathology, as confounding effects of concomitant medical conditions or the use of alcohol or other drugs cannot be readily discerned. Indeed, hepatitis and portal triad infiltration have been frequently observed in intravenous injectors of other drugs of abuse. However, alpha adrenergic stimulation has demonstrated hepatotoxic effects, which may account uniquely for liver pathology observed in conjunction with MA and other stimulant drug use (Karch, 2002). Prior literature has supported the link between other amphetamine-like drugs and hepatotoxicity, including pemoline, methylphenidate (Ritalin), and MDMA ("Ecstasy") (e.g., Mehta et al., 1984; Pratt & Dubois, 1990; de Man et al., 1993). Thus the etiology of MA-associated hepatic injury is likely multifaceted; proposed mechanisms include direct hepatocellular toxicity, indirect damage from catecholamine-mediated vasoconstriction and ischemia, and necrotizing vasculitis (Jones et al., 1994; Albertson et al., 1999).

Additional gastrointestinal complications reported in relation to MA use include giant gastroduodenal ulcers (Pecha et al., 1996), ischemic colitis (Johnson & Berenson, 1991), and hemorrhagic pancreatitis (Pecha et al., 1996). Literature to date suggests a stronger association between ulcer formation and cocaine than with MA use, but shared mechanisms involving catecholamine excess and ischemia have been suggested (Karch, 2002). Although hemorrhagic pancreatitis may be only infrequently associated with MA abuse with limited case reports to date, the relationship has been reproduced in animal studies after chronic MA administration (Ito et al., 1997).

Genitourinary Effects

The relationship between MA use and rhabdomyolysis, a potentially life-threatening condition associated with kidney function compromise, has been increasingly recognized in the literature. Rhabdomyolysis is characterized by muscle tissue injury and subsequent release of myocyte contents, including creatine phosphokinase (CPK) and myoglobin, into the circulatory system. Several of these byproducts are nephrotoxic, and their accumulation may lead to acute renal failure, particularly if treatment is delayed. Nephrotoxicity may also be exacerbated during this process by the release of intracellular potassium and other electrolytes, resulting in fluid shifts, hypotension, and diminished oxygen supply to kidney tissue (Karch, 2002).

The causes of rhabdomyolysis are numerous and include physical trauma, metabolic disturbances, infection, excess muscle activity, hyperthermia, and direct toxicity from medications, alcohol, or illicit substances (Knochel, 1993; Karch, 2002). Literature supporting the link between stimulant use and rhabdomyloysis has focused primarily on cocaine, but case reports involving MA use have also been published (e.g., Scandling & Spital, 1982; Terada et al., 1988). In a retrospective study of ED visits at a large public hospital, MA use was identified in a substantial proportion of patients diagnosed with rhabdomyolysis and was implicated as a potential risk factor for this condition. Moreover, MA-positive subjects presented with significantly elevated CPK values relative to those with rhabdomyolysis who did not test positive for MA (Richards et al., 1999b).

Varied mechanisms specific to rhabdomyolysis in MA users have been proposed, including muscle tissue damage from hyperthermia, agitation, or hyperkinetic movements during MA intoxication, which may be exacerbated by other sympathomimetic effects of the drug. Sleep deprivation and dehydration associated with MA use may also confer elevated risk of rhabdomyolysis. Direct drug-related myotoxicity has been suggested and has been shown to occur following cocaine use. In addition, concomitant alcohol ingestion is a known risk factor for rhabdomyolysis; ethanol has myotoxic effects, and electrolyte deficiencies present in many chronic users may also facilitate muscle injury (Richards et al., 1999b; Karch, 2002).

Other renal complications of MA use are uncommon (Karch, 2002); in a large autopsy review of MA-related deaths, the prevalence rate of renal pathology was less than 2%. The majority of lesions were of the nephrosclerotic type typically found in association with hypertension; a causal relationship with MA use is also possible but could not be determined (Karch et al., 1999). Ginsberg et al. (1970) first reported on reversible renal failure associated with hyperthermia and coagulopathy after amphetamine ingestion. Cases of renal failure associated with cardiovascular shock and acute tubular necrosis have also been described (Albertson et al., 1999). In one case of acute interstitial nephritis and renal failure after amphetamine use, common secondary mediators such as rhabdomyolysis, hyperthermia, or shock were absent, suggesting that amphetamine use alone may be sufficient to induce renal toxicity (Foley et al., 1984).

Oral Health Effects

Recent evidence suggests that use of MA is associated with a variety of oral health deficits. The term "meth mouth" has been used to denote the deleterious effects of MA on dental health (Shaner, 2002; Davey, 2005), although in the clinical research literature it has been recently argued that this term overgeneralizes the expected direct effects of MA on dentition (Donaldson & Goodchild, 2006; Goodchild et al., 2007). The most commonly observed oral health problems reported by MA users include rampant caries and tooth fracture (e.g., Curtis, 2006; Shaner, 2002; Shaner et al., 2006) as well as periodontal disease (e.g., gingivitis, periodontitis) (see Shaner, 2002; Shaner et al., 2006), and a considerable debate concerning the etiology of these problems and their clinical consequences is ongoing.

One of the most frequently cited mechanisms for tooth decay and caries development in individuals who use MA is xerostomia, or dry mouth (Donaldson & Goodchild, 2006; Lewis, 2005; Saini et al., 2005), a common complaint in MA users. Xerostomia-related deficits in the quantity of saliva production can, in turn, mediate tooth decay (Saini et al., 2005). Although the precise mechanism underlying MA-related xerostomia is not known, the link between MA use and xerostomia can be explained by both pharmacological and behavioral factors. Given that salivary secretion is mediated by the autonomic nervous system, the pharmacological action of MA, in facilitating sympathetic nervous system activity, can stimulate alpha-2-receptors, causing inhibition of salivary secretion (see Saini et al., 2005). Behaviorally, in the context of appetite suppression coupled with substantial increases in psychomotor activity and metabolism induced by use of the drug, MA users often display anorexia during acute intoxication, resulting in generalized dehydration and consequent reductions in saliva secretion. A related behavioral account of xerostomia has been identified in case reports, in which MA users have reported consumption of unusually large quantities of caffeinated, carbohydrate-rich soft drinks to counteract thirst and sugar cravings (Donaldson & Goodchild, 2006; Shaner et al., 2006; Richards & Brofeldt, 2000).

The compromised saliva production associated with xerostomia deprives the oral environment of the protective effects of saliva on tooth enamel, rendering the MA user vulnerable to caries development. As a result of the binge–crash pattern typical of MA users, periods of poor oral hygiene during active MA use are thought to be interspersed with periods of abstinence and corresponding improvements in oral hygiene, resulting in a gradual overall progression of tooth decay (Rhodus & Little, 2005). Likewise, the extent to which poor oral hygiene, observed in individuals with broad-ranging substance abuse problems (e.g., Araujo et al., 2004; Friedlander et al., 2003), contributes to accumulation of bacterial dental plaque and progression of caries observed in MA users has yet to be understood, relative to MA-specific factors.

Bruxism, or tooth clenching and/or grinding, has also been observed in MA users and is thought to contribute to tooth wear. The tendency of MA using individuals to clench their jaws and grind their teeth may be secondary to the anxiety and restlessness often reported during acute withdrawal (Curtis, 2006). In addition to tooth wear, bruxism in MA users is associated with myofacial pain and related conditions such as temporomandibular joint (TMJ) syndrome (Richards & Brofeldt, 2000).

Finally, the acidic content of MA itself is an often cited but controversial putative mechanism underlying tooth decay and wear (American Dental Association, 2005). While it has been argued that the corrosive contaminates in MA (e.g., phosphoric, sulfuric, or muriatic acid), when smoked, facilitate enamel erosion and demineralization, Shaner et al. (2006) propose that caries cannot be explained by this mechanism alone, given that caries is a complex and bacterially mediated disease, coupled with evidence that carious lesions are observed in MA users who do not use smoking as the route of administration (Howe, 1995; Mooney et al., in press).

In summary, dental problems observed in MA-using populations include caries, tooth fracture and loss, and periodontal disease. Hypothesized mediating mechanisms include xerostomia secondary to generalized dehydration and sympathetic nervous system activation, frequent consumption of carbonated beverages with high sugar concentration, poor oral hygiene practices, bruxism, and the acidic nature of the drug.

Dermatological Effects

Dermatological manifestations of MA abuse are most often the result of self-inflicted injury during intoxication, infection from repeated injection, or accidental burns related to the process of drug manufacture. When experiencing distressing physical or psychiatric symptoms, MA users may repeatedly scratch or pick at their skin, generating visible excoriations or cutaneous ulcers. These behaviors are typically observed as a consequence of drug-induced perceptual disturbances such as formication, which is the sensation of bugs crawling on or underneath the skin (MacKenzie & Heischober, 1997; Bostwick & Lineberry, 2006).

Serious self-injurious behaviors have also been reported in association with amphetamine-related psychosis, including severe and repetitive self-mutilation. In a case series described by Kraftofil and colleagues (1996), self-mutilation was most commonly witnessed in the context of chronic MA abuse and psychosis, and such behaviors were observed in patients both with and without psychiatric comorbidity. Observed injuries included self-inflicted stab wounds and severing of extremities. In related case reports, repeated acts of genital self-mutilation during MA intoxication have also been described (Israel & Lee, 2002), and self-injurious behaviors have been demonstrated in rodents after administration of high doses of amphetamine-type compounds (Gorea & Lombard, 1984; Mueller et al., 1986). A cited putative mechanism underlying self-mutilation associated with MA use is dopaminergic agonism, which likely contributes in a similar manner to motor stereotypies and hyperkinetic movements in humans and animals (Israel & Lee, 2002).

Skin and soft-tissue infections may also occur as a consequence of intravenous drug administration. Damage to skin tissue may facilitate the formation of abscesses, or collections of pus, at injection sites. Injection directly into muscle or skin, also known as "skin popping," confers even greater risk for this type of infection than intravenous administration. Cellulitis, another type of skin infection that may develop in injection drug users, poses risk of spread to deeper tissues, lymph nodes, and the bloodstream, rapidly becoming life threatening if left untreated (Murphy et al., 2001; Ebright & Pieper, 2002).

Potentially hazardous and volatile chemicals are mixed together during MA manufacture, causing burns from explosions, fires, and chemical injuries (Danks et al., 2004; Santos et al., 2005). In a retrospective analysis of burn unit admissions, patients with MA-associated injuries required greater volumes of fluid resuscitation than those with burns unrelated to MA production. Furthermore, all subjects with burns covering greater than 40% of their body surface area died; notably, this death rate far exceeded the expected fatality rate for this sample in light of the extent of their burn-related injuries and age. It was speculated that direct MA toxicity as well as chemical inhalation injury were responsible for the elevated morbidity and mortality demonstrated in these subjects (Warner et al., 2003).

Conclusion

MA use is associated with a host of medical, psychiatric, and neurocognitive impairments. The medical sequelae of this drug can have profoundly deleterious effects at both the individual and public health levels, given its association with increased transmission of infectious diseases. The health-related consequences of MA use span numerous organ systems, as reviewed in this chapter, with particularly prominent effects on the CNS and cardiovascular system. Although the mechanisms of action underlying various MA-related pathologies vary, toxicity induced by MA is most consistently associated with its sympathomimetic effects, particularly the facilitation of excess catecholamine release. Further research is needed to understand the epidemiology of medical illnesses in MA-using populations, the mechanisms underlying disease pathogenesis, and the clinical course of these conditions in relation to that of MA abuse and/or dependence.

References

Albertson TE, Derlet RW, Van Hoozen BE. (1999). Methamphetamine and the expanding complications of amphetamines. *West J Med* 170:214–219.

Albertson TE, Walby WF, Derlet RW. (1995). Stimulant-induced pulmonary toxicity. *Chest* 108:1140–1149.

Allcott JV, 3rd, Barnhart RA, Mooney LA. (1987). Acute lead poisoning in two users of illicit methamphetamine. *JAMA* 258(4):510–511.

American Dental Association. (2005). For the dental patient ... methamphetamine use and oral health. *J Am Dent Assoc* 136(10):1491.

Araujo MW, Dermen K, Connors G, et al. (2004). Oral and dental health among inpatients in treatment for alcohol use disorders: A pilot study. *J Int Acad Periodontol* 6(4):125–130.

Bailey DN, Shaw RF. (1989). Cocaine- and methamphetamine-related deaths in San Diego County (1987): Homicides and accidental overdoses. *J Forensic Sci* 34(2):407–422.

Baselt RC, Cravey RH. (1995). Amphetamine. In RC Baselt, RH Cravey (Eds), *Disposition of toxic drugs and chemicals in man* (pp. 44–47). Foster City, CA: Chemical Toxicology Institute.

Bostwick JM, Lineberry TW. (2006). The "meth" epidemic: Managing acute psychosis, agitation, and suicide risk. *Current Psychiatry* 5(11):47–62.

Brennan K, Shurmur S, Elhendy A. (2004). Coronary artery rupture associated with amphetamine abuse. *Cardiol Rev* 12:282–283.

Burgess JL. (2001). Phosphine exposure from a methamphetamine laboratory investigation. *Clin Toxicol* 39:165–168.

Caligiuri MP, Buitenhuys C. (2005). Do preclinical findings of methamphetamine-induced motor abnormalities translate to an observable clinical phenotype? *Neuropsychopharmacology* 30:2125–2134.

Call TD, Hartneck J, Dickinson WA, et al. (1982). Acute cardiomyopathy secondary to intravenous amphetamine abuse. *Ann Internal Med* 97(4):559–560.

Centers for Disease Control and Prevention. (1989). Lead poisoning associated with intravenous-methamphetamine use: Oregon, 1988. *MMWR Morb Mortal Wkly Rep* 38(48):830–831.

Centers for Disease Control and Prevention. (2006). Methamphetamine use and HIV risk behaviors among heterosexual men: Preliminary results from five northern California counties, December 2001–November 2003. *MMWR Morb Mortal Wkly Rep* 55(10):273–277.

Chang L, Ernst T, Speck O, et al. (2002). Perfusion MRI and computerized cognitive test abnormalities in abstinent methamphetamine users. *Psychiatry Res* 114(2):65–79.

Chen JP. (2007). Methamphetamine-associated acute myocardial infarction and cardiogenic shock with normal coronary arteries: Refractory global coronary microvascular spasm. *J Invasive Cardiol* 19(4):E89–E92.

Chen CK, Lin SK, Sham PC, et al. (2003). Pre-morbid characteristics and co-morbidity of methamphetamine users with and without psychosis. *Psychol Med* 33(8):1407–1414.

Chen CK, Lin SK, Sham PC, et al. (2005). Morbid risk for psychiatric disorder among the relatives of methamphetamine users with and without psychosis. *Am J Med Genet B Neuropsychiatr Genet* 136(1):87–91.

Chin KM, Channik RN, Rubin LJ. (2006). Is methamphetamine use associated with idiopathic pulmonary arterial hypertension? *Chest* 130(6):1657–1663.

Cho AK, Melega WP, Kuczenski R, et al. (2001). Relevance of pharmacokinetic parameters in animal models of methamphetamine abuse. *Synapse* 39(2):161–166.

Copeland AL, Sorensen JL. (2001). Differences between methamphetamine users and cocaine users in treatment. *Drug Alcohol Depend* 62(1):91–95.

Cretzmeyer M, Sarrazin MV, Huber DL, et al. (2003). Treatment of methamphetamine abuse: Research findings and clinical directions. *J Subst Abuse Treat* 24(3):267–277.

Cruz, R, Davis M, O'Neil H, et al. (1998). Pulmonary manifestations of inhaled street drugs. *Heart & Lung* 27(5):297–305.

Curtis EK. (2006). Meth mouth: A review of methamphetamine abuse and its oral manifestations. *Gen Dent* 54(2):125–129.

Danks RR, Wibbenmeyer LA, Farcher LD, et al. (2004). Methamphetamine-associated burn injuries: A retrospective analysis. *J Burn Care Rehabil* 25:425–429.

Davey M. (2005, 11 June). Grisly effect of one drug: "Meth mouth." *The New York Times,* 242:A1.

Davidson C, Gow AJ, Lee TH, et al. (2001). Methamphetamine neurotoxicity: Necrotic and apoptotic mechanisms and relevance to human abuse and treatment. *Brain Res Brain Res Rev* 36(1):1–22.

Davis GG, Swalwell CI. (1994). Acute aortic dissections and ruptured berry aneurysms associated with methamphetamine abuse. *J Forensic Sci* 39:1481–1485.

Davis GG, Swalwell CI. (1996). The incidence of acute cocaine or methamphetamine intoxication in deaths due to ruptured cerebral (berry) aneurysms. *J Forensic Sci* 41(4):626–628.

Delaney P, Estes M. (1980). Intracranial hemorrhage with amphetamine abuse. *Neurology* 30(10):1125–1128.

de Man RA, Wilson JH, Tjen HS. (1993). Acute liver failure caused by methylene-dioxymethamphetamine ("ecstasy"). *Ned Tijdschr Geneeskd* 137:727–729.

Derlet RW, Horowitz BZ. (1995). Cardiotoxic drugs. *Emerg Med Clinic North Am* 13:771–779.

Derlet RW, Rice P, Horowitz BZ, et al. (1989). Amphetamine toxicity: Experience with 127 cases. *J Emerg Med* 7:157–161.

Donaldson M, Goodchild JH. (2006). Oral health of the methamphetamine abuser. *Am J Health Syst Pharm* 63(21):2078–2082.

Ebright JR, Pieper B. (2002). Skin and soft tissue infections in injection drug users. *Infec Dis Clin North Am* 16(3):697–712.

Farnsworth TL, Brugger CH, Malters P. (1997). Myocardial infarction after inhalation of methamphetamine. *Am J Health Syst Pharm* 54:586–587.

Foley RJ, Kapatkin K, Verani R, et al. (1984). Amphetamine-induced acute renal failure. *South Med J* 77:258–260.

Friedlander AH, Marder SR, Pisegna JR, et al. (2003). Alcohol abuse and dependence: Psychopathology, medical management, and dental implications. *J Am Dent Assoc* 134(6):731–740.

Furst SR, Fallon SP, Reznik GN, et al. (1990). Myocardial infarction after inhalation of methamphetamine. *N Engl J Med* 323:1147–1148.

Ginsberg MD, Hertzman M, Schmidt-Nowara WW. (1970). Amphetamine intoxication with coagulopathy, hyperthermia, and reversible renal failure: A syndrome resembling heatstroke. *Ann Intern Med* 73(1):81–85.

Glasner-Edwards S, Marinelli-Casey P, Hillhouse M, et al. (2007). *Psychiatric illness as a predictor of post-treatment methamphetamine use.* Paper presented at the 69th annual meeting of the College on Problems of Drug Dependence, Quebec City, Canada.

Gonzales R, Marinelli-Casey P, Shoptaw S, et al. (2006). Hepatitis C infection among methamphetamine-dependent individuals in outpatient treatment. *J Substance Abuse Treatment* 31(2):195–202.

Goodchild JH, Donaldson M, Mangini DJ. (2007). Methamphetamine abuse and the impact on dental health. *Dent Today* 26(5):124, 126, 128–131; quiz 131.

Gorea E, Lombard, MC. (1984). The possible participation of a dopaminergic system in mutilation behavior in rats with forelimb differentiation. *Neurosci Lett* 48:75–80.

Gospe SM Jr. (1995). Transient cortical blindness in an infant exposed to methamphetamine. *Ann Emerg Med* 26:380–382.

Haning W, Goebert D. (2007). Electrocardiographic abnormalities in methamphetamine abusers. *Addiction* 102(Suppl. 1):70–75.

Harris D, Batki SL. (2000). Stimulant psychosis: Symptom profile and acute clinical course. *Am J Addict* 9(1):28–37.

Hart CL, Ward AS, Haney M, et al. (2001). Methamphetamine self-administration by humans. *Psychopharmacology* 157(1):75–81.

He SY. (1995). Methaphetamine-induced toxicity in cultured rat cardiomyocytes. *Jpn J Legal Med* 49:175–186.

He SY, Matoba R, Fujitani N, et al. (1996). Cardiac muscle lesions associated with chronic administration of methamphetamine in rats. *Am J Forensic Med Pathol* 17:155–162.

Hendrickson RG, Cloutier R, McConnell KJ. (2008). Methamphetamine-related emergency department utilization and cost. *Acad Emerg Med* 15:23–31.

Hong R, Matsuyama E, Nur K. (1991). Cardiomyopathy associated with the smoking of crystal methamphetamine. *JAMA* 265(9):1152–1154.

Howe AM. (1995). Methamphetamine and childhood and adolescent caries. *Aust Dent J* 40(5):340.

Imanishi M, Sakai T, Nishimura A, et al. (2007). Cerebral infarction due to bacterial emboli associated with methamphetamine abuse. *No To Shinkei* 49(6):537–540.

Islam MN, Kuroki H, Hongcheng B, et al. (1995). Cardiac lesions and their reversibility after administration of methamphetamine. *Forensic Sci Int* 75(1):29–43.

Israel JA, Lee K. (2002). Amphetamine useage and genital self-mutilation. *Addiction* 97:1215–1218.

Ito Y, Jono H, Shojo H. (1997). A histopathological study of pancreatic lesions after chronic administration of methamphetamine to rats. *Kurume Med J* 44(3):209–215.

Iwanami A, Sugiyama A, Kuroki N, et al. (1994). Patients with methamphetamine psychosis admitted to a psychiatric hospital in Japan: A preliminary report. *Acta Psychiatr Scand* 89(6):428–432.

Iyo M, Sekine Y, Mori N. (2004). Neuromechanism of developing methamphetamine psychosis: A neuroimaging study. *Ann NY Acad Sci* 1025:288–295.

Jacobs LJ. (1989). Reversible dilated cardiomyopathy induced by methamphetamine. *Clin Cardiol* 12:725–727.

Johnson TD, Berenson MM. (1991). Methamphetamine-induced ischemic colitis. *J Clin Gastroenterol* 91:2523–2527.

Jones AL, Jarvie DR, McDermid G, et al. (1994). Hepatocellular damage following amphetamine intoxication. *J Toxicol Clin Toxicol* 32:435–444.

Kaku DA, Lowenstein DH. (1990). Emergence of recreational drug abuse as a major risk factor for stroke in young adults. *Ann Intern Med* 113:821–827.

Karch SB. (2002). Synthetic stimulants. In SB Karch (Ed), *Karch's pathology of drug abuse* (3rd ed., pp. 230–280). Boca Raton, FL: CRC Press.

Karch SB, Stephens BG, Ho CH. (1999). Methamphetamine-related deaths in San Francisco: Demographic, pathologic, and toxicologic profiles. *J Forensic Sci* 44(2):359–368.

Kaye S, McKetin R, Duflou J, et al. (2007). Methamphetamine and cardiovascular pathology: A review of the evidence. *Addiction* 102:1204–1211.

Kneehans S, Sziegoleit W, Krause M, et al. (1975). Clinical-pharmacological studies on the effect of mephentermine and methamphetamine on the hemodynamics of the lung circulation. *Z Gesamte Inn Med* 30(6):227–230.

Knochel JP. (1993). Mechanisms of rhabdomyolysis. *Curr Opin Rheumatol* 5(6):725–731.

Kratofil PH, Baberg HT, Dimsdale JE. (1996). Self-mutilation and severe self-injurious behavior associated with methamphetamine psychosis. *Gen Hosp Psychiatry* 18(2):117–120.

King GE, Everett HE Jr. (2005). Amphetamines and other stimulants. In JH Lowinson, P Ruiz, RB Millman, JG Langrod (Eds), *Substance abuse: A comprehensive textbook* (4th ed., pp. 277–302). Philadelphia: Lippincott Williams & Wilkins.

Kuczenski R, Segal DS. (2001). Caudate–putamen and nucleus accumbens extracellular acetylcholine response to methamphetamine binges. *Brain Res* 923:32–38.

Lan KC, Lin YF, Yu FC, et al. (1998). Clinical manifestations and prognostic features of acute methamphetamine intoxication. *J Formos Med Assoc* 97:528–533.

Lessing MP, Hyman NM. (1989). Intracranial haemorrhage caused by amphetamine abuse. *J R Soc Med* 82(12):766–767.

Lewis DM. (2005). Xerostomia: A clinical approach. *J Okla Dent Assoc* 97(2):22–25.

Logan BK, Fligner CL, Haddix T. (1998). Cause and manner of death in fatalities involving methamphetamine. *J Forensic Sci* 43(1):28–34.

Lundh H, Tunving K. (1981). An extrapyramidal choreiform syndrome caused by amphetamine addiction. *J Neurol Neurosurg Psychiatry* 44:728–730.

MacKenzie RG, Heischober B. (1997). Methamphetamine. *Pediatr Rev* 18(9):305–309.

Maeno Y, Iwasa M, Inoue H, et al. (2000a). Direct effects of methamphetamine on hypertrophy and microtubules in cultured rat ventricular myocytes. *Forensic Sci Int* 113:239–243.

Maeno Y, Iwasa M, Inoue H, et al. (2000b). Methamphetamine induces an increase in cell size and reorganization of myofibrils in cultured adult rat cardiomyocytes. *Int J Legal Med* 113:201–207.

Matoba R, Onishi S, Shimizu Y, et al. (1984). Sudden death in methamphetamine abusers: A histological study of the heart. *Jpn J Legal Med* 38:199–205.

Matoba R, Shikata I, Fujitani N. (1986). Cardiac lesions in methamphetamine abusers. *Acta Med Leg Soc* 36(1):51–55.

Mattson R, Calvery JR. (1968). Dextro-amphetamine-sulfate-induced dyskinesias. *JAMA* 204:108–110.

Maulik N, Engelman RM, Wei Z, et al. (1995). Drug-induced heat-schock preconditioning improves postischemic ventricular recovery after cardiopulmonary bypass. *Circulation* 92(9 Suppl.):II381–II388.

McGregor C, Srisurapanont M, Jittiwutikarn J, et al. (2005). The nature, time course, and severity of methamphetamine withdrawal. *Addiction* 100(9):1320–1329.

McKetin R, McLaren J, Lubman DI, et al. (2006). The prevalence of psychotic symptoms among methamphetamine users. *Addiction* 101(10):1473–1478.

Mehta H, Murray B, LoIudice TA. (1984). Hepatic dysfunction due to intravenous abuse of methylphenidate hydrochloride. *J Clin Gastroenterol* 6(2):149–151.

Mendelson J, Jones RT, Upton R, et al. (1995). Methamphetamine and ethanol interactions in humans. *Clin Pharm Ther* 57:559–568.

Meredith CW, Jaffe C, Ang-Lee K, et al. (2005). Implications of chronic methamphetamine use: A literature review. *Harv Rev Psych* 13(3):141–154.

Monterosso JR, Aron AR, Cordova X, et al. (2005). Deficits in response inhibition associated with chronic methamphetamine abuse. *Drug Alcohol Depend* 79(2):273–277.

Mooney, LJ, Glasner-Edwards S, Marinelli-Casey P, et al. (in press). Medical illness in methamphetamine-dependent patients 3 years post-treatment. *J Addiction Med.*

Mueller K, Hollingsworth E, Pettit H. (1986). Repeated pemoline produces self-injurious behavior in adult and weaning rats. *Pharmacol Biochem Behav* 25:933–938.

Murphy EL, DeVita D, Liu H, et al. (2001). Risk factors for skin and soft-tissue abscesses among injection drug users: A case-control study. *Clin Infec Dis* 33(1):35–40.

Nestor TA, Tamamoto WI, Kam TH, et al. (1989). Crystal methamphetamine-induced acute pulmonary edema: A case report. *Hawaii Med J* 48:457–460.

Newton, TF, De La Garza R 2nd, Kalechstein AD, et al. (2005). Cocaine and methamphetamine produce different patterns of subjective and cardiovascular effects. *Pharmacol Biochem Behav* 82:90–97.

Newton TF, Kalechstein AD, Duran S, et al. (2004). Methamphetamine abstinence syndrome: Preliminary findings. *Am J Addict* 13(3):248–255.

Nishida N, Ikeda N, Kudo K, et al. (2003). Sudden unexpected death of a methamphetamine abuser with cardiopulmonary abnormalities: A case report. *Med Sci Law* 43(3):267–271.

Numachi Y, Ohara A, Yamashita M, et al. (2007). Methamphetamine-induced hyperthermia and lethal toxicity: Role of the dopamine and serotonin transporters. *Eur J Pharmacol* 572(2–3):120–128.

O'Neill ME, Arnolda LF, Coles DM, et al. (1983). Acute amphetamine cardiomyopathy in a drug addict. *Clin Cardiol* 6(4):189–191.

Packe GE, Garton MJ, Jennings K. (1990). Acute myocardial infarction caused by intravenous amphetamine abuse. *Br Heart J* 64:23–24.

Pecha RE, Prindiville T, Pecha BS, et al. (1996). Association of cocaine and methamphetamine use with giant gastroduodenal ulcers. *Am J Gastroenterol* 91(12):2523–2527.

Perez JA Jr, Arsura EL, Strategos S. (1999). Methamphetamine-related stroke: Four cases. *J Emerg Med* 17(3):469–471.

Perez-Reyes M, White WR, McDonald SA, et al. (1991). Clinical effects of daily methamphetamine administration. *Clin Neuropharmacol* 14:352–358.

Pratt DS, Dubois RS. (1990). Hepatotoxicity due to pemoline (Cylert): A report of two cases. *J Pediatr Gastroenterol Nutr* 10(2):239–241.

Rhee KJ, Albertson TE, Douglas JC. (1988). Choreoathetoid disorder associated with amphetamine-like drugs. *Am J Emerg Med* 6:131–133.

Rhodus NK, Little JW. (2005). Methamphetamine abuse and "meth mouth." *Northwest Dent* 84(5):29, 31, 33–37.

Richards JR, Bretz SW, Johnson EB, et al. (1999a). Methamphetamine abuse and emergency department utilization. *Western J Med* 170(4):198–202.

Richards JR, Brofeldt BT. (2000). Patterns of tooth wear associated with methamphetamine use. *J Periodontol* 71(8):1371–1374.

Richards JR, Johnson EB, Stark RW, et al. (1999b). Methamphetamine abuse and rhabdomyolysis in the ED: A 5-year study. *Am J Emerg Med* 17(7):681–685.

Rippeth JD, Heaton RK, Carey CL, et al. (2004). Methamphetamine dependence increases risk of neuropsychological impairment in HIV-infected persons. *J Int Neuropsychol Soc* 10(1):1–14.

Robertson CH Jr, Reynolds RC, Wilson JE III. (1976). Pulmonary hypertension and foreign body granulomas in intravenous drug abusers: Documentation by cardiac catheterization and lung biopsy. *Am J Med* 61:657–664.

Rothrock JF, Rubenstein R, Lyden PD. (1988). Ischemic stroke associated with methamphetamine inhalation. *Neurology* 38(4):589–592.

Saini T, Edwards PC, Kimmes NS, et al. (2005). Etiology of xerostomia and dental caries among methamphetamine abusers. *Oral Health Prev Dent* 3(3):189–195.

Salanova V, Taubner R. (1984). Intracerebral haemorrhage and vasculitis secondary to amphetamine use. *Postgrad Med J* 60:429–430.

Santos AP, Wilson AK, Hornung CA, et al. (2005). Methamphetamine laboratory explosions: A new and emerging burn injury. *J Burn Care Rehabil* 26:228–232.

Scandling J, Spital A. (1982). Amphetamine-associated myoglobinuric renal failure. *South Med J* 75(2):63–68.

Schaiberger PH, Kennedy TC, Miller FC, et al. (1993). Pulmonary hypertension associated with long-term inhalation of "crank" methamphetamine. *Chest* 104:614–616.

Schmidt R, Glenny R, Godwin J, et al. (1991). Panlobular emphysema in young intravenous Ritalin abusers. *Am Rev Respir Dis* 143:649–656.

Scott JC, Woods SP, Matt GE, et al. (2007). Neurocognitive effects of methamphetamine: A critical review and meta-analysis. *Neuropsychol Rev* 17(3):275–297.

Shaner JW, Kimmes N, Saini T, et al. (2006). "Meth mouth": Rampant caries in methamphetamine abusers. *AIDS Patient Care and STDs* 20(3):146–150.

Shaner JW. (2002). Caries associated with methamphetamine abuse. *J Mich Dent Assoc* 84(9):42–47.

Shibata S, Mori K, Sekine I, et al. (1991). Subarachnoid and intracerebral hemorrhage associated with necrotizing angiitis due to methamphetamine abuse: An autopsy case. *Neurol Med Chir* 31(1):49–52.

Shoptaw S, Reback CJ. (2007). Methamphetamine use and infectious disease-related behaviors in men who have sex with men: Implications for interventions. *Addiction* 102(Suppl. 1):130–135.

Shoptaw S, Peck J, Reback CJ, et al. (2003). Psychiatric and substance dependence comorbidities, sexually transmitted diseases, and risk behaviors among methamphetamine-dependent gay and bisexual men seeking out-patient drug abuse treatment. *J Psychoactive Drugs* 35(Suppl. 1):161–168.

Simon SL, Dacey J, Glynn S, et al. (2004). The effect of relapse on cognition in abstinent methamphetamine abusers. *J Subst Abuse Treat* 27(1):59–66.

Simon SL, Domier C, Carnell J, et al. (2000). Cognitive impairment in individuals currently using methamphetamine. *Am J Addict* 9(3):222–231.

Smith HJ, Roche AH, Jausch MF, et al. (1976). Cardiomyopathy associated with amphetamine administration. *Am Heart J* 91:792–797.

Soetens E, Casaer S, D'Hooge R, et al. (1995). Effect of amphetamine on long-term retention of verbal material. *Psychopharmacology* 119(2):155–162.

Sommers I, Baskin D, Baskin-Sommers A. (2006). Methamphetamine use among young adults: Health and social consequences. *Addictive Behav* 31(8):1469–1476.

Sperling LS, Horowitz JL. (1994). Methamphetamine-induced choreoathetosis and rhabdomyolysis. *Ann Int Med* 121:986.

Stern EJ, Frank MS, Schmutz JF, et al. (1994). Panlobular pulmonary emphysema caused by i.v. injection of methylphenidate (Ritalin): Findings on chest radiographs and CT scans. *Am J Raoentgenol* 162(3):555–560.

Substance Abuse and Mental Health Services Administration. (2004). *Drug Abuse Warning Network, 2004. National estimates of drug-related emergency department visits* (DAWN series D-28, DHHS Publication No. [SMA] 06-4143). Rockville, MD: Department of Health and Human Services.

Swalwell CI, Davis GG. (1999). Methamphetamine as a risk factor for acute aortic dissection. *J Forensic Sci* 44:23–26.

Terada Y, Shinohara S, Matui N, et al. (1988). Amphetamine-induced myoglobinuric acute renal failure. *Jpn J Med* 27(3):305–308.

Turnipseed SD, Richards JR, Kirk JD, et al. (2003). Frequency of acute coronary syndrome in patients presenting to the emergency department with chest pain after methamphetamine use. *J Emerg Med* 24:369–373.

Ujike H, Harano M, Inada T, et al. (2003). Nine or fewer repeat alleles in VNTR polymorphism of the dopamine transporter gene is a strong risk factor for prolonged methamphetamine psychosis. *Pharmacogenomics J* 3(4):242–247.

Ujike H, Sato M. (2004). Clinical features of sensitization to methamphetamine observed in patients with methamphetamine dependence and psychosis. *Ann NY Acad Sci* 1025:279–287.

Varner KJ, Ogden BA, Delcarpio J, et al. (2002). Cardiovascular responses elicited by the "binge" administration of methamphetamine. *Pharmacol Exp Ther* 301(1):152–159.

Volkow ND, Chang L, Wang GJ, et al. (2001a). Association of dopamine transporter reduction with psychomotor impairment in methamphetamine abusers. *Am J Psychiatry* 158(3):377–382.

Volkow ND, Chang L, Wang GJ, et al. (2001b). Loss of dopamine transporters in methamphetamine abusers recovers with protracted abstinence. *J Neurosci* 21(23):9414–9418.

Volkow ND, Wang GJ, Fowler JS, et al. (2007). Stimulant-induced enhanced sexual desire as a potential contributing factor in HIV transmission. *Am J Psychiatry* 164(1):157–160.

Vongpatanasin W, Mansour Y, Chavoshan B, et al. (1999). Cocaine stimulates the human cardiovascular system via a central mechanism of action. *Circulation* 100:497–502.

Wallace TL, Gudelsky GA, Vorhees CV. (1999). Methampetamine-induced neurotoxicity alters locomotor activity, stereotypic behavior, and stimulated dopamine response in the rat. *J Neurosci* 19:9141–9148.

Wang GJ, Volkow ND, Chang L, et al. (2004). Partial recovery of brain metabolism in methamphetamine abusers after protracted abstinence. *Am J Psychiatry* 161(2):242–248.

Warner P, Connolly JP, Gibran NS, et al. (2003). The methamphetamine burn patient. *J Burn Care Rehab* 24(5):275–278.

Welder AA. (1992). A primary culture system of postnatal rat heart cells for the study of cocaine and methamphetamine toxicity. *Toxicol Lett* 60:183–196.

Westover AN, McBride S, Haley RW, (2007). Stroke in young adults who abuse amphetamines or cocaine: A population-based study of hospitalized patients. *Arch Gen Psych* 64(4):495–502.

Westover AN, Nakonezny PA, Haley RW. (2008). Acute myocardial infarction in young adults who abuse amphetamines. *Drug Alcohol Depend* 96(1–2):49–56.

Wijetunga M, Bhan R, Lindsay J, et al. (2004). Acute coronary syndrome and crystal methamphetamine use: A case series. *Hawaii Med J* 63:8–13.

Wijetunga M, Seto T, Lindsay J, et al. (2003). Crystal methamphetamine-associated cardiomyopathy: Tip of the iceburg? *J Toxicol Clini Toxicol* 41:981–986.

Willers-Russo LJ. (1999). Three fatalities involving phosphine gas, produced as a result of methamphetamine manufacturing. *J Forensic Sci* 44:647–652.

Yen DJ, Wang SJ, Ju TH, et al. (1994). Stroke associated with methamphetamine inhalation. *Eur Neurol* 34(1):16–22.

Yui K, Ikemoto S, Goto K. (2002). Factors for susceptibility to episode recurrence in spontaneous recurrence of methamphetamine psychosis. *Ann NY Acad Sci* 965:292–304.

Zweben JE, Cohen JB, Christian D, et al. (2004). Psychiatric symptoms in methamphetamine users. *Am J Addict* 13(2):181–190.

Chapter 7

Public Health Issues Surrounding Methamphetamine Dependence

Steven Shoptaw, William D. King, Evan Landstrom,
Michelle A. Bholat, Keith Heinzerling, Gregory D. Victorianne,
and John M. Roll

Use of methamphetamine (MA) at levels that meet criteria for abuse or dependence typically reflects serious behavioral disorganization in the social, occupational, and legal domains that results in clinical distress. Both acute high doses and chronic use of MA exact high tolls on the physical health of the user and of the general public. The scope of the problem is quite large. In the United States of an estimated 1.2 million adults who reported use of amphetamine-type stimulants in the previous month, 50% used MA (Substance Abuse and Mental Health Services Administration [SAMHSA], 2006). More than *five* times as many of these individuals reside in the Western United States compared with the Northeast and more than twice as many as the Southern United States. Although the absolute numbers of Americans who reported MA use in the prior month decreased 14.3% between 2002 and 2005 (the number peaked in 2003), the percent of current MA users who meet criteria for abuse or dependence has doubled and remained stable over the same period (10.6% in 2002, 15.2% in 2003, 22.5% in 2004, 20.1% in 2005). These indicators suggest that although the absolute numbers of Americans initiating MA use are not increasing nationwide, the severity of use among current users has increased significantly in the past few years.

MA abuse and its consequences have emerged as some of the most serious public health problems worldwide; its use is linked to the spread of HIV and other sexually transmitted diseases, acute and chronic psychosis, violence, and family and social disruptions. The drug is popular in many subgroups of Americans, including middle-class shift workers, men who have sex with men, women, and youth (Rawson et al., 2005). In the first year of California's Proposition 36, which mandates treatment instead of incarceration for drug-abusing offenders, more than half of those eligible for treatment (some 37,000) named MA abuse as their number-one drug problem (Longshore et al., 2005).

The literature is consistent in describing serious physical effects from chronic abuse of MA that involve many major body systems (see Mooney et al., Chapter 6 this volume). Perhaps greater than the physical effect of the drug on the body, however, regular abuse of MA corresponds with impaired impulse control, which can correspond with individuals who engage in extreme sexual behaviors that carry risks for transmission of infectious diseases. Finally, MA-associated impairments in cognition and impulse control can contribute to occurrence of personal and vehicular accidents, leading to care-seeking at emergency departments and urgent care settings. This chapter reviews the public health issues common to MA users.

Often, the consequences from MA abuse can be linked to the route of administration for the drug. MA powder can be ingested orally or by inhaling via the nostrils. MA powder or crystal can be made into a solution and injected. MA can also be inserted in the anus and absorbed via the anal mucosa. Each of these methods carry different pharmacokinetic properties. For example subjective effects of MA peak about 90 minutes after oral administration (Hart et al., 2001), which compares with about 15 minutes for peak subjective effects to be measured for intranasal, smoked, and injection administration of MA (Harris et al., 2003; Newton et al., 2005). Peak plasma levels for MA also vary according to the method of administration. Peak levels for oral administration are reached about 3 hours post ingestion, which compares with 15 minutes for levels to reach 80% of peak for smoked administration and about 2 hours to reach the peak after smoking (Cook, 1991).

A novel method of drug administration associated often associated with overdose is "parachuting." Parachuting involves wrapping MA in plastic, perforating, and then swallowing the plastic-wrapped package. This is a variant of "body stuffing," which is commonly used to transport quantities of MA by packaging and sealing the drug into finger-size plastic bags and then having the packages ingested by individuals (Hendrickson et al., 2006). In body stuffing, the packages are not perforated, but both methods of administration present exceptionally high risks for overdose.

Overdose

Overdose remains one of the most pressing medical consequences of MA abuse. Compared with other drugs, MA carries significant risks for overdose. In a cohort study of drug injectors in Vancouver, Canada, those who reported use of crystal MA were more likely to report nonfatal overdose experiences (Fairbairn et al., 2008). Toxicity from overdose due to MA is marked by hyperthermia (up to 40°C), a condition that facilitates rhabdomyolysis and multiorgan failure; neurological symptoms of coma or stroke (particularly in young patients); psychiatric symptoms of uncontrolled agitation and altered consciousness (paranoia, delusions, hallucinations); and cardiac symptoms including tachycardia, hypertension, vasoconstriction, and arrhythmias (White, 2002).

Neurobiological and Cognitive Consequences

MA accumulates at high levels in the brain following ingestion, likely due to the drug's highly lipophilic property (Fowler et al., 2007). Once MA is ingested, users experience immediate effects that include profound feelings of euphoria and well-being, sharpening of attention, and increasing levels of energy (Meredith et al., 2005). There is a growing literature that addresses specific initial (acute) and long-term (chronic) effects to neurobiology and is reviewed in greater detail in other chapters. But a general understanding of the neurological bases of MA, particularly at acute, high doses, is likely related to observed reductions in the number of dopamine transporters in striatum in humans (Volkow et al., 2001; White & Kalivas, 1998). MA use also leads to downregulation of D_2 dopamine receptors in the striatum (Chang & Haning, 2006) and areas in the nucleus accumbens and anterior cingulate cortex (Paulus et al., 2002; Leland et al., 2008). As well, there is some indication that one of the neurobiological consequences of MA abuse is changes in brain volume (Jernigan et al., 2005), a finding that is consistent with volumetric increases in laboratory animals exposed to MA. MA is toxic to 5-HT terminals in forebrain regions (Armstrong & Noguchi, 2004), which also may contribute to protracted neurobiological changes and cognitive deficits observed in MA abusers. An outstanding meta-analysis of the cognitive deficits for MA abusers compared with controls is provided by Scott and colleagues (2007). In their meta-analysis of neurocognitive outcomes from 18 studies and 951 subjects (487 with MA abuse or dependence; 464 normal controls), the effect sizes of MA on performance was in the medium-large range for tests measuring learning

(–0.66), executive functioning (–0.63), memory (–0.59), speed of information processing (–0.52), and motor skills (–0.48).

Depression

Although acute use of MA typically brightens mood, lifts fatigue, and
increases energy, a hallmark of chronic use is clinically significant levels
of depression (see Homer et al., 2008, for a review). Levels of depression associated with MA use are sufficiently severe that fully 28% of
females and 13% of males reported suicidal ideation at some point during their lifetime at entry to treatment for MA dependence (Zweben et
al., 2004). When making a differential diagnosis between the contributions of MA use to depression symptoms, the directive is to assume that
the symptoms are substance induced until some period of observation
off-drug can be made. Evidence exists to show abnormalities in brain
regions implicated in mood disorders for MA abusers undergoing initial abstinence from MA that may explain consistent linkages between
symptoms of depression with MA discontinuation (London et al., 2004).
Although depressive symptoms that accompany the presentation of MA
abuse and dependence can cause severe distress and can even be dis-
abling, a growing number of studies show a profound antidepressant
effect from sustained abstinence from MA (Jaffe et al., 2007; Peck et al.,
2005; Shoptaw et al., 2008).

Psychosis

One of the most salient psychiatric consequences to MA abuse is the
development of a paranoid-type psychotic process that can be sufficiently
severe to be clinically indistinguishable from paranoid schizophrenia.
Sources of information that describe prevalence include admission data
to emergency departments (where patients experiencing severe psychosis
symptoms present) and surveys of active users. Approximately 1.2% of
13,125 emergency department admissions to a Perth Australia tertiary
care hospital over 3 months in 2005 involved amphetamine use (Gray
et al., 2007). The most common presentation involved psychiatric problems that included MA-induced delirium and acute psychosis. Of these,
16% had prior episodes of MA-induced psychosis, as compared with
8.3% who had known diagnoses of schizophrenia. Informal estimates
of psychiatric facilities in Thailand indicate that approximately 10% of
admissions are due to MA-related psychosis (Farrell et al., 2002).

Surveys of current users of amphetamines indicate that psychosis
symptoms are common and are directly associated with extent of use

of the drug. McKetin's group (2006) recruited 309 individuals actively using amphetamines in Sydney, Australia, and reported that 13% screened positive for acute psychosis in the past year and 23% reported "clinically significant suspiciousness, unusual thought content or hallucinations, with hallucinations and suspiciousness more common than delusional thoughts." When excluding participants with schizophrenia or other psychotic disorders, prevalence of clinically significant symptoms was 18%. Moreover, participants with MA dependence were 3.1 times more likely to report significant psychosis symptoms than those who did not have MA dependence. In a sample of 180 MA-using youth in Canada, similar associations were observed between length of MA use and prevalence of auditory hallucinations (Martin et al., 2006).

Among those who experience MA-induced psychotic symptoms, resolution, although it may be incomplete, usually occurs with abstinence and increases risks for drug relapse (Ujike & Sato, 2004). Psychotic symptoms due to MA abuse generally resolve with medications used to treat schizophrenia (Leucht et al., 1999) for those seen in emergency departments and psychiatric units, including antipsychotic or benzodiazepine medications. Similarities in clinical presentation between those with MA-induced psychosis and with schizophrenia complicate understanding the underlying mechanisms regarding MA-induced psychoses: Psychotic symptoms of individuals with MA-induced psychosis may be due exclusively to heavy use of the drug, or heavy use of the drug may exacerbate an underlying vulnerability to schizophrenia. Indications of genetic links support this assumption. Relatives of MA users with a lifetime history of MA psychosis are 5 times more likely to have schizophrenia than MA users without a history of MA psychosis (Chen et al., 2005; Liu et al., 2004). Biomarkers for the two conditions are also similar. Patients with schizophrenia and with MA-induced psychosis show significantly increased peripheral plasma levels of norepinephrine (NE) than levels in MA users who do not have psychosis and non-MA-using controls (Yui et al., 1997, 2000). In both conditions, patients present for treatment with psychiatric manifestations that include hallucinations, delusions of reference, and intense suspiciousness and paranoia in the setting of clear consciousness (Dore & Sweeting, 2006; Srisurapanont et al., 2003). In MA-induced psychosis, persecutory delusions are most frequent, followed by auditory and visual hallucinations. A minority of patients experience negative symptoms (Srisurapanont et al., 2003). The similarities shared by MA-induced psychosis and schizophrenia raise questions of whether MA-induced psychosis is a unique presentation or whether MA-induced symptoms actually represent an underlying vulnerability to schizophrenia. Distinguishing between these disorders is most often determined by quick resolution of symptoms in MA-induced psychosis, which is not a likely outcome of schizophrenia (McIver et al., 2006).

Chronic MA-induced psychosis is even more enigmatic and disturbing. In Japanese reports, about "82 percent of patients with MA psychosis recover from the paranoid psychotic state within a month after withdrawal" (Sato et al., 1992, p. 118). The psychotic state recurs promptly with subsequent MA use, however, even with a small dose, suggesting an MA-induced mechanism that triggers such symptoms. Exposure to psychosocial stressors can also exacerbate the risks for relapse to MA-induced psychosis (Yui et al., 2002), in some cases without actual re-exposure to the drug.

Oral Health

The consequences to oral health from using MA can be immediately apparent, as in users suffering with "meth mouth" (see Mooney et al., Chapter 6, this volume; Shaner et al., 2006). Patients with severe cases of "meth mouth" may be candidates for dentures. The factors responsible for the extensive tooth decay and gum damage observed in some individuals who abuse MA are thought to include dry mouth (xerostomia), frequent use of sugary soft drinks, lack of oral hygiene (Shaner, 2002), and bruxism (Donaldson & Goodchild, 2006). Questions about whether exposure of the teeth and gums to the drug and/or its constituents when smoking, inhaling, or orally using the drug are the primary factors explaining dry mouth, tooth erosion, and damage to the gums are yet unanswered. Yet it does not appear that xerostomia is caused by direct effects of MA on the secretory acini (Saini et al., 2005). Instead, causes for dry mouth/xerostomia may better be attributed to a general state of dehydration frequent to MA use. It may be that the decreased rate of salivary flow contributes to the high frequency of dental caries observed in MA users, but there is as yet no strong evidence linking MA abuse and prevalence of dental caries.

Accidents/Emergency Visits

Perhaps reflecting problems in decision making, MA users are frequent consumers of emergency room visits. When they arrive to the emergency room, MA abusers are significantly more likely to arrive in an ambulance (Richards et al., 1999) or with police (Bunting et al., 2007) than are other types of patients. Presentation at the emergency room is marked by significantly higher levels of agitation, aggression, and violence than other admits (Bunting et al., 2007), and the vast majority of these patients (83.7%) have engaged two or more visits to the emergency room in the previous 12 months (Richards et al., 1999). These MA users are significantly more likely to be males, more likely to be white, less likely to be African American, and more likely to have no health insurance than non-MA-using patients (Richards et al., 1999). A variety of accidents typically are responsible for emergency room presentations, including blunt trauma (e.g., auto/truck crashes, assault, falls), altered levels of consciousness (e.g., hallucinations, delusions), abdomen pain, suicide attempt, chest pain, skin infection, penetrating trauma, miscarriage, and ingestion of MA. Among those who appear at the emergency room with abscesses or cellulitis from injection use of MA, the majority of these will insist that their condition is due to a spider bite (Richards et al., 1999).

Infectious Disease

MA is a drug that facilitates sexual transmission behaviors in both men who have sex with men (MSM; see Shoptaw et al., 2007, for a review) and in heterosexual men and women (Semple et al., 2006; Zule et al., 2007). Characteristics of the drug that facilitate high-risk sex behaviors include a long half-life (9–12 hours) as well as heightened libido (Peck et al., 2005). The impact of MA on HIV transmission is particularly acute among MSM, especially in urban areas of the United States. In this country, the burden of HIV is disproportionately borne by MSM, who account for fully 52.6% of the total cases of HIV/AIDS cases and for 68% of cases among all men. This indicates that MSM who engage in drug-associated sexual risk behaviors face substantially higher risks for encountering HIV during that episode than do heterosexual men or women (Centers for Disease Control and Prevention, 2005, p. 12). While heterosexual men and women may experience heightened libido and engage in unprotected sex as a result of MA use, their partners are unlikely to be HIV-infected unless they also have sex with MSM. Among MSM, use of MA has been shown to significantly predict HIV seroconversion in two separate studies (Drumright et al., 2006; Plankey et al., 2007). Consistent with this, HIV prevalence is exceptionally high (~60%) among MSM seeking outpatient treatment for MA dependence (Shoptaw & Reback, 2006; Shoptaw et al., 2008), but is rare among heterosexual males and females seeking outpatient treatment (Twitchell et al., 2002). In urban areas of the United States, MSM who engage high-risk sexual behaviors concomitant to MA use are more likely to risk exposure to HIV from their male partners than heterosexuals who experience similar MA-associated increases in libido and in high-risk behaviors. The mechanism underlying increased risks for HIV transmission enhanced by MA use among MSM includes potential drying of the mucosa and reducing the sensitivity of the rectal and genital areas. This can facilitate longer and rougher sexual episodes and contribute to increased likelihood of bruising and tearing in the region and to increase opportunities for transmission of infectious disease.

Among HIV-infected individuals, MA use has been shown to produce measureable neurocognitive deficits above those that can be attributed to HIV and to hepatitis C (Letendre et al., 2005). Chronic use of MA causes some MSM to experience erectile dysfunction, or "crystal dick," although sildenafil, vardenafil, or tadalafil are successfully used to counter this problem. Combining sildenafil and amyl nitrite in the presence of recreational use of MA and other club drugs has been reported to cause death (Smith & Romanelli, 2005).

MA is also associated with transmission of other infectious diseases. Among MSM, MA use significantly increases likelihood of early syphilis (Wong et al., 2005). Factors that associated significantly with syphilis infection included being of nonwhite race (odds ratio [OR] = 2.1, 95% confidence interval [CI] = 1.1–4.4), being HIV infected (OR = 3.9, 95% CI = 2.0–7.7), using MA with sildenafil (OR = 6.2, 95% CI = 2.6–14.9), using MA alone (OR = 3.2, 95% CI = 1.3–7.6), stronger gay community affiliation (OR = 2.3, 95% CI = 1.2–4.6), and having recent Internet sex partners (OR = 2.1, 95% CI = 1.0–4.3). Linkages between MA and infectious disease in this high-risk group have led some to call for including MA and other drug use in comprehensive HIV prevention plans (Shoptaw & Reback, 2006).

Social and Financial Costs

MA is a Schedule II drug with high potential for abuse and dependence (psychological and physical) and is derived from common over-the-counter (OTC) products. Primary precursors—ephedrine and pseudoephedrine—are key ingredients of such OTC drugs as Tylenol Cold and Sudafed. Researchers and law enforcement officers once considered these products to have low potential for abuse. However, the Drug Enforcement Agency (DEA) became aware of legally imported ephedrine and pseudoephedrine products to local clandestine labs. In response, federal legislative measures were implemented to help control the availability of these precursors. Key legislation includes the Domestic Chemical Diversion Control Act, which requires distributors, importers, and exports of List I chemicals to register with the DEA. This act also allows the DEA to deny or revoke a company's registration without proof of criminal intent.

Additional key federal legislation limited the availability of active precursor ingredients. In 1996 the Methamphetamine Control Act regulated access to OTC medicines containing ephedrine. In the following year another Methamphetamine Control Act regulated products containing pseudoephedrine or phenylpropanolamine with or without active ingredients over which time a slight decrease in production was observed. In July 2000 the Methamphetamine Anti-Proliferation Act established thresholds for pseudoephedrine drug products. Most recently, in 2005, the Combat Methamphetamine Epidemic Act placed limits on retail OTC sales of products containing ephedrine, pseudoephedrine, and phenylpropanolamine.

MA production was only partially affected despite these attempts by the U.S. federal government to significantly control the market. MA abuse and dependence have increased greatly in recent years, and until recently much of the MA purchased in the United States was produced locally in clandestine laboratories. A correlated increase in methamphetamine lab-related burns have been observed as a consequence of the increase in local labs, due in large part to the volatile manufacturing process. A larger proportion of individuals injured in MA lab fires suffer third-degree burns, which often result in longer hospital stays, increased frequency of complications, and increased morbidity and rehabilitation (Santos et al., 2005). Mean treatment costs per incident over $75,000, coupled with the fact that most burn-unit patients are either underinsured or uninsured, results in a significant cost burden on the community (health care providers, hospitals, and tax payers). Burn units are also faced with the challenge of patients who become violent and need assistance with detoxification, which is an added expense. With the elimination of many of the "mom-and-pop" labs, however, manufacture of MA has shifted to superlabs in countries developed in the second or third world, such as Mexico and Myanmar. With existing drug distribution networks such as mafias and gangs, disruption in the availability of MA for individuals who seek the drug has not been disrupted (United Nations Office on Drugs and Crime, 2007).

Conclusion

MA users frequently experience issues related to a range of public health problems due not only to the direct effects of the drug, but also due to indirect but potent health threats caused by behavioral disorganization from using the drug. MA-associated behavioral disorganization can lead drug users to neglect health regimens (e.g., nonadherence to medications used to treat various diseases) and can result in impulsive behaviors that carry risks for disease transmission (e.g., engaging in unprotected sexual behaviors with multiple and/or unknown sexual partners). The medical consequences outlined in this chapter provide substantial significance both for continuing to develop effective prevention strategies across the nation and to identify effective medication and behavior therapies for those affected by MA abuse and dependence.

References

Armstrong BD, Noguchi KK. (2004). The neurotoxic effects of 3,4-methylene-dioxymethamphetamine (MDMA) and methamphetamine on serotonin, dopamine, and GABA-ergic terminals: An in-vitro autoradiographic study in rats. *Neurotoxicology* 25(6):905–914.

Bunting PJ, Fulde GW, Forster SL. (2007). Comparison of crystalline meth-amphetamine ("ice") users and other patients with toxicology-related problems presenting to a hospital emergency department. *Med J Aust* 187(10):564–566.

Centers for Disease Control and Prevention. (2005). *HIV/AIDS Surveillance Report 2005*. Vol 17. Retrieved March 5, 2008, from *www.cdc.gov.hiv/surveillance/resources/reports.com.*

Chang L, Haning W. (2006). Insights from recent positron emission tomo-graphic studies of drug abuse and dependence. *Curr Opin Psychiatry* 19(3):246–252.

Chen CK, Lin SK, Pak CS, et al. (2005). Morbid risk for psychiatric disorder among the relatives of methamphetamine users with and without psycho-sis. *Am J Med Genet B: Psychiatr Genet* 136B:87–91.

Cook CE. (1991). Pyrolytic characteristics, pharmacokinetics, and bioavail-ability of smoked heroin, cocaine, phencyclidine, and methamphetamine. *NIDA Res Monogr* 115:6–23. Review. No abstract available.

Donaldson M, Goodchild JH. (2006). Oral health of the methamphetamine abuser. *Am J Health Syst Pharm* 63(21):2078–2082. Erratum in *Am J Health Syst Pharm* 63(22):2180.

Dore G, Sweeting M. (2006). Drug-induced psychosis associated with crystal-line methamphetamine. *Australas Psychiatry* 14(1):86–89.

Drumright LN, Little SJ, Strathdee SA, et al. (2006). Unprotected anal inter-course and substance use among men who have sex with men with recent HIV infection. *J Acquir Immune Defic Syndr* 43(3):344–350.

Fairbairn N, Wood E, Stoltz JA, et al. (2008). Crystal methamphetamine use associated with non-fatal overdose among a cohort of injection drug users in Vancouver. *Public Health* 122(1):70–78.

Farrell M, Marsden J, Ali R, et al. (2002). Methamphetamine: Drug use and psychoses becomes a major public health issue in the Asia Pacific region. *Addiction* 97(7):771–772.

Fowler JS, Kroll C, Ferrieri R, et al. (2007). PET studies of *d*-methamphetamine pharmacokinetics in primates: Comparison with *l*-methamphetamine and cocaine. *J Nucl Med* 48(10):1724–1732.

Gray SD, Fatovich DM, McCoubrie DL, et al. (2007). Amphetamine-related presentations to an inner-city tertiary emergency department: A prospective evaluation. *Med J Aust* 186:336–339.

Harris DS, Boxenbaum H, Everhart ET, et al. (2003). The bioavailability of intranasal and smoked methamphetamine. *Clin Pharmacol Ther* 74(5):475–486.

Hart CL, Ward AS, Haney M, et al. (2001). Methamphetamine self-administration by humans. *Psychopharmacology* 157(1):75–81.

Hendrickson RG, Horowitz BZ, Norton RL, et al. (2006). "Parachuting" meth: A novel delivery method for methamphetamine and delayed-onset toxicity from "body stuffing." *Clin Toxicol* 44(4):379–382.

Homer BD, Solomon TM, Moeller RW, et al. (2008). Methamphetamine abuse and impairment of social functioning: A review of the underlying neurophysiological causes and behavioral implications. *Psychol Bull* 134(2):301–310.

Jaffe A, Shoptaw S, Stein J, et al. (2007). Depression ratings, reported sexual risk behaviors, and methamphetamine use: Latent growth curve models of positive change among gay and bisexual men in an outpatient treatment program. *Exp Clin Psychopharmacol* 15(3):301–307.

Jernigan TL, Gamst AC, Archibald SL, et al. (2005). Effects of methamphetamine dependence and HIV infection on cerebral morphology. *Am J Psychiatry* 162(8):1461–1472. Erratum in *Am J Psychiatry* 162(9):1774.

Leland DS, Arce E, Miller DA, et al. (2008). Anterior cingulate cortex and benefit of predictive cueing on response inhibition in stimulant dependent individuals. *Biol Psychiatry* 63(2):184–190.

Letendre SL, Cherner M, Ellis RJ, et al. (2005). The effects of hepatitis C, HIV, and methamphetamine dependence on neuropsychological performance: Biological correlates of disease. *AIDS* 19(Suppl. 3):S72–S78.

Leucht S, Pitschel-Walz G, Abraham D, et al. (1999). Efficacy and extrapyramidal side effects of the new antipsychotics olanzapine, quetiapine, risperidone, and sertindole compared to conventional antipsychotics and placebo: A meta-analysis of randomized controlled trials. *Schizophr Res* 35(1):51–68.

Liu HC, Lin SK, Liu SK, et al. (2004). DAT polymorphism and diverse clinical manifestations in methamphetamine abusers. *Psychiatr Genet* 14(1):33–37.

London ED, Simon SL, Berman SM, et al. (2004). Mood disturbances and regional cerebral metabolic abnormalities in recently abstinent methamphetamine abusers. *Arch Gen Psychiatry* 61:73–84.

Longshore D, Annon J, Anglin MD, et al. (2005). Levo-alpha-acetylmethadol

(LAAM) versus methadone: Treatment retention and opiate use. *Addiction* 100(8):1131–1139.

Martin I, Lampinen TM, McGhee D. (2006). Methamphetamine use among marginalized youth in British Columbia. *Can J Public Health* 97(4):320–324.

McIver C, McGregor C, Baigent M, et al. (2006). *Guidelines for the medical management of patients with methamphetamine-induced psychosis.* Canberra, Australia: Drug and Alcohol Services.

McKetin R, McLaren J, Lubman DI, et al. (2006). The prevalence of psychotic symptoms among methamphetamine users. *Addiction* 101(10):1473–1478.

Meredith CW, Jaffe C, Ang-Lee K, et al. (2005). Implications of chronic methamphetamine use: A literature review. *Harv Rev Psychiatry* 13(3):141–154.

Newton TF, De La Garza R, 2nd, Fong T, et al. (2005). A comprehensive assessment of the safety of intravenous methamphetamine administration during treatment with selegiline. *Pharmacol Biochem Behav* 82(4):704–711.

Paulus MP, Hozack NE, Zauscher BE, et al. (2002). Behavioral and functional neuroimaging evidence for prefrontal dysfunction in methamphetamine-dependent subjects. *Neuropsychopharmacology* 26(1):53–63.

Peck JA, Shoptaw S, Rotheram-Fuller E, et al. (2005). HIV-associated medical, behavioral, and psychiatric characteristics of treatment-seeking, methamphetamine-dependent men who have sex with men. *J Addict Dis* 24(3):115–132.

Plankey MW, Ostrow DG, Stall R, et al. (2007). The relationship between methamphetamine and popper use and risk of HIV seroconversion in the multicenter AIDS cohort study. *J Acquir Immune Defic Syndr* 45(1):85–92.

Rawson RA, Gonzales R, Obert JL, et al. (2005). Methamphetamine use among treatment-seeking adolescents in Southern California: Participant characteristics and treatment response. *J Subst Abuse Treat* 29(2):67–74.

Richards JR, Bretz SW, Johnson EB, et al. (1999). Methamphetamine abuse and emergency department utilization. *West J Med* 170(4):198–202.

Saini T, Edwards PC, Kimmes NS, et al. (2005). Etiology of xerostomia and dental caries among methamphetamine abusers. *Oral Health Prev Dent* 3(3):189–195.

Santos AP, Wilson AK, Hornung CA, et al. (2005). Methamphetamine laboratory explosions: A new and emerging burn injury. *J Burn Care Rehabil* 26(3):228–232.

Sato M, Numachi Y, Hamamura T. (1992). Relapse of paranoid psychotic state in methamphetamine model of schizophrenia. *Schizophr Bull* 18(1):115–122.

Scott JC, Woods SP, Matt GE, et al. (2007). Neurocognitive effects of methamphetamine: A critical review and meta-analysis. *Neuropsychol Rev*17(3):275–297.

Semple SJ, Grant I, Patterson TL. (2006). Perceived behavior of others and AIDS risk behavior among heterosexually identified methamphetamine users. *J Psychoactive Drugs* (Suppl. 3):405–413.

Shaner JW. (2002). Caries associated with methamphetamine abuse. *J Mich Dent Assoc* 84(9):42–47.

Shaner JW, Kimmes N, Saini T, et al. (2006). "Meth mouth": Rampant caries in methamphetamine abusers. *AIDS Patient Care STDS* 20(3):146–150.

Shoptaw S, Reback CJ. (2007). Methamphetamine use and infectious disease-related behaviors in men who have sex with men: Implications for interventions. *Addiction* 102(Suppl. 1):130–135.

Shoptaw S, Reback CJ. (2006). Associations between methamphetamine use and HIV among men who have sex with men: A model for guiding public policy. *J Urban Health* 83(6):1151–1157.

Shoptaw S, Reback CJ, Larkins S, et al. (2008). Outcomes using two tailored behavioral treatments for substance abuse in urban gay and bisexual men. *J Subst Abuse Treat* 35(3):285–293.

Smith KM, Romanelli F. (2005). Recreational use and misuse of phosphodiesterase 5 inhibitors. *J Am Pharm Assoc* 45(1):63–72; quiz 73–75.

Srisurapanont M, Ali R, Marsden J, et al. (2003). Psychotic symptoms in methamphetamine psychotic inpatients. *Int J Neuropsychopharmacol* 6(4):347–352.

Substance Abuse and Mental Health Services Administration. (2006). *National Survey on Drug Use & Health*. Retrieved March 5, 2008, from *www.oas.samhsa.gov/nsduhLatest.htm*.

Twitchell G, Huber A, Reback C, et al. (2002). Comparison of general and detailed HIV risk assessments among methamphetamine abusers. *AIDS and Behavior* 6(2):153–162.

Ujike H, Sato M. (2004). Clinical features of sensitization to methamphetamine observed in patients with methamphetamine dependence and psychosis. *Ann NY Acad Sci*1025:279–287.

United Nations Office on Drugs and Crime. (2007). *World Drug Report*. Retrieved March 5, 2008, from *www.unodc.un.or.th/publications/default.htm*.

Volkow ND, Chang L, Wang GJ, et al. (2001). Low level of brain dopamine D_2 receptors in methamphetamine abusers: Association with metabolism in the orbitofrontal cortex. *Am J Psychiatry* 158(12):2015–2021.

White SR. (2007). Amphetamine toxicity. *Semin Respir Crit Care Med*23(1):27–36.

White FJ, Kalivas PW. (1998). Neuroadaptations involved in amphetamine and cocaine addiction. *Drug Alcohol Depend* 51(1–2):141–153.

Wong W, Chaw JK, Kent CK, et al. (2005). Risk factors for early syphilis among gay and bisexual men seen in an STD clinic: San Francisco, 2002–2003. *Sex Transm Dis* 32(7):458–463.

Yui K, Ishiguro T, Goto K, et al. (1997). Precipitating factors in spontaneous recurrence of methamphetamine psychosis. *Psychopharmacology* 134(3):303–308.

Yui K, Ikemoto S, Goto K. (2002). Factors for susceptibility to episode recurrence in spontaneous recurrence of methamphetamine psychosis. *Ann NY Acad Sci* 965:292–304.

Yui K, Ishiguro T, Goto K, et al. (2000). Susceptibility to subsequent episodes in spontaneous recurrence of methamphetamine psychosis. *Ann NY Acad Sci* 914:292–302.

Zule WA, Costenbader EC, Meyer WJ, Jr, et al. (2007). Methamphetamine use and risky sexual behaviors during heterosexual encounters. *Sex Transm Dis* 34(9):689–694.

Zweben JE, Cohen JB, Christian D, et al. (2004). Methamphetamine treatment project: Psychiatric symptoms in methamphetamine users. *Am J Addict* 13(2):181–190.

Chapter 8

Methamphetamine and Crime

David Farabee and Angela Hawken

According to the National Drug Intelligence Center Drug Threat Survey, 40% of state and local law enforcement agencies now consider methamphetamine (MA) to pose the greatest drug threat in their areas, surpassing cocaine/crack (36%), and well above marijuana (12%) and heroin (9%). About one third of these agencies identify MA as the drug that contributes most to the commission of property and/or violent crimes (National Drug Intelligence Center [NDIC], 2005). But what is the actual relationship between MA and crime? Can we be sure that the former causes the latter? And, if so, will treatment-induced reductions in MA use result in commensurate declines in criminality?

Such questions are not unique to MA. Indeed, they reflect long-standing controversies in the broader literature concerning drug use and criminal behavior. Over the most recent decade, however, some important strides have been made toward defining the relationship between MA and crime with greater precision. In this chapter we summarize this growing literature, describe current treatment and intervention approaches for MA-dependent offenders, and identify a set of unanswered questions that we believe should be priorities for future research in this area.

Review of the Literature

Because the association between drug use and crime is complex, Goldstein's conceptual framework for the various types of drug–crime relationships deserves some discussion here (Goldstein, 1985). Although originally proposed to explain the relationships between drug use, the drug trade, and violence, this framework can be applied more generally to include property offenses as well. Goldstein argues that drug use can be associated with other forms of criminality because of economic–compulsive, pharmacological, and systemic models of use and/or distribution. These are briefly summarized below:

- *Economic–compulsive model.* This model suggests that some drug users resort to criminal behavior to support their drug use. This category includes property crimes to obtain money for drugs, selling drugs to support one's habit, or having sex with someone in exchange for drugs or money for drugs.
- *Pharmacological model.* According to the pharmacological model, some drug users engage in irrational or violent behavior as a result of the acute and/or chronic psychological or physiological effects of a drug. For example, certain offenders might use, or threaten to use, violence because they are intoxicated and are not aware of what they are doing; in some cases, an offender might use drugs or alcohol expressly to reduce the fear of danger prior to engaging in a criminal act.
- *Systemic model.* This model holds that a large share of drug-related crime is the result of illegal drug trafficking and sales. This class of crime ranges from selling drugs to using violence, or the threat of violence, to protect a drug operation.

Empirical research provides strong support for these three models of the drug–crime relationship. In an analysis of survey data collected from youths entering the Texas Youth Commission, Fredlund et al. (1995) demonstrated the applicability of all three of these models, with 41% of substance-dependent offenders reporting crimes attributable to the economic–compulsive model, 40% to the pharmacological model, and 60% to the systemic model. Thus there is some indication that certain types of substance-using offenders actively engage in crimes directly related to their substance use while, for others, substance use and crime appear to coexist somewhat independently.

Below, using Goldstein's categorization of the various routes of influence of drug use on criminal behavior, we provide a summary of the MA literature as it relates to crime.

Economic–Compulsive Model

To link MA with crime from the perspective of the economic–compulsive model, it must first be established that (1) for many users, the cost of acquiring the drug using licit income is prohibitive, and (2) the typical patterns of MA use occur at a relatively high frequency. Indeed, prior analyses of these variables in offender populations have shown substantial variation. For example, using data from the Arrestee Drug Abuse Monitoring program, Golub and Johnson (2004) found that, among arrestees in New York City (in 2000–2002), median drug expense in the past 30 days varied widely with frequency of use and drug-user type. Infrequent marijuana-only users spent as little as $5, while daily marijuana-only users spent about $600. Arrestees who used both heroin and cocaine spent over $1,000 (data regarding MA use were not available at the time of the study).

With regard to the first criterion, available data on typical MA users indicate that the majority are in their 20s or 30s, have at least a high school education, and are employed (either full- or part-time; National Institute of Justice, 2006). Consequently, many MA users are likely to be able to support their habits without resorting to income-generating crime.

Assessing the cost criterion is more complex. Because a single "hit" of MA produces a substantially longer-lasting high than a single dose of cocaine, it is possible that this further reduces the strength of the MA–crime relationship attributable to the economic–compulsive model. Indeed, Rawson et al. (2000) found that, among patients receiving treatment for stimulant dependence, MA users reported spending less than cocaine users to maintain their habits. On the other hand, current market changes suggest that the rather ironic benefit of MA's low cost and high purity may be short lived. During the first 6 months of 2007, the average price per gram of pure MA purchased in the United States increased 37%, from $141.72 to $194.25, while purity fell 24%, from 57% to 43% (Drug Enforcement Administration, 2007). Consequently, as MA use expands to less-affluent sectors of society and prices increase while the duration of the effect decreases, the economic–compulsive link between MA and crime may grow stronger.

Pharmacological Model

As indicated above, some drug users engage in violent behavior because of the physiological effects of a drug. Drug-induced psychosis occurs more commonly with amphetamine/MA abusers than among abusers of other stimulants such as cocaine probably because MA has a longer half-life than other stimulants do (Kosten & Singha, 1999). For instance, smoking MA produces a high that lasts 8–24 hours, compared with 20–30 minutes for smoking cocaine (National Institute on Drug Abuse, 1998). Although psychosis does not necessarily lead to acts of violence, some clinical studies have supported the hypothesis that MA increases the likelihood of attack behaviors and aggression in humans (Pihl & Hoaken, 1997; Reiss & Roth, 1993), leading to the concern that public safety may be threatened by high-level MA users whose irritability and paranoia may prompt a violent reaction when they are in contact with others, especially medical or law enforcement personnel (Dillon et al., 2000).

In another study of MA users admitted to treatment in Los Angeles, nearly two thirds of the participants cited violent behavior as an outcome of their usage (von Mayrhauser et al., 2002). Wright and Klee (2001) found that nearly half of their MA-using subjects reported being involved in violent crime, and 24% reported that their involvement in violent crime was a direct result of their MA use. Another study, specific to MA use in five western cities, found that one third of MA-using arrestees cited violent behavior as a consequence of their use. Moreover, MA-using arrestees were more likely to have been arrested and incarcerated previously than their non-MA-using peers (Pennell et al., 1999).

Although MA users' attributions of the causes of their behaviors may not be entirely accurate, a study conducted by Sokolov et al. (2004) suggests that the relationship between chronic MA use and violence may, indeed, be causal. These investigators compared certain fighting behaviors (number of initiated bite attacks and latency before attacks) between mice that had received a single injection of MA (6 mg/kg) versus chronic injections (over 8 weeks). The authors found that the single injection did not increase fighting, but chronic injections were associated with increased attacks and decreased latencies.

Systemic Model

The relationship between MA and drug-trade-related ("systemic") crimes has changed considerably over the past decade. Although production of MA is a relatively simple process, crackdowns on domestic production have led to a surge in the number—and size—of MA production laboratories outside the United States, especially in Mexico, where criminal organizations are able to acquire large quantities of pseudoephedrine and ephedrine from China and other countries (NDIC, 2005).

MA production and trafficking have been demonstrated to be strongly associated with violent behavior and have forced local law enforcement agencies in jurisdictions with high levels of MA production to establish task forces specifically trained to interdict the production and distribution of the drug and cope with the associated violence (National Drug Intelligence Center, 2001).

Cartier et al. (2006) examined data from 641 state prison parolees in California to examine the associations between MA use and three measures of criminal behavior: (1) self-reported violent criminal behavior, (2) return to prison for a violent offense, and (3) return to prison for any reason during the first 12 months of parole. The purpose of the study was to test the hypothesis that, *even after controlling for drug-trade involvement* (i.e., sales, distribution, manufacturing), MA use would predict violent crime and recidivism among adult male parolees during their first 12 months of parole. They found that drug-trade involvement was statistically significant across all outcomes. That is, self-reported drugs sales, distribution, and manufacturing predicted self-reported violent crime, general recidivism, and recidivism for a violent offense. This finding is important because it suggests that involvement in drug-trade activities has a stable relationship with violence. However, after controlling for drug-trade involvement, MA use was still significantly predictive of self-reported violent crime and general recidivism.

Many of the studies described here suffer from one of the chief difficulties in linking substance use to criminal behavior. Fewer than half of all crimes are ever reported to the police (Levitt, 1998), and even lower rates of reporting have been found for violent victimization (Conaway & Lohr, 1994) and sexual assault (Kilpatrick et al., 1987). As a result, studies that operationalize criminal behavior outcomes in terms of arrest or conviction records require enormous sample sizes in order to overcome the error inherent in their dependent measures.

Relation to Treatment

To date, there is little evidence in the correctional treatment literature that treatment interventions are being developed or modified to meet the needs of the growing number of MA abusers. Nor, for that matter, is it clear whether new or modified programs will prove necessary.[1] In this section we describe the most prominent treatment approaches for drug-involved criminal justice populations, which reflect the treatments offered to MA users as well. They are therapeutic communities, contingency management, cognitive behavioral therapy, and drug court and other diversion models.

---

[1]In a study comparing treatment performance of cocaine and MA users in a community-based outpatient treatment program, Rawson et al. (2000) found that treatment responses of the two groups were similar.

Therapeutic Communities

Among prison-based substance abuse treatment programs, the most commonly evaluated is the therapeutic community (TC). The TC philosophy holds that substance abuse is not the main cause of the offender's problems. Rather, it is a symptom of a larger problem: the disorder of the whole person. Thus the goal of a TC is to "habilitate" clients in a holistic fashion, emphasizing personal responsibility. Rather than attempting to change offenders through counselor-led, didactic presentations, TCs rely primarily on the residents themselves to effect change on the individual. After reviewing 11 evaluations of prison-based TCs, Phipps et al. (1999) reported that two of the TC programs showed clear evidence of an effect, three showed some evidence of an effect, three showed no effect, and three were inconclusive. However, the reviewers recommended caution in interpreting this literature because the individual studies varied considerably in terms of their quality and conclusions.

Our review of the literature for this chapter revealed no controlled studies of the impact of TCs on MA users specifically. One noteworthy effort at the Southwest Illinois Correctional Center (SWICC) to adapt the traditional prison-based TC model to meet the needs of MA users does merit describing here—although it should be pointed out that this modified program has not yet been evaluated. Operated by CiviGenics, the SWICC Meth Program has made the following modifications to better suit the needs of MA-dependent clients:

- Smaller "informational bites" than would be used in normal treatment program presentations because of the reduced attention span of MA addicts in early recovery.
- Supplementation of presentations with the use of visual aids to further engage this population.
- A delivery style based on simplified, clear, and concrete concepts and examples.
- Program materials that focus on the use of "role play" from early on to further engage the MA addicts in the treatment process, to keep them focused, and to provide a means for them to relate the information conveyed to their personal experience.
- The use of structured exercise and relaxation techniques to offset the higher levels of anxiety often experienced by MA addicts in early recovery.
- Greater emphasis on the issue of sexual practices and a "safer sex plan."
- Intensive focus on anger management and violence reduction.

Although outcomes from the SWICC Meth Program are not yet available, these modifications serve as an example of how curricula and settings of existing treatment modalities might be adapted to overcome the cognitive and other behavioral challenges common among MA-dependent offenders, should future research indicate that such tailoring is necessary.

Contingency Management

Contingency management (CM) has strong support in the research literature, particularly with regard to its impact on substance use while the contingencies are in place (Lussier et al., 2006; Roll et al., 2006). Our review of the literature revealed only one experimental test of CM on substance-abusing offenders (the majority of whom reported MA as their primary drug). In this study Prendergast et al. (2007) randomly assigned drug court clients to one of four conditions: (1) standard treatment, (2) earned vouchers for negative drug tests, (3) earned vouchers for completing treatment plan activities (e.g., photocopies of completed job applications), and (4) a combined group in which clients could earn vouchers for either clean drug tests or completing treatment plan activities. In contrast to the consistently positive findings for CM among other populations of substance abusers, Prendergast and his colleagues found no statistically significant differences among the four study conditions. The researchers concluded that the influence of the judge eclipsed the impact of the relatively low-value vouchers awarded to reinforce drug abstinence and treatment plan compliance.

Outside of the criminal justice system, however, CM has been repeatedly shown to produce among the largest effect sizes found in the substance abuse treatment literature (Prendergast et al., 2006). Consequently, the dearth of studies specifically testing the impact of CM on substance-abusing offenders should not be construed as suggesting that this would not be an effective approach; rather, it is the result of the difficulty in mounting such studies in correctional environments (due to logistics and philosophical resistance). The development of an expanded set of nonmonetary incentives that carry sufficient valence to shape offenders' behaviors will be critical to overcoming some of these barriers.

Cognitive-Behavioral Therapy

Over the past 15 years, cognitive-behavioral therapy (CBT) has grown in popularity as a means to address a range of behavioral problems, including substance abuse. CBT is based on the theory that self-destructive thinking styles are learned and, therefore, can be unlearned or restructured. Although our review of the literature did not reveal any large-scale meta-analyses addressing the specific impact of CBT on drug use, a number of meta-analyses have shown that CBT/criminal thinking programs for offenders are associated with significant reductions in recidivism. Pearson and colleagues (2002) conducted a meta-analysis of 69 primary research studies on the effectiveness of a heterogeneous set of psychosocial treatments for offenders and found that the overall effect size was primarily due to the cognitive-behavioral interventions such as reasoning and rehabilitation. A separate systematic review of 14 cognitive-behavioral evaluations conducted by Lipsey et al. (2001) found a weighted mean recidivism rate of .26 for participants in CBT, compared with .38 for controls. Unfortunately, drug use outcomes were not reported, although recidivism may serve as a proxy for relapse.

Drug Court

Drug courts were established in the late 1980s in response to tougher drug laws and the resulting rise in drug-related caseloads. These programs capitalize on the courts' authority to reduce crime by providing close judicial monitoring combined with sanctions for drug use or treatment noncompliance. Defendants can choose to be diverted to drug court programs in exchange for the possibility of expunged records, dismissed charges, or reduced sentences.

As described by Rawson et al. (2002), drug courts are based upon the swift and certain application of sanctions and rewards based on the behavior of the drug user. Drug court clients who comply with their treatment plan and goals (e.g., treatment attendance and clean urinalyses) can earn their way to progressively less demanding treatment requirements and ultimately to removal of legal sanctions. Those who fail to comply are required to move to more intensive levels of care or are subject to periods of incarceration. The combination of the MA user's ambivalence and drug court judges' decrees appear to have a tremendous potential for synergy (Burdon et al., 2001).

One of the most rigorous reviews of drug courts was conducted by the U.S. Government Accountability Office (GAO, 2005). The GAO based their analysis on a subset (n = 23) of the most rigorous program evaluations available at the time. Among their conclusions were (1) participation in a drug court was associated with reduced recidivism, (2) the observed recidivism reductions occurred for participants who had committed a range of different offenses, and (3) it was unclear which of the two basic components of the drug court model—judicial monitoring versus the treatment received—accounted for more of the variance in outcomes. Evidence regarding the effectiveness of drug court programs on drug use was limited to a smaller subset (n = 8) of program evaluations. Evaluations of these eight drug court programs reported mixed results on substance use relapse.

To date, there is little information available regarding the impact of drug court treatment on MA users specifically. Marinelli-Casey et al. (2008) compared outcomes of a group of 57 MA-dependent patients receiving outpatient treatment under drug court supervision with a group of comparable MA-dependent patients (n = 230) receiving similar outpatient drug treatment but without drug court supervision. Patients in the drug-court-supervised group were more likely than the non-drug-court participants to remain in treatment for at least 30 days (80% vs. 57%) and complete treatment (56% vs. 32%), and less likely to report using MA at discharge, as well as at the 6- and 12-month follow-ups.

Other Community Supervision Models

Two important tests of community supervision models involving primarily MA-dependent offenders are under way: California's treatment in lieu of incarceration initiative (Proposition 36), and Hawaii's swift and certain sanctions program (HOPE).

California's Proposition 36 Initiative

In November 2000, California voters approved the Substance Abuse and Crime Prevention Act of 2000, also known as "Proposition 36." This act allowed adults convicted of nonviolent drug possession offenses the option of participating in drug treatment in the community in lieu of incarceration or probation without treatment.

Arizona was the first state to implement drug policy reform to provide treatment in lieu of incarceration with the passage of the Drug Medicalization, Prevention, and Control Act of 1996 (Proposition 200), but the enormous scale of California's initiative was unprecedented. Proposition 36 provided the option of treatment to many habitual drug users who had never participated in treatment before (more than half of the Proposition 36 participants had no prior treatment history). More than 54,000 offenders are referred to the program each year, and more than half report MA as their primary drug (Urada & Longshore, 2007).

Although there was evidence that Proposition 36 clients were more likely to be rearrested for a drug crime than other criminal-justice-referred treatment participants (Farabee et al., 2004) or similar pre-Proposition 36 offenders (Urada et al., 2007), the statewide evaluation of Proposition 36 showed substantial savings to the state ($2.50 was saved for every $1 invested in the program), primarily owing to reduced prison costs (Hawken et al., 2007). But one of the most important findings to emerge from these evaluations was the apparent interaction effect between addiction severity and treatment intensity. Residential treatment beds in California are scarce, and inappropriate treatment matching has affected the treatment and criminal justice outcomes of the program (Hawken & Anglin, 2007). Across the primary drugs, the underutilization of residential treatment was of greatest consequence for primary MA users. Heavy-user Proposition 36 participants who reported MA as their primary drug and who were given a residential placement had significantly higher treatment completion rates (and therefore compliance with the terms of their Proposition 36 probation) and significantly lower arrest and conviction rates than similar participants who were placed into outpatient care.

Another important finding from this large initiative concerns the role of criminal justice sanctions. Twenty-five percent of offenders who accept the Proposition 36 bargain never appear for treatment, and of those who do enter treatment, only about one third complete it (Urada & Longshore, 2007). Even California treatment providers have expressed frustration with the lack of clients' compliance with the terms of Proposition 36 treatment and the limited ability of the criminal justice system to intervene (Hawken & Poe, 2008). Indeed, there is growing evidence that the application of swift and cetain graduated sanctions might lead to improved outcomes in drug use and crime. Some of the most compelling evidence comes from Hawaii's HOPE program.

HOPE Probation

Hawaii Opportunity Probation with Enforcement (HOPE) was implemented as a pilot program in 2004, the brainchild of Judge Steven S. Alm of the Honolulu First Circuit, who had grown frustrated with inept probation supervision, particularly in the management of MA abusers. Honolulu's probation officers were overwhelmed with high caseloads (often over 180:1), were struggling to manage their workloads, and had limited ability to detect and respond to violations. These difficulties led to long delays in responses to probation violations and high rates of noncompliance. The typical noncompliant offender accumulated a long list of violations before action was taken. The judge was convinced that the long delay between the probationers' violations and the response was key to the failed management of his primarily MA-using caseload; it fostered noncompliance and, ultimately, high rates of probation revocation.

HOPE was the product of Alm's effort to design a probation program based on theories of behavior modification. The swift and certain sanctions model that resulted was designed to reinforce a strong and immediate relationship between probationers' actions and their consequences, sending consistent messages to probationers about personal responsibility and accountability. HOPE probationers are brought to court for a formal-warning hearing and given clear instructions on the content and implications of the rules of the probation program. Offenders who violate any of the terms of probation are immediately arrested and brought before a judge (typically the same day, but always within 48 hours). *Every* violation of probation terms is met with a sanction, but a key feature of the program is *parsimonious* use of punishment. HOPE offenders are sentenced to very brief jail stays (typically only a few days) for each violation of the terms of their probation, but the program sanctions are progressive in that continued violations result in increasingly stringent responses.

Sentencing judges who employ the HOPE model maintain close relationships with local drug treatment providers. But whereas treatment diversion programs typically mandate treatment for all participants (as is the case with Proposition 36), the HOPE model relies on regular drug-testing results as a signal for treatment need. This "behavioral triage model" economizes on treatment resources, because offenders who are able to remain drug free on their own are not required to enter a treatment program, allowing for more intensive service provision for those who need help.

Preliminary data on outcomes under HOPE are extremely promising. Data gathered by the Hawaii Attorney General's Office show impressive reductions in no-show rates (down 88% for probationers who had 12 months of HOPE exposure compared with their own pre-HOPE performance) and in positive tests for illicit drug use (down 90%). The data also show evidence of a HOPE "dose" effect. That is, although impressive improvements were found with short-term exposure, reductions in no-shows and positive urines were greater for those offenders with longer exposure to HOPE. These results contrast with those for a comparison group of similar offenders not assigned to the HOPE program, for which no-show rates and positive urine analyses were significantly higher in the short term and became progressively worse over time. Stark differences were also found for recidivism. Arrest and conviction rates for HOPE participants over a 1-year follow-up period were 66% lower than for the comparison group. In response to these positive findings, the Hawaii legislature increased funding for the HOPE program. The program has been adopted by all of the 10 First Circuit Court judges and has expanded to include 1,200 offenders.

HOPE provides evidence that re-engineering the probation-enforcement process can yield good results in terms of compliance with all types of probation conditions, including abstaining from drug use, among even strongly drug-involved MA users.

Conclusion

Most of the lingering questions concerning the association of MA use and crime are similar to those concerning the drug–crime nexus generally. Although we have summarized evidence in this chapter that suggests certain causal influences of MA use on other forms of criminal behavior—particularly with regard to the pharmacological and systemic pathways—it is difficult to rule out the possibility that, for many offenders, MA use may simply be another facet of a criminal lifestyle. In fact, some criminologists view excessive alcohol use, illicit drug use, and engagement in risky sexual practices as "analogous behaviors" that often co-occur with other criminal behavior as a result of reduced self-control and the absence of certain environmental controls (Gottfredson & Hirschi, 1990). Unfortunately, arguments advanced for either of these perspectives (or variations thereof) are difficult to test experimentally.

On a much brighter note, regarding the unanswered questions regarding the effectiveness of various treatments designed to reduce MA use among offenders, the vetting process could be much more systematic. Although it is virtually impossible to rule out all but one of the competing theories of the causes of MA (and other drug) dependence and crime, it is within our power to assess whether an *intervention* designed to address one of these presumed causes actually produces the intended results. The gold standard for measuring the efficacy of an intervention is the randomized controlled trial (RCT). Our review of the literature revealed no experimental studies of MA treatment in criminal justice settings. If, in fact, the MA–crime links described earlier in this chapter are causal, the need to employ RCTs to identify effective interventions for this population cannot be overstated.

The final unanswered question we propose relates to MA specifically. As indicated earlier in this chapter, the fact that a single dose of MA produces a much longer-lasting high than a single dose of cocaine, it is possible that the economic–compulsive impact of MA use may be relatively low. However, in light of recent evidence that MA prices are surging while purity is declining, it is possible that the causal role of MA use on crime via the economic–compulsive link will strengthen. This potential growth in MA-related crime assumes, among other factors, that current pricing and purity trends continue. If so, this is a trend that bears watching.

References

Burdon W, Prendergast M, Roll J, et al. (2001). The role of contingency management in drug courts. *J Drug Iss* 31:73–90.

Cartier J, Farabee D, Prendergast ML. (2006). Methamphetamine use, violence, and recidivism among California parolees. *J Interpers Violence* 21:435–445.

Conaway MR, Lohr SL. (1994). A longitudinal analysis of factors associated with reporting violent crimes to the police. *J Quant Criminol* 10(1):23–39.

Dillon H, Fritz L, Blanton L, et al. (2000). *A look at methamphetamine use among three populations* (Department of Health and Human Services Publication No. (SMA) 00-3423). Rockville.

Drug Enforcement Administration. (2007). *Methamphetamine price/purity analysis of STRIDE data.* Retrieved June 3, 2008, from *www.usdoj.gov/dea/concern/meth_prices_purity.html.*

Farabee D, Hser YH, Anglin MD, et al. (2004). Recidivism among an early cohort of California's Proposition 36 offenders. *Criminol Public Policy* 3(4):501–522.

Fredlund EV, Farabee D, Blair LA, et al. (1995). *Substance use and delinquency among youths entering Texas Youth Commission Facilities: 1994.* Austin, TX: Texas Commission on Alcohol and Drug Abuse.

Goldstein PJ. (1985). The drugs/violence nexus: A tripartite conceptual framework. *J Drug Iss* 15:493–506.

Golub A, Johnson BD. (2004). How much do Manhattan arrestees spend on drugs? *Drug Alcohol Depend* 3(7):235–246.

Gottfredson M, Hirshci T. (1990). *A general theory of crime.* Palo Alto, CA: Stanford University Press.

Government Accountability Office. (2005). *Adult drug courts: Evidence indicates recidivism reductions and mixed results for other outcomes* (Report No. GAO 05-219). Washington, DC: Author.

Hawken A, Anglin D. (2007). Treatment differences. In *Evaluation of the Substance Abuse and Crime Prevention Act: Final report* (pp. 81–93). Sacramento: California Department of Alcohol and Drug Programs.

Hawken A, Longshore D, Urada D, et al. (2007). SACPA benefit–cost analysis. In *Evaluation of the Substance Abuse and Crime Prevention Act: Final report* (pp. 94–125). Sacramento: California Department of Alcohol and Drug Programs.

Hawken A, Poe A. (2008). Testing and sanctions for Proposition 3L probation violations. In *Evaluation of the Substance Abuse and Crime Prevention Act: 2007 Final report* (pp. 185–200). Sacramento: California Department of Alcohol and Drug Programs.

Kilpatrick DG, Saunders BE, Veronen LJ, et al. (1987) Criminal victimization: Lifetime prevalence, reporting to police, and psychological impact. *Crime Del* 33(4):479–489.

Kosten TR, Singha AK. (1999). Stimulants. In M Galanter, HD Kleber (Eds), *Textbook of substance abuse treatment* (2nd ed, pp. 183–193). Washington, DC: American Psychiatric Press.

Levitt SD. (1998). The relationship between crime reporting and police: Implications for the use of uniform crime reports. *J Quant Criminol* 14(1):1573–7799.

Lipsey MW, Chapman GL, Landenberger NA. (2001). Cognitive-behavioral programs for offenders. *Ann Amer Acad Pol Soc Sci* 578:144–157.

Lussier JP, Heil SH, Mongeon JA, et al. (2006). A meta-analysis of voucher-based reinforcement therapy for substance use disorders. *Addiction* 101:192–203.

Marinelli-Casey P, Gonzales R, Hillhouse M, et al. (2008). Drug court treatment for methamphetamine dependence: Treatment response and post-treatment outcomes. *J Subst Abuse Treat* 34(2):242–248.

National Drug Intelligence Center. (2001). *National Drug Threat Assessment, 2001.* Washington, DC: U.S. Department of Justice.

National Drug Intelligence Center. (2005). *Methamphetamine drug threat assessment.* Washington, DC: U.S. Department of Justice.

National Institute of Justice. (2006). *Methamphetamine abuse: Challenges for law enforcement.* Washington, DC: U.S. Department of Justice.

National Institute on Drug Abuse. (1999). Methamphetamine abuse alert. *NIDA Notes* 13(6).

Pearson FS, Lipton DS, Cleland CM, et al. (2002). The effects of behavioral/cognitive-behavioral programs on recidivism. *Crime Del* 48(3):476–496.

Pennell S, Ellett J, Rienick C, et al. (1999). *Meth matters: Report on methamphetamine users in five western cities.* Washington, DC: U.S. Department of Justice.

Phipps P, Korinek K, Aos S, et al. (1999). *Research findings on adult corrections programs: A review.* Olympia: Washington State Institute for Public Policy.

Pihl RO, Hoaken P. (1997). Clinical correlates and predictors of violence in patients with substance use disorders. *Psychiatric Ann* 27(11):735–740.

Prendergast ML, Hall EH, Roll J, et al. (2007). Use of vouchers to reinforce abstinence and positive behaviors among clients in a drug court treatment program. *J Subst Abuse Treat* 35(2):125–136.

Prendergast ML, Podus D, Finney J, et al. (2006). Contingency management in the treatment of substance abuse disorders: A meta-analysis. *Addiction* 101:1546–1560.

Rawson R, Anglin MD, Ling W. (2002). Will the methamphetamine problem go away? *J Addict Dis* 21(1):5–19.

Rawson R, Huber A, Brethen P, et al. (2000). Methamphetamine and cocaine users: Differences in characteristics and treatment retention. *J Psych Drugs* 32(2):233–238.

Reiss A, Roth J. (Eds). (1993). *Understanding and preventing violence.* Washington, DC: National Academy Press.

Roll JM, Petry NM, Stitzer ML, et al. (2006). Contingency management for the treatment of methamphetamine use disorders. *Am J Psychiatry* 163:1993–1999.

Sokolov BP, Schindler CW, Cadet JL. (2004). Chronic methamphetamine increases fighting in mice. *Pharmacol Biochem Behav* 77:319–326.

Urada D, Longshore D. (2007). SACPA offenders. In *Evaluation of the Substance Abuse and Crime Prevention Act: Final report* (pp. 12–32). Sacramento: California Department of Alcohol and Drug Programs.

Urada D, Longshore D, Hawken A. (2007). Re-offending. In *Evaluation of the Substance Abuse and Crime Prevention Act: Final report* (pp. 57–67). Sacramento: California Department of Alcohol and Drug Programs.

von Mayrhauser C, Brecht M, Anglin MD. (2002). Use ecology and drug use motivation of methamphetamine users admitted to substance abuse treatment facilities in Los Angeles: an emerging profile. *J Addict Dis* 21(1):45–60.

Wright S, Klee H. (2001). Violent crime, aggression and amphetamine: What are the implications for drug treatment services? *Drugs: Ed Prev Policy* 8(1):73–89.

Chapter 9

Effects of Methamphetamine on Communities

Linda J. Thompson, Sharon Sowell, and John M. Roll

It is well documented that manufacturers and users of methamphetamine (MA) place themselves at physical, psychosocial, socioeconomic, and legal risk, and efforts focusing on these hazards are ongoing. It is also imperative to focus on the effects of MA on a larger scale, as increased MA use and manufacture in recent years has profoundly affected communities. The two objectives of this chapter are (1) to integrate recent literature on MA-related community-level costs and (2) to provide an in-depth case report on how community members in Spokane, Washington, have united and persevered to lessen the burdens that MA has inflicted on their community. The rationale of the case report is to elucidate some potentially overlooked scenarios that arise when communities are threatened by MA use and production and to provide a heightened understanding of the challenges and opportunities for other at-risk communities.

Who Is Affected by MA at the Community Level?

MA impacts communities in multiple ways, often affecting those who have no intentional contact with it and those whose professions involve keeping it at bay. In various ways, MA use and production diminishes the quality of life of children, property owners and renters, emergency responders, health and child care providers, retailers, and government employees. Just as children cannot control their parents' behaviors or the environment in which they reside, property owners or renters cannot be certain that their home's walls and carpeting have not previously been saturated with hazardous chemicals. When emergency responders (e.g., law enforcement, firefighters, paramedics) rush to emergency scenes, they often have little forewarning of the environment they are stepping into—the noxious fumes, booby traps (Mecham & Melini, 2002), explosive chemicals, and/or potentially paranoid and violent MA users (Maxwell, 2005; Rawson et al., 2002). According to data collected through the Hazardous Substances Emergency Events Surveillance system, which described "acute hazardous substance-releasing events" in 16 states over a 4-year period (2000–2004), emergency responders comprised 60% of all individuals who required decontamination after being exposed to MA toxins (Centers for Disease Control and Prevention [CDC], 2005). If not properly decontaminated, others who come into contact with them are also at risk. Those threatened by secondary contamination include health care providers (McFadden et al., 2006; Sheridan et al., 2006), child welfare providers, foster care caseworkers, and perhaps even schoolteachers, acquaintances, and unrelated passersby.

MA affects far more than just the physical health of community members; it also imposes an economic burden on the community. The theft of MA precursors (the ingredients commonly used to manufacture the drug) has been a substantial problem for community members who regularly have them in their possession (e.g., retailers, farmers, ranchers, veterinarians). Government programs, such as foster care agencies and Child Protective Services, are challenged by the influx of neglected and abused children entering the systems because of their parents' involvement with MA. On a different but equally disconcerting note, MA endangers communities by fueling the spread of infectious diseases, some of which may be treatment resistant. Finally, each person in a community is affected by the MA problem when he or she pays taxes to provide funding for MA-related issues.

As the large-scale impact of MA has become more apparent in recent years, community leaders have come together to regain a sense of safety and security. The next section identifies several subpopulations of communities that are affected by MA and examples of the problems it has caused them.

Drug-Endangered Children and the Adults Who Protect Them

Children's small bodies and developing minds make them especially vulnerable to physical, emotional, and sexual maltreatment (Mecham & Melini, 2002; Connell-Carrick, 2007). They reside in roughly one third of all MA manufacture sites (National Drug Intelligence Center, 2002) and are often maltreated, neglected, and physically/sexually abused (Altshuler, 2005; Connell-Carrick, 2007; Ostler et al., 2007) by parents whose criminal activities are not conducive to positive parenting. The younger a child is, the more time he or she likely spends at home and, consequently, the more likely it is that he or she will be exposed to the direct and indirect consequences of MA (Mecham & Melini, 2002). Some MA-endangered children seen at Primary Children's Medical Center Emergency Department (Salt Lake City, UT) experienced toxicological symptoms ranging from agitation and hyperactivity to seizures (Mecham & Melini, 2002). Emotional and behavioral problems are commonly reported in this population of children; for this reason, classroom and foster home situations can be difficult (Ostler et al., 2007). Other individuals whose professions involve helping these children, such as foster care and child welfare providers, place themselves at significant risk when inadvertently making home visits to volatile manufacturing sites (Connell-Carrick, 2007). In short, MA use and manufacture affects not only its users, but also their children and the community members who help care for their children.

Renters/Homeowners

While it is reasonable to assume that renters/homeowners should not have to worry about their homes being contaminated with MA, unfortunately this is not the case. Therefore, various states have passed legislation establishing the maximum amount of residual MA that can remain in homes or apartments following decontamination. In general, the maximum allowable MA residual ranges from 0.1 to 0.5 mg MA per 100 cm^2. The state of Colorado set the maximum post-cleanup MA residue level at the less stringent level (i.e., 0.5 mg/100 cm^2) after researchers found that the health risks associated at 0.1 and 0.5 mg residual MA per 100 cm^2 (both extremes of the range) are qualitatively the same (Hammon & Griffon, 2007). This is noteworthy because decontamination of a three-bedroom home at the 0.1 mg/100 cm^2 level costs $45,000 more than at the 0.5 mg/100 cm^2 level, while failing to significantly minimize the associated health risks (Hammon & Griffon, 2007). MA decontamination statutes have also been created in some states to rid renters/homeowners of the responsibility of decontaminating their homes (Krause, 2008). At the federal level, the Methamphetamine Remediation Act of 2007 (H.R. 365) requires the Environmental Protection Agency to work on establishing guidelines to ensure that former MA manufacture sites are "safe and livable"; it also funds research that investigates how best to clean such sites and a longitudinal study to better understand the longer term effects of secondary MA exposure (Govtract.us, 2007).

Trauma and Burn Centers, Hospitals, and Health Care Workers

MA-related accidents, injuries, and emergency room visits take a significant financial toll on hospitals, trauma centers, and burn centers throughout the nation. Over a 10-year period from 1992 to 2002, MA-related emergency admissions increased 420% (Gettig et al., 2006).

In 1995 the level I trauma center of Scripps Mercy Hospital, San Diego, California, spent almost $1,500,000 on MA-related accidents—a 70% increase from 2002 (Swanson et al., 2007). Upon further investigation, MA-related injuries were found to cost an average of 9% more to treat than non-MA-related injuries (Swanson et al., 2007). In Portland, Oregon, MA-related emergency room visits cost one hospital an estimated $6.9 million each year (Hendrickson et al., 2008). Because fires and explosions are not unusual during MA production, burn centers frequently serve MA manufacturers as well. MA-related burns cost Vanderbilt University Burn Center $5 million to $10 million each year. As can be expected, such high costs pose significant burdens for hospitals (Bersch, 2005).

The physical and emotional suffering associated with MA can be severe. The causes of MA-related injuries treated in Scripps Mercy Hospital trauma I center were found to be much more violent in nature (i.e., assault, gunshot, and stab wounds) than non-MA injuries (Swanson et al., 2007). As many as 90% of MA-related psychiatric emergency visits require hospitalization (Szuster, 1990). Amphetamine-related crises are 35% more likely to result in hospitalization than those related to cocaine (Leamon et al., 2002).

Law Enforcement and Emergency Responders

It is understandable that police officers and other emergency responders might feel ill prepared to handle this unpredictable and often violent population (Sekine et al., 2006, Szuster, 1990). MA users in Scripps Mercy Hospital level I trauma center were much more likely to have had previous altercations with law enforcement officials than non-MA users (Swanson et al., 2007). In one study, 43% of the patients who received emergency care for MA-related reasons had a history of outward aggression (Szuster, 1990).

In addition to being at risk of assault, law enforcement and emergency responders jeopardize their health by being exposed to toxic chemicals and fumes when entering MA manufacturing sites (CDC, 2005). About 70% of law enforcement agents have indicated that they have developed an array of physical symptoms after exposure to MA laboratories, including headache, sore throat, rapid heartbeat, chest pain or tightness, and respiratory, skin, eye, central nervous system, and gastro-intestinal symptoms. Those who have been exposed to more than 30 MA manufacturing sites tend to experience far more severe symptoms than those who have been exposed to fewer than 30 MA manufacturing sites; nonetheless, even those with very little exposure to toxins also report a variety of symptoms, which last from an hour to months after exposure (Witter et al., 2008). Secondary contamination is even a possibility for those in close proximity to individuals who have been directly exposed. One social worker sought medical care after giving her client, whose clothes were saturated with fumes, a ride in her car (Bersch, 2005).

Other Community Members

As previously mentioned, there is a risk that individuals who are going about their day-to-day business might be exposed to mishandled, flammable precursors of MA or its toxic byproducts. Although this some-times occurs through secondary contamination (e.g., the social worker mentioned above), it also takes place because MA can be produced almost anywhere—in cars, vans, apartments, motel rooms, and so on (Mecham & Melini, 2002). Many of these manufacturing sites are in, or very close to, public settings, placing community members at risk. Furthermore, 5 to 7 pounds of toxic waste are produced along with each pound of MA (Mecham & Melini, 2002). The byproducts contaminate the environment (e.g., soil, water supplies, farmland) and are often carelessly dis-carded in places where community members might encounter them (e.g., on the side of the road; Sexton et al., 2006; Connell-Carrick, 2007).

Agricultural communities are particularly affected by the theft and mishandling of anhydrous ammonia, a corrosive fertilizer commonly used in the manufacturing of MA. When untrained individuals attempt to steal the volatile chemical from high-pressure steel containers where it is stored, explosions resulting in injury or death have been known to occur (Bloom et al., 2007). In Kentucky, a number of anhydrous ammo-nia thefts resulted in explosions that required nearby residential and business properties to be evacuated (Sexton et al., 2006).

Case Study: Spokane, Washington

Washington State

In 2001 a statewide group of community leaders met to discuss the increasing presence of MA in their communities. Representatives from King, Pierce, and Spokane counties lobbied Washington's legislative del-egation in an effort to obtain funding necessary to help lessen their com-munities' MA-related burdens. MA crimes were depleting the resources of law enforcement agencies as manufacturing sites spread rampantly throughout the state. Financial support was needed to augment both the treatment and prevention of MA abuse and dependency, as well as to provide for drug-endangered children. Ongoing collaboration between county officials and members of the U.S. Congress led Washington to become one of the first states in the nation to receive federal funding to combat MA. Development of the Washington State Methamphetamine Initiative provided community leaders the capacity and motivation to more effectively battle the drug that was spreading throughout their communities.

In 2001 community representatives from the 15 counties in Washington with the highest concentration of reported MA laboratories were invited to Bellevue for the Washington State Methamphetamine Summit. Each county independently assembled a Methamphetamine Action Team, which focused on developing a community-tailored strategy to lessen the impact of MA in its region. The following community members were included in each team's initial meeting: the county's sheriff, a Community Mobilization Against Substance Abuse coordinator, a county prosecutor, a treatment provider, a health district representative (responsible for MA manufacturing site cleanup), and a K–12 educator.

Representatives from Spokane County were invited to the summit and awarded a $15,000 grant. In an attempt to provide a specific illustrative example, the remaining portion of this chapter will focus on Spokane as a case study on the effects of MA at the community level.

Spokane Methamphetamine Action Team Meetings

At each regularly scheduled meeting, individuals representing diverse sectors of the community collectively provided one another with a keen awareness of their ongoing burdens related to MA. Law enforcement officers (i.e., detectives from the Spokane County Sheriff's Office, Spokane Police Department, and Washington State Patrol) expressed the need for MA-specific policing strategies, one official stating that "[MA had been] the only drug that really united [them] in the fight against substance abuse." They underscored the crucial role of community partnerships in their undertaking. Spokane firefighters, dealing with hazardous byproducts of and decontamination processes linked to MA, were concerned about being repeatedly exposed to such toxic environments (and potential chemical reactions). MA also posed a problem to members of Spokane's housing authority, as MA manufacturing sites often contaminated their properties. Making matters worse, renters were frequently fleeing MA manufacturing dump sites without paying rent. Landlords who participated in the Methamphetamine Action Team meetings offered newsletters and tenant meetings as a means of public education.

Initially, members of the justice system (i.e., county prosecutors and the representative of Washington's Attorney General) informed the group that there were 2,000 backlogged MA-related cases in the county because caseworkers were struggling and often unable to close users' initial cases before repeat cases were filed. The Methamphetamine Action Team responded to this burden by obtaining funding that successfully increased the caseworkers' resources and diminished the backlog. The State Attorney General's office representative was assigned to assist in termination of MA-involved parents' rights. Later, during the second year of the initiative, a Family Treatment Court was established and served to help parents complete substance rehabilitation, which led to many families' reestablishing cohesiveness. City council members worked directly with members of Congress and state legislators to elaborate on pressing issues. Foster care providers (including Child Protective Services) were strained with the increasing numbers of drug-endangered children rescued from manufacturing sites.

Members of the business community (e.g., retailers) told of financial difficulties that stemmed from the large-scale theft of MA precursors (i.e., ephedrine) from their stores. Educators (from the K–12 system) in several districts disclosed stories of hungry and disheveled children who smelled of chemicals. They wanted to find ways to help these children and were also curious about how other children in the classroom were being affected. Chemical dependency treatment providers shared history, data, and navigation tools for treatment availability in the community. Professors from surrounding universities informed the team about MA addiction and treatment options; in addition, the Director of Government Relations for Consumer Health Products educated the group about potential technological advances in the area of substance abuse. Finally, those personally touched by MA (e.g., family members and friends) often attended the meetings, both to seek help for their loved ones and to advocate for others who found themselves in similar situations. Although family members often minimized the importance of their contribution to the team, the insight they provided was often invaluable.

Spokane's community issues were similar to those in many other communities; they felt that the MA epidemic was (1) compromising their safety, (2) taking the freedom or lives of far too many community members, and (3) straining community businesses (e.g., store owners), nonprofits (e.g., foster care), and law enforcement/emergency care providers.

Examples of Typical Meeting Topics and Discussions

Finding Clothes for Children Who Lived at MA Sites

The decontamination of MA manufacturing sites required firefighters to remove and dispose of everything within the location—even the inhabitants' clothing. The firefighters were disconcerted because they had no choice but to clothe young drug-endangered children in their adult-size jumpsuits. When this issue was raised in a meeting, a Child Protective Services worker offered them a large number of backpacks filled with clothes, toys, and necessities for children of all ages and sizes, which were stored in their offices. The outcome of this interagency connection demonstrated that some ongoing problems may have relatively simple solutions.

Training for Local and State Law Enforcement

Community-oriented policing efforts were developed and found to be instrumental in preparing officers for MA-related incidences. The sheriff's Community-Oriented Policing Effort, community-oriented policing stations, and the Neighborhood Watch Program each provided large numbers of volunteers who served as conduits for neighborhood trainings. Resources were shared to provide regional training for all area officers.

Spokane Methamphetamine Action Team Goals

The group established two main goals: (1) to reduce MA manufacture and sales in Spokane County, and (2) to reduce MA use in Spokane County.

The Methamphetamine Action Team strove to achieve the first goal by reducing the availability of MA precursors through legislative acts[1] and community awareness. Common ingredients used to manufacture MA include the following: anhydrous ammonia (a fertilizer), ether (an automotive starting fluid), hydrochloric acid (an industrial acid), iodine

---

[1] Laws limiting the availability of precursors were enacted as early as the 1980s (Gettig et al., 2006). The bulk sales of the powder forms of pseudoephedrine and ephedrine were regulated in 1988 (Chemical Diversion and Trafficking Act). Between 1995 and 1997, the distribution of marketed products containing ephedrine (Domestic Chemical Diversion and Control Act), pseudoephedrine, and phenylpropanolamine also became more closely scrutinized (Comprehensive Methamphetamine Control Act). Penalties for manufacturing or selling any of these products increased during this time. In 2000 federal legislation limited the amount of pseudoephedrine that an individual could purchase over the counter, raised penalties for MA-related crimes once again, enhanced law enforcement, and intensified preventative and treatment efforts (Methamphetamine Antiproliferation Act of 2000). In 2005 pseudoephedrine-containing products were deemed Schedule V controlled substances (Combat Meth Bill), meaning that they must be kept behind the counter and thus more strictly monitored (Gettig et al., 2006).

Iowa was one of the first states to limit the availability of the precursors to MA. In doing so, the number of MA-related incidents and burns was drastically reduced. Retailers' sales of over-the-counter cold products actually increased, rather than the opposite, because shoplifting was not as prevalent (Burke, 2008).

(an over-the-counter extract), lithium (found in batteries), methanol (antifreeze), petroleum distillate (fuel), pseudoephedrine (in over-the-counter cold medications), red phosphorous (plates on matchbox strikers), sodium chloride (table salt), and sodium hydroxide (drain cleaner; McFadden et al., 2006). Clearly, many of these components of MA are not difficult to obtain.

Spokane decided to focus its efforts on limiting the accessibility of ephedrine, iodine, gasoline additives, and anhydrous ammonia. The team's policy makers successfully advocated for legislation that restricted the amount of ephedrine products consumers could purchase. In 2002 the Spokane Methamphetamine Action Team initiated the Washington State METH WATCH, a replication of a model previously implemented in Kansas. Collaboration between local retailers, the initiative's Methamphetamine Technical Assistance Team, and a Spokane County Precurser Detective, as well as funding through a High-Intensity Drug Trafficking Area grant allowed the program to come to fruition. Members of the Washington State METH WATCH used a variety of program materials (e.g., window decals, retailer report forms, training materials, and informational packets) to recruit other retailers to join them in their efforts to share information, report suspicious sales, and provide their employees with MA awareness. Retailers were enthusiastic that shoplifting of ephedrine products in their stores had decreased; consequently, their enthusiasm boosted the campaign's success as they encouraged other retailers to adopt the program as well.

The training team helped implement the Washington State METH WATCH program in counties statewide. Veterinarians, automotive-parts store owners, and those in the ranching/farming community became involved. Educational talks about the potential uses of anhydrous ammonia were conducted at events (e.g., Spokane's Northwest Agriculture Show), and signage was manufactured to reinforce the campaign's message. With continued collaboration between the Spokane Methamphetamine Action Team and METH WATCH retailers, the number of reported MA manufacturing sites began to decrease.

The team's second goal was addressed by focusing on improving educational resources for youth and other at-risk individuals, equipping them with information about the risks and consequences of MA prior to their first exposure to the substance. Spokane's public information campaign aimed to provide resources to help answer the many questions that surfaced from various sectors of the community. Team representatives spoke at speakers bureaus that covered requests across the county, from school groups to rotary clubs.

A major accomplishment of Spokane's Methamphetamine Action Team was the development of the Spokane County Methamphetamine

Family Treatment Court. As one of three such courts in the state, the Family Treatment Court provided care (e.g., resources, supportive programs, and MA treatment) to users and their children. Although only a limited number of families qualified for these treatment services, the impact on those families who did take advantage of the court was monumental. Upon completion of the program, all but one of the families were reunited with their children. The Methamphetamine Action Team also made progress toward its second goal by collaborating with the Spokane Addiction Recovery Center and the Greater Spokane Substance Abuse Council's Community Coalition in an effort to reduce the stigma of MA treatment and promote recovery.

Discrepancies among Methamphetamine Action Team Members' Stances on MA-Related Issues

Guidelines for Rescuing Children from Drug-Related Environments

Spokane County established a Drug-Endangered Children program, which provided the community with guidelines for rescuing children from situations in which they might be affected by drugs. The broad definition of such situations included conditions in which alcohol had led to abuse of the child, neglect was evident by the lack of care by a substance-using parent, or when a MA manufacturing site was discovered. Although most Drug-Endangered Children programs had only included MA as the drug that necessitated intervention (i.e., when to "rescue" a child), Spokane successfully persuaded other counties throughout the state to reconsider their definition of a hazardous environment and include all illicit drugs in the category. Spokane's role in changing such a widely used definition reflects the positive influence that dedicated communities can have on their community and society on a much larger scale.

Following Protocols or Guidelines

Across the state, colleagues differed in opinion concerning procedures for assisting children found in substance-involved environments. The documents generated to describe appropriate courses of action in situations involving drug-endangered children were initially known as "protocols"; however, legal experts of the Spokane Methamphetamine Action Team argued that, semantically, the use of the word "protocol" could potentially lead to problems. The word's legal definition entails the exact implementation of the protocol and would not allow modifications based on situational needs. Although mandated protocols may work in counties with abundant resources, small rural counties often do not have the financial or other resources necessary to comply with state protocols at every level (e.g., urine/drug testing). In addition, if "protocols" are violated in any way, cases could be lost in the court system due to procedural error. For these reasons, Spokane's team members suggested to state leaders that the word "guideline" may be a more appropriate descriptor than "protocol." At first, their proposed modification was deemed unnecessary; however, the distinction was eventually recognized and the semantic transition was made.

Varying Ideas on Efficacy of MA Treatment

Many community leaders believed that treatment for MA abuse and dependence is futile. It was crucial for Spokane treatment provider partners to provide education and awareness to other community and team members to bolster their confidence regarding the efficacy of MA treatment. To do so, a public education forum was organized. At the forum, national experts in the area described successful treatment modalities and research suggesting that reaching and maintaining recovery is possible for individuals addicted to MA. Spokane team members gained confidence by being well informed about the research on the treatment of addiction. During the forum, topics such as the importance of using appropriate scientific methodology and data analysis were discussed, because having some understanding of these areas would be necessary before accurately advocating for such an expensive community program. This type of leadership from academics provided guidance and motivation to the Spokane Methamphetamine Action Team, helping them make well-informed recommendations.

Conclusion

In summary, drug-endangered children, foster care workers, child protective agencies, renters, homeowners, health care workers, retail store owners, veterinarians, farmers, ranchers, law enforcement officers, and emergency responders are among the groups of individuals within communities who are unintentionally exposed to the hazards associated with MA use and manufacture. While members of many of these groups, in Spokane and elsewhere, certainly have diverse pursuits and priorities, they have demonstrated a common drive to shield one another and the greater public from the threat of MA. Obtaining funding to achieve this goal has been an ongoing challenge; however, community members continue to collaborate across agencies to find viable solutions to this problem. Reflection on their efforts emphasizes the importance of both community connectedness and dynamic policies that address different needs (e.g., prevention, law enforcement, treatment) at different stages in the MA crisis (Caulkins, 2007). Understanding their particular objectives, struggles, and achievements can be useful in guiding other communities that are facing similar challenges.

References

Altshuler SJ. (2005). Drug-endangered children need a collaborative community response. *Child Welfare* 84(2):171–190.

Bersch C. (2005). From the editor: What a meth. *Medical Laboratory Observer* 37(11):4.

Bloom GR, Suhail F, Hopkins-Price P, et al. (2007). Acute anhydrous ammonia injury from accidents during illicit methamphetamine production. *J Int Soc Burn Inj* 34:713–718.

Burke BA, Lewis RW, Latenser BA, et al. (2008). Pseudoephedrine legislation decreases methamphetamine laboratory-related burns. *J Burn Care Res* 1:138–140.

Caulkins JP. (2007). Editorial: The need for dynamic drug policy. *Addiction* 102:4–7.

Centers for Disease Control and Prevention (CDC). (2005). Acute public health consequences of methamphetamine laboratories—16 states, Jan 2000–June 2004. *Morb Mort Weekly Rep* 356–359.

Connell-Carrick K. (2007). Methamphetamine and the changing face of child welfare: Practice principles for child welfare workers. *Child Welfare* 86(3):125–144.

Gettig JP, Grady SE, Nowosadzka I. (2006). Methamphetamine: Putting the brakes on speed. *J School Nursing* 22(2):66–73.

GovTrack.us. (2007). *Methamphetamine Remediation Research Act of 2007* (H.R. 365). Retrieved June 25, 2008, from *www.govtrack.us/congress/bill.xpd?bill=h110–365&tab=summary.*

Hammon TL, Griffin S. (2007). Support for selection of a methamphetamine cleanup standard in Colorado. *Reg Toxicol Pharmacol* 48:102–114.

Krause EI. (2006). Comment: Take my property please! Who should bear the burden of cleaning up toxic methamphetamine lab waste? *Catholic Univ Law Rev* 56(1):187–226.

Leamon MH, Gibson DR, Canning RD, et al. (2002). Hospitalization of patients with cocaine and amphetamine use disorders from a psychiatric emergency service. *Psychiatric Serv* 53(11):1461–1466.

Maxwell J. (2005). *Implications of research for treatment: Methamphetamine.* Austin, TX: Gulf Coast Addicton Technology Transfer Center, U.T. Center for Social Work Research.

McFadden D, Kub J, Fitzgerald S. (2006). Occupational health hazards to first responders from clandestine methamphetamine labs. *J Addict Nursing* 17:169–173.

Mecham N, Melini J. (2002). Unintentional victims: Development of a protocol for the care of children exposed to chemicals at methamphetamine laboratories. *Pediatric Emerg Care* 18(4):327–332.

National Drug Intelligence Center. (2002). *Children at risk* (2002-LO424-001). Johnstown, PA: U.S. Department of Justice.

Ostler T, Haight W, Black J, et al. (2007). Case series: Mental health needs and perspectives or rural children reared by parents who abuse methamphetamine. *J Am Acad Child Adol Psychiatry* 46(4):500–507.

Rawson R, Gonzales R, Brethen P. (2002). Treatment of methamphetamine use disorders: An update. *J Subst Abuse Treat* 23:145–150.

Sekine Y, Ouchi Y, Takei N, et al. (2006). Brain serotonin transporter density in abstinent methamphetamine users. *Arch Gen Psychiatry* 63(1):90–100.

Sexton RL, Carlson RG, Leukefeld CG, et al. (2006). Patterns of illicit methamphetamine production ("cooking") and associated risks in the rural South: An ethnographic exploration. *J Drug Iss* 36:853–876.

Sheridan J, Bennett S, Coggan C, et al. (2006). Injury associated with methamphetamine use: A review of the literature. *Harm Red J* 3:14.

Siegal HA, Faick RS, Wang J, et al. (2006). Emergency department utilization by crack-cocaine smokers in Dayton, Ohio. *Am J Drug Alcohol Abuse* 32:55–68.

Swanson SM, Sack MJ, Holbrook GM, et al. (2007). The scourge of methamphetamine: Impact on a level I trauma center. *J Trauma* 63(3):531–537.

Szuster RR. (1990). Methamphetamine in psychiatric emergencies. *Hawaii Med J* 49:389–391.

Witter RZ, Martyny JW, Mueller K, et al. (2008). Symptoms experienced by law enforcement personnel during methamphetamine lab investigations. *J Occ Env Hygiene* 4:895–902.

Chapter 10

Psychosocial and Behavioral Treatment of Methamphetamine Dependence

Steven Shoptaw, Richard A. Rawson, Matthew Worley, Sarah Lefkowith, and John M. Roll

Although the search for medications is ongoing, there are currently no medications approved for the treatment of methamphetamine (MA) dependence. There are, however, a range of behavioral and psychosocial treatments that are effective in helping individuals to quit using MA (achieve abstinence) and to return to abstinence should lapse or relapse occur (relapse prevention). This chapter opens with a discussion of the clinical presentation of MA abuse and dependence and reviews the evidence regarding the efficacy of these treatments. We close with a proposed algorithm by which clinicians can help individuals meet their goals of ceasing MA use and achieving abstinence.

What Is MA Abuse and Dependence?

Case Example

José is a 37-year-old Hispanic male who appears in your office seeking help for his MA problem. He initially started using MA about 10 years ago to have the energy to work 12-hour days in the construction business and to complete his increasing load of household responsibilities to his wife and three (now teenage) children. He uses about a quarter of a gram daily. He started using by snorting MA, but now smokes it because the drug was irritating his nose and causing frequent nosebleeds. José's use of MA has been consistent for some time. His first use of the day is right after he prepares for work (about 5:15 A.M.) and a second use occurs during lunchtime. José tells you that when he first started using MA, he would get high, which helped him deal with the stresses of a demanding job and having a young and growing family, but he hasn't gotten euphoric from his drug use for as long as he can remember. On the other hand, if he misses a day of drug use, he immediately experiences withdrawal and becomes irritable and sleepy. He's seeking treatment now because the financial and physical costs of maintaining his consistent use of MA are too great. His employer, who runs a religious-based workplace, learned of José's MA use by catching him smoking the glass pipe during lunch. José will have to submit to random drug screening to keep his job, and his employer is working with him to get his problem under control. His wife knows little of the extent of José's drug use, and there is no way the family will be able to sustain the loss of his income. José tells you he is seeking treatment now so that he "can get his life back" and that he's tired of facing the daily risks of obtaining and using the drug just to finish his daily responsibilities. He knows the first days without MA will be difficult to hide from his employer and his family, and he's wondering what advice you might have to help him initiate and sustain abstinence.

Definitional Issues Regarding MA Dependence

Individuals with MA abuse and dependence often present for treatment with complex, interrelated problems. For this and other reasons, it can be important to consider relevant definitional issues before adopting a treatment approach. Moreover, the clinician's understanding of the disorder is crucial to guiding selection of the specific treatment approach. José's case demonstrates multiple ways that MA dependence threatens his and his family's well-being and illustrates the multiple points at which a clinician might intervene. Moreover, José expresses distress about his situation, which contributes to the immediacy of the need for treatment. But the question of what exactly is being "treated" is left unanswered. Is José's MA dependence truly a disease? Some would hold that José's problem is not a disease, but instead a seemingly unending series of poor choices. The concept of "disease" can be defined as

> an impairment, interruption, disorder, or cessation of the normal state of the living body or of any of its components that interrupts or modifies the performance of its vital functions, being a response to environmental factors, to specific infective agents, to inherent defects of the organism

(e.g., genetic anomalies), or to combinations of these factors. (Koplan et al., 2005, p. 333)

Contrasting with understandings of MA dependence as a moral or character defect, neurobiological evidence supports the contention that dependence stems from the accumulation of the brain's repeated, concurrent exposures to MA and to environmental factors that modify the performance of its vital functions. Brain-imaging studies of MA-dependent individuals show irregularities in the function of specific areas, including structures in the midbrain (Thompson et al., 2004) and the orbitofrontal cortex (Paulus, et al., 2002). Some neurocognitive impairments in MA abusers persist over time, even after periods of sustained abstinence (Kalechstein et al., 2003; Simon et al., 2004). Although information is advancing to suggest the disease concept is apt, no current characterization of "dependence" fully accommodates all of the changes in brain and in behavior. Thus MA dependence is relegated to the status of a disorder, "a clinically significant behavioral or psychological syndrome or pattern that occurs in an individual and that is associated with present distress or disability or with a significantly increased risk of suffering death, pain, disability, or loss of freedom" (American Psychiatric Association, 2000, p. xxxi). In addition, the disorder must currently be considered "a manifestation of a behavioral, psychological, or biological dysfunction in the individual."

Whether understood as a disease or a disorder, to warrant a diagnosis of MA dependence the treatment provider must be able to specify a minimum threshold of behavioral criteria (i.e., a set of symptoms expressed within the past 12 months) that result in clinically significant distress. This definition recognizes that the common course is for the disorder to develop almost imperceptibly until a series of events occur that cause significant distress (e.g., fear of being fired after being caught using MA at work). Neurobiological changes that occur with the brain's repeated exposure to MA develop slowly and may culminate in reorganization of select brain structures and functions (Thompson et al., 2004). Concomitant reorganization of the composition and qualities of the individual's social environment also occur. The decision to enter treatment happens relatively rarely. In a 12-month period, only about 30% of Americans with drug dependence and about 6% of those with drug abuse enter treatment voluntarily (Compton et al., 2007), typically after one or more critical events or a reappraisal of one's situation occurs.

For those seeking treatment for MA dependence, interventions with demonstrated efficacy are entirely psychosocial and behavioral because there are no approved medications, which may contribute to the relatively low engagement into treatment. Although these psychosocial and behavioral treatments may not directly influence the underlying neuro-biological mechanisms of MA dependence, they are sufficiently potent to help many treatment-seeking individuals organize their psychology and behavior to achieve important and sustained reductions in drug use.

Treatment Targets

When developing a treatment approach, identification of treatment goals is an important first step. Effective treatments can address a variety of targets, including biological, psychological, and social aspects of the individual's dependence. Hence most current treatments adopt a synthetic model that can incorporate approaches to these complex and inter-related problems, such as the bio-psycho-social model (Donovan, 1988). "Bio" emphasizes treatment targets that refer to biological aspects of dependence, such as genetic factors (including a family history of substance abuse or dependence), gender of the individual, and physiological changes that may occur due to chronic exposure, withdrawal, or sustained abstinence from the substance. "Psycho" refers to the complex psychological, cognitive, and emotional needs that are usually manifest in the intake session with MA-abusing or MA-dependent individuals. Cognitive and behavioral treatments can aid individuals in reducing disruptions and distress due to marked mood symptoms (e.g., depression, anxiety), interference with cognitive functioning (e.g., impaired decision making, impulsive behaviors) in individuals under the age of 21, and to unique psychological factors. "Social" refers to treatment targets pertaining to the individual's relation with the social, work, cultural, and criminal justice environments that are affected by MA abuse.

Individuals presenting for treatment with a range of problems often have difficulties selecting which ones need to be addressed first, and many of them may be sufficiently severe to distract focus from the primary purposes of drug abuse treatments: (1) to instill abstinence, (2) to sustain abstinence, and (3) to regain abstinence upon lapse or relapse. It can be difficult for the client and clinician to maintain focus on abstinence goals, especially when immediate legal, medical, and social problems resulting from chronic drug use require attention.

In addition to abstinence targets, many patients require assistance in improving mood and cognition and in reducing drug craving. These psychological, emotional, and craving factors frequently become more severe during initial abstinence periods, and MA use provides immediate but temporary relief. In contrast to many other drugs of abuse, MA often serves important functional purposes. In the case of José, it provides the physical and psychological energy he needs to sustain his standard of living and to meet the needs of his family. Other functional aspects of MA dependence include restriction of diet and enhancement of sexual experience. When attempting to help the individual instill abstinence, the clinician must address functional aspects that were previously addressed by MA. Failure to do so can impinge directly on the quality of life of the individual and the family. Without the energy provided by MA to work long hours, individuals increasingly require assistance to reduce economic commitments to allow them to pay the bills within the amount of energy and money available. As well, issues regarding weight gain and enhanced sexual experiences facilitated by MA require attention.

Even with selection of appropriate targets for treatment and the individual's progression toward his or her goals, treatment cannot "cure" the individual, as one might cure an infection or other type of biological disease. Once MA dependence develops, it is a condition that an individual must manage for the rest of his or her life. Long-term abstinence is defined as being "in remission" in contrast with a state of resolution. Hence selection of the targets for treatment will enable the patient to focus on specific desirable outcomes (i.e., achieve initial abstinence, improve social problems) over a time frame (i.e., immediate treatment targets will likely be replaced by other targets with time), always recognizing the central function of maintaining abstinence from MA use as the foundation for longer-term treatment goals.

Treatments for MA Dependence

Several effective behavioral and psychosocial treatments have been applied in management of MA use disorders. These interventions include behavioral interventions (community reinforcement approach, contingency management, motivational incentives), psychosocial therapies (motivational interviewing, cognitive-behavioral therapy, matrix model), and abstinence-oriented treatments (detoxification, residential rehabilitation, 12-step programs). This balance of this chapter presents evidence supporting use of these approaches and describes the components and goals of each treatment approach.

Brief Interventions

There is a robust database supporting and practice guidelines describing use of brief screening interventions by general clinicians in order to screen their patients and to provide brief, directed advice to those who admit to using cigarettes (Fiore et al., 2000) and problem levels of alcohol use (Whitlock et al., 2004). Patients screened and identified as using cigarettes or alcohol at levels approximating abuse or dependence are provided with facilitated referrals to treatment. One randomized clinical trial of a condition containing two 20-minute brief intervention sessions (n = 24) compared with one 15-minute psychoeducation session (n = 24) for MA-dependent Thai youth ages 14–19 showed statistically significant reductions in the reported number of days of MA use for the brief intervention condition (Srisuraponont et al., 2007). Findings from a clinical trial of brief cognitive-behavioral and motivational interviewing interventions compared with standard care conditions in Australia (Baker et al., 2005) indicated that benefits are measured in reductions in MA use from receiving brief, self-help-oriented interventions for all users, with heavier users benefiting in direct association with their extent of involvement with formal treatment interventions. While screening and brief interventions are able to alter the progression of a potential MA use disorder for patients seen in general health care settings, the evidence suggests that patients with frank MA abuse or dependence should be offered effective treatments in order to address their substance use goals.

The essential component identifies individuals with substance use at levels substantially lower than abuse or dependence in general health care and community settings followed by medical professionals providing direct advice to quit and guidance to find help in quitting. Interrupting the progression of inconsistent drug use to regular or daily use carries the potential for being a low-cost, high-impact intervention for preventing development of drug dependence. Although evidence substantially supports screening and brief intervention for cigarette smokers and alcohol drinkers, evidence is currently being collected to evaluate this intervention approach for drug users.

Behavioral Therapies

Research in behavioral therapy for MA abuse has focused on the community reinforcement approach and contingency management. These two behavioral approaches have been assessed as stand-alone treatments but are often used as a combination therapy.

Community Reinforcement Approach

The community reinforcement approach (CRA) is a multifaceted approach that incorporates biological, psychological, and social elements of treatment (Azrin et al., 1982) that seek to reduce the availability of substance-related reinforcers and increase the alternative reinforcers unrelated to substance use (Roozen, et al., 2004). CRA-type therapy helps patients by conducting a functional analysis of their behavior repertoire to identify the factors that sustain drug dependence. Sessions focus on identifying and avoiding the antecedents of drug use and on finding alternative, non-drug-related behaviors that are incompatible with drug use. CRA sessions also focus on relationship counseling, vocational guidance, and education on skills relating to recreation, to developing a non-addict social network, and to practicing drug refusal skills. CRA often incorporates the behavioral therapy of contingency management.

Although there are no efficacy trials of CRA for treating MA dependence, Steve Higgins and his group at the University of Vermont initially validated the efficacy of various elements of CRA for cocaine dependence more than 15 years ago (Higgins et al., 1991). In one randomized controlled trial (RCT), outcomes for 60 cocaine-dependent patients assigned to receive 24 weeks of CRA plus the behavioral therapy of contingency management (CM; providing vouchers of increasing value in exchange for successive urine samples documenting drug abstinence), compared with 60 patients assigned to receive only CM, showed better substance use and psychosocial functioning during treatment, but both conditions showed similar reductions in cocaine use at distal follow-up evaluations (Higgins et al., 2003). CRA plus CM has been demonstrated to work similarly with cocaine-dependent outpatients compared with standard treatment in Spain (Secades-Villa et al., 2007), with superior outcomes at 6-month evaluations. Although there are no efficacy studies supporting use of CRA applied to the treatment of MA dependence, substantial efficacy for its use with cocaine-dependent individuals supports generalizing this approach to MA users.

Contingency Management

Although CM programs can be part of CRA, the behavioral therapy has been demonstrated to work by itself to reduce stimulant use (Higgins et al., 2003; Rawson et al., 2006; Shoptaw et al., 2005a). The goals of CM incentive-based programs are to attract stimulant users into treatment and to promote initial abstinence from stimulants. CM strategies achieve this objective by providing vouchers or similar incentives in exchange for urine samples documenting abstinence; thus the approach is also called motivational incentives therapy. Given the 3-day limit of the sensitivity of urine drug screening tests to detect metabolites of amphetamine and MA, CM schedules require frequent clinic visits. Most schedules provide patients with incentives of increasing value with successive urine samples testing negative for MA metabolite in order to shape behavior toward sustained abstinence. For patients who provide a sample positive for MA metabolites, no incentive is earned, and the value of the next incentive typically returns to the initial value. Because lapses to MA use are common early in the abstinence process, most CM schedules employ a "rapid reset" procedure to nurture motivation to continue working toward the goal of sustained abstinence (Roll & Shoptaw, 2006). The rapid reset is a procedure in which patients can prove a brief period of abstinence to return to the point in the reinforcement schedule prior to the drug lapse or relapse.

Several studies demonstrate efficacy for using CM for treating MA dependence. In a 16-week outpatient trial of 171 stimulant-dependent patients randomly assigned to CM, cognitive-behavioral therapy (CBT), or CM plus CBT conditions, patients randomly assigned to a condition containing CM produced significant reductions in MA use and improvements in retention during treatment compared with the CBT-only condition, but all conditions performed similarly at 1-year follow-up evaluations (Rawson et al., 2006). In a multisite trial incorporating CM into standard treatment compared with standard treatment alone in 415 patients with cocaine or MA dependence (Petry et al., 2005), patients randomly assigned to receive CM with standard care produced significantly greater improvements in retention, in completed counseling sessions, and produced more urine samples that documented stimulant abstinence. Analysis of only the MA-dependent patients from the Petry study (Roll et al., 2006) showed that both CM plus standard care and standard care only produced similar outcomes for retention in treatment and for reductions in MA use, although standard care plus CM produced significantly longer stretches of sustained abstinence from amphetamines (5 weeks vs. 3 weeks).

CM has also been validated for use with gay and bisexual male MA-dependent patients, a group at extremely high risk for HIV (Shoptaw et al., 2005a). In this study, outcomes for 162 gay and bisexual male MA-dependent patients randomly assigned to one of four conditions for 16 weeks (CM, CBT, CM + CBT, or a CBT condition specially tailored to gay male culture) were similar to the Rawson trial: Conditions containing CM produced significant reductions in MA use and increases in retention during treatment, but conditions showed similar levels of drug use reductions at 1-year follow-up visits. Of interest, however, was the observation that these behavioral therapies also significantly reduced reported HIV-related sexual risk behaviors, particularly unprotected anal intercourse, reductions that were observed during treatment and that were sustained to 1-year follow-up evaluations.

Interest is growing for using CM only in clinical settings to address the syndemics of MA abuse and HIV infection in gay and bisexual male populations, with outcomes in uncontrolled trials being similar to those seen in controlled treatment studies (Strona et al., 2006).

Psychosocial Therapies

In contrast to behavioral therapies, effective psychosocial therapies typically manipulate elements of education and the social environment to help patients meet their stimulant use goals. Psychosocial therapies with evidence supporting their efficacy include CBT (including the matrix model) and motivational interviewing.

Cognitive-Behavioral Therapy

CBT is an almost ubiquitous form of psychosocial treatment that teaches patients about their disorder and trains them in the cognitive and behavioral skills necessary to instill abstinence, to return to abstinence following lapse or relapse, and to prevent relapse (Marlatt & Gordon, 1985). CBT is compatible with other behavior therapies and 12-step approaches. One of the elements of CBT involves functional analysis, a procedure by which the patient and therapist identify specific persons, places, things, thoughts, and emotions associated with drug use. The goal of this procedure is to identify behaviors and thoughts that the patient may use to avoid drug use and to improve mood. In addition, CBT focuses on training patients how to prevent a lapse to drug use from becoming a full-blown relapse (i.e., how to reinstate abstinence following brief-episodic lapse to drug use). The procedure is highly didactic, with the therapist seen as a teacher or coach. Patients typically are given extra-session skills implementation (homework) and engage within-session skills practice. Findings of one trial with cocaine-dependent patients showed that completion of homework assignments significantly correlated with reductions in cocaine use at 1-year follow-up visits compared with patients who did not complete their homework (Carroll et al., 2005).

Research shows CBT is effective in treating MA dependence. A high-quality model of CBT is freely available for download and use for cocaine dependence. That intervention that can be easily tailored for use with patients with MA dependence (Carroll, 1998). CBT is frequently the comparison condition in controlled clinical trials of behavior therapies for stimulant dependence owing to its consistent ability to produce sustained reductions in drug use. Principles of CBT also have been used in 12-step groups (McKay et al., 1997). One advantageous feature of CBT is its flexibility, as it retains efficacy when being tailored to work with other approaches or to special treatment populations. For example, the matrix model (Rawson et al., 1995) is a synthetic model that incorporates elements of social learning, psychological education, and social support with standard CBT principles. In the largest trial of a treatment for MA-dependent patients (Rawson et al., 2004), patients randomly assigned to receive matrix model treatment demonstrated superior ability for retention in treatment, in producing more metabolite-free urine samples and in achieving longer periods of abstinence compared with patients assigned to receive "treatment as usual." The matrix model tailored for use with gay and bisexual male MA-dependent patients is available for download (Shoptaw et al., 2005b) and shows comparable efficacy to CM and to standard matrix model CBT when used in this special population (Shoptaw et al., 2005a).

Motivational Interviewing

Motivational interviewing (MI) is another popular form of psychosocial treatment. MI is designed to engage patients into long-term treatment and promote specific behavior change. The MI treatment platform has been described as a "client-centered, directive method for enhancing intrinsic motivation to change by exploring and resolving ambivalence" (Miller & Rollnick, 2002, p. 25). It is based on the central assumption that the organizing psychological principle underlying dependence is ambivalence about having and not having a substance abuse problem. According to MI theory, people change their thinking and behaviors along a series of stages (Prochaska et al., 1992; Miller et al., 2003) that moves from *contemplation* (ambivalence and inaction), through *preparation* (change options are explored), to *action* and *maintenance* of change. *Relapse* occurs when patients return to substance use followed by re-engagement of a prior stage. One key concept of MI is that the therapy is designed for patients to progress along the stages of change, assuming sole responsibility for their decisions about substance use (Bux & Irwin, 2006). Using this model, resistance indicates that the counselor is ahead of the patient, which is counterproductive. Confronting resistance is also counterproductive and potentially harmful. Instead, counselors are trained to "roll with resistance," and to explore the ambivalence with the patient rather than feel the need to resolve the resistance.

Clinical application of MI involves the use of four basic principles: (1) expressing empathy through techniques such as reflective listening, (2) developing and exaggerating a discrepancy between the patient's self-image as a drug user and ideal self-image, (3) avoiding argumentation (i.e., rolling with resistance), and (4) supporting the patient's self-efficacy. MI can be delivered in two phases: the first seeks to increase the patient's motivation to enter treatment, and the second aims to strengthen the patient's adherence to the chance process (Zweben & Zuckoff, 2002).

There exist two similar versions of MI, FRAMES (Miller & Rollnick, 2002) and BRENDA (Volpicelli et al., 2001). FRAMES is an acronym for *F*eedback, *R*esponsibility, *A*dvice, *M*enu of options, *E*mpathy and *Self*-efficacy. BRENDA is an acronym for *Bio*-psycho-social, *Reporting*, *Empathy*, *Needs* assessment, *Direct* advice, and *Assessment* of progress. Although there have been no RCTs of MI to treat MA-using populations exclusively, studies have demonstrated the beneficial effects of MI among general substance-using populations. A meta-analysis of MI studies published in 2003 revealed moderate effect sizes in drug dependence (alcohol and drug dependence) when comparing MI with no-treatment or placebo control groups (Burke et al., 2003). In one multisite RCT of MI for drug users (18% MA users), MI was integrated into the intake procedure of community drug treatment programs, not as a stand-alone treatment (Carroll et al., 2006). Compared with a non-MI intake, MI led to increased retention at 1 month but no differential improvement in measures of substance use. Two studies have assessed brief MI with treatment for cocaine users. Stotts et al. (2001) found that provision of MI during an initial detox program led to less use of cocaine during a subsequent relapse-prevention treatment. This effect was strongest for patients with low initial motivation. Another study replicated this "matching" finding and revealed that among patients with high initial motivation, MI actually led to more frequent cocaine use during the following year (Rohsenow et al., 2005). One study of amphetamine users compared a brief cognitive-behavioral intervention (with one MI session) to a self-help booklet condition, with the brief intervention condition demonstrating more abstinence at 6-month follow-up (Baker et al., 2001). This group replicated their original report showing that abstinence outcomes increased when treatment-seeking amphetamine-abusing individuals received two or more CBT sessions (Baker et al., 2005). More recently, McKee et al. (2007) revealed that an enhanced MI + CBT condition, compared with CBT only, led to more sessions attended, but no difference in cocaine use. Results from these studies indicate that MI is best implemented as an early intervention designed to increase patient motivation to change and increase treatment adherence, unless patients already are highly motivated. Further research is needed to understand the effect of MI interventions when the population is restricted to patients with MA dependence.

Residential Rehabilitation

Residential rehabilitation offers longer-term maintenance of abstinence within a contained residential setting. Residential rehabilitation programs are often based on 12-step principles and use a social or family model to catalyze change of individual behavior (Shearer, 2007). Elements of CBT (group and individual) are often incorporated, as are strictly enforced behavioral norms and clearly defined roles and responsibilities with concomitant rewards or punishments (Platt, 1997). Due to logistical and ethical considerations, there are few RCTs of residential rehabilitation for MA dependence. Most of the evidence supporting the effectiveness of residential rehabilitation programs comes from treatment cohort studies, and there are no studies that focus specifically on MA dependence. Gossop et al. (2000) found that primary stimulant users enrolled in a drug treatment cohort study who received residential rehabilitation significantly reduced drug use at 1-year follow-up visits. Another cohort study found that among patients enrolled in long-term residential treatment, cocaine use had decreased at a 1-year follow-up but had increased significantly from 1 year to 5 years posttreatment (Hubbard et al., 2003). Given the lack of consistency and experimental control of rehabilitation programs in these cohort studies, it is not clear whether all patients would benefit from residential rehabilitation. In the absence of controlled evidence, it still seems reasonable that the containment, supervision, structure, and stability offered in residential rehabilitation may be essential for MA-dependent patients who consistently fail outpatient treatments.

12-Step Programs

A recent review of the literature regarding the role of 12-step self-help activities in recovery from MA use disorders suggests that the integration of this approach into treatment processes is associated with reduced substance use and improved outcomes for patients (Donovan & Wells, 2007). The broadly prevalent 12-step self-help groups are advantageous for being readily accessible and available at low or no cost (Room & Greenfield, 1993). Even though there have been no studies to isolate the role of 12-step involvement specifically with MA users, studies of 12-step involvement with cocaine users reveal potential benefits, since treatments for cocaine abuse are generally also effective for MA abuse (Copeland & Sorensen, 2001; Rawson et al., 2000).

Comparison of the Previously Discussed Therapies

The matrix model retains more participants than other standard treatments do. Participants in the matrix model were 38% more likely to stay in treatment than were patients in opposing studies. Matrix model patients were also 27% more likely to complete treatment than patients at other sites where the condition was "treatment as usual." Both of these statistics exclude a scenario in which a drug court is involved. Matrix-treated patients tended to provide more drug-free urine samples than their counterparts in non-matrix treatments, and they also experienced longer mean periods of abstinence. MA-free urine samples increased from the baseline in both conditions, and abstinence was maintained in 69% of those treated in both categories (from results at a 6-month follow-up; Rawson et. al., 2004).

CM produces many more alcohol-negative and stimulant-negative samples from patients, and CM produces longer mean periods of abstinence than matrix model therapy alone. In a study conducted from 2001–2003, 17.6% of patients within a subgroup receiving CM therapy remained abstinent throughout the entire study, as opposed to only 6.5% being treated only with the matrix model (Roll et al., 2006)

CM also appears to be superior to CBT, although both are effective in treatment. In a study published in 2001, patients receiving either CM alone or a combination of CM and CBT stayed in treatment significantly longer than those patients receiving CBT alone (with the mean for CM and CM+CBT at around 12 weeks and the mean for CBT alone at 9 weeks). Patients in the CM and CM+CBT studies provided more stimulant-free samples than the CBT group during the trial. During treatment, those who received a form of CM seemed to benefit most, but the rates of return to substance use became equivalent at follow-up visits as time progressed. All three treatments were characterized as effective (Rawson et al., 2006).

Conclusion

The clinician treating a client with MA dependence is faced with key decisions regarding the type of treatment to engage in with the patient and how to respond depending on the client's progress. While many clinicians generally feel comfortable using one model of treatment with all of their clients, there is increased interest in use of an algorithm that guides treatment decisions based on client presentation and response to that treatment. This interest is founded on a growing acceptance that, for many affected individuals, drug dependence is a chronic health condition and that treatments are best guided by understanding the current episode in context of past and likely future treatments (McLellan et al., 2005). There are no evidence-based "algorithms" for guiding selection or timing of specific treatments for individuals with MA dependence. But there are logical patient-placement criteria as guides, such as those of the American Society of Addiction Medicine (ASAM, 2001), with treatment decisions ranging from least-intensive interventions, for those with emerging disorders or disorders that carry mild subjective distress, through most-intensive interventions, for those with recurrent disorders or severe subjective distress.

Future research will determine the appropriateness of applying chronic disease models for managing MA and other drug dependencies, but there is a growing body of literature that describes evidence-based interventions for treating MA dependence. Moreover, there is a strong indication that evidence-based interventions can be adapted successfully to a variety of specialty populations, such as gay and bisexual men, in ways that retain elements of efficacy for the treatment approach, yet are also culturally sensitive and relevant. As the variety of treatments with demonstrated evidence continues to grow for MA dependence, clinicians will have more options for implementing logical algorithms to guide treatments.

References

American Psychiatric Association. (2000). *Diagnostic and statistical manual of mental disorders* (4th ed, text rev). Washington, DC: American Psychiatric Association Press.

American Society of Addiction Medicine. (2001). *ASAM patient placement criteria, second revision (ASAM PPC 2R)*. Chevy Chase, MD: Author.

Azrin NH, Sisson RW, Meyers R, et al. (1982). Alcoholism treatment by disulfiram and community reinforcement therapy. *J Behav Ther Exp Psychiatry* 13:105–102.

Baker A, Boggs TG, Lewin TJ. (2001). Randomized controlled trial of brief cognitive-behavioral interventions among regular users of amphetamine. *Addiction* 96:1279–1287.

Baker A, Lee NK, Claire M, et al. (2005). Brief cognitive-behavioral interventions for regular amphetamine users: A step in the right direction. *Addiction* 100(3):367–378

Burke B, Arkowitz H, Menchola M. (2003). The efficacy of motivational interviewing: A meta-analysis of controlled clinical trials. *J Consult Clin Psychol* 71:843–861.

Bux DA, Irwin TW. (2006). Combining motivational interviewing and cognitive-behavioral skills training for the treatment of crystal methamphetamine abuse/dependence. *J Gay Lesbian Psychotherapy* 10:143–152.

Carroll KM. (1998). *A cognitive-behavioral approach: Treating cocaine addiction*. (NIH Publication No. 98-4308). Retrieved October 9, 2007, from *www.nida.nih.gov/TXManuals/CBT/CBT1.html*.

Carroll KM, Ball SA, Nich C, et al. (2006). Motivational interviewing to improve treatment engagement and outcome in individuals seeking treatment for substance abuse: A multisite effectiveness study. *Drug Alcohol Depend* 81:301–312.

Carroll KM, Nich C, Ball SA. (2005). Practice makes progress? Homework assignments and outcome in treatment of cocaine dependence. *J Consult Clin Psychol* 73:749–755.

Compton WM, Thomas YF, Stimson FS, et al. (2007). Prevalence, correlates, disability, and comorbidity of DSM-IV drug abuse and dependence in the United States: Results from the National Epidemiologic Survey on Alcohol and Related Conditions. *Arch Gen Psychiatry* 64:566–576.

Copeland AL, Sorenson JA. (2001). Differences between methamphetamine users and cocaine users in treatment. *Drug Alcohol Depend* 62(1):92–95.

Donovan DM. (1988). Assessment of addictive behaviors: Implications of an emerging biopsychosocial model. In DM Donovan, GA Marlatt (Eds), *Assessment of Addictive Behaviors* (pp. 3–48). New York: Guilford Press.

Donovan DM, Wells EA. (2007). 'Tweaking 12-step': The potential role of 12-step self-help group involvement in methamphetamine recovery. *Addiction* 102:121–129.

Fiore MC, Bailey WC, Cohen SJ, et al. (2000). *Treating tobacco use and dependence: Clinical practice guideline.* Rockville, MD: U.S. Department of Health and Human Services, Public Health Service.

Gossop M, Marsden J, Stewart D. (2000). Treatment outcomes of stimulant misusers: One-year follow-up results from the National Treatment Outcome Research Study (NTORS). *Addict Behav* 25(4):509–522.

Higgins ST, Delaney DD, Budney AJ, et al. (1991). A behavioral approach to achieving initial cocaine abstinence. *Am J Psychiatry* 148:1218–1224.

Higgins ST, Sigmon ST, Wong CJ, et al. (2003). Community reinforcement therapy for cocaine-dependent outpatients. *Arch Gen Psychiatry* 60:1043–1052.

Hubbard R, Craddock S, Anderson J. (2003). Overview of 5-year follow-up outcomes in the Drug Abuse Treatment Outcome Studies (DATOS). *J Subst Abuse Treat* 25 125–134.

Kalechstein AD, Newton TF, Green M. (2003). Methamphetamine dependence is associated with neurocognitive impairment in the initial phases of abstinence. *J Neuropsychiatry Clin Neurosci* 15:215–220.

Koplan JP, Liverman CT, Kraak VA. (2005). *Preventing childhood obesity: Health in the balance.* Washington, DC: National Academies Press.

Marlatt GA, Gordon JR (Eds). (1985). *Relapse prevention: Maintenance strategies in the treatment of addictive behaviors.* New York: Guilford Press.

McKay JR, Alterman AI, Cacciola JS, et al. (1997). Group counseling versus individualized relapse prevention aftercare following intensive outpatient treatment for cocaine dependence: Initial results. *J Consult Clin Psychol* 65(5):778–788.

McKee SA, Carroll KM, Sinha R, et al. (2007). Enhancing brief cognitive-behavioral therapy with motivational enhancement techniques in cocaine users. *Drug Alcohol Depend* 91:97–101.

McLellan AT, McKay JR, Forman R, et al. (2005). Reconsidering the evaluation of addiction treatment: From retrospective follow-up to concurrent recovery monitoring. *Addiction* 100:447–458.

Miller W, Rollnick S. (2002). *Motivational interviewing: Preparing people for change.* New York: Guilford Press.

Miller W, Yahne EY, Tonigan JS. (2003). Motivational interviewing in drug abuse services: A randomized trial. *J Consult Clin Psychology* 71:754–763.

Paulus MP, Hozack NE, Zauscher BE, et al. (2002). Behavioral and functional neuroimaging evidence for prefrontal dysfunction in methamphetamine-dependent subjects. *Neuropsychopharmacology* 26(1):53–63.

Petry NM, Peirce JM, Stitzer ML, et al. (2005). Effect of prize-based incentives on outcomes in stimulant abusers in outpatient psychosocial treatment programs: A national drug abuse treatment clinical trials network study. *Arch Gen Psychiatry* 62:1148–1156.

Platt J. (1997). *Cocaine addiction: Theory, research, and treatment.* Cambridge, MA: Harvard University Press.

Prochaska JO, DiClemente CC, Norcross JC. (1992). In search of how people change: Applications to addictive behavior. *Am Psychologist* 47:1102–1114.

Rawson RA, Obert JL, McCann MJ. (1995). *The matrix intensive outpatient program therapist manual.* Los Angeles, CA: The Matrix Center, Inc.

Rawson R, Marinelli-Casey P, Anglin M, et al. (2004). A multisite comparison of psychosocial approaches for the treatment of methamphetamine dependence. *Addiction* 99:708–717.

Rawson R, McCann M, Flammino F, et al. (2006). A comparison of contingency management and cognitive-behavioral approaches for stimulant-dependent individuals. *Addiction* 101:267–274.

Rawson RA, McCann MJ, Hasson AJ, et al. (2000). Addiction pharmacotherapy 2000: New options, new challenges. *J Psychoactive Drugs* 32(4):371–378.

Roll JM, Petry NM, Stitzer ML, et al. (2006). Contingency management for the treatment of methamphetamine use disorders. *Am J Psychiatry* 163:1993–1999.

Roll JM, Shoptaw S. (2006). Contingency management for the treatment of methamphetamine abuse: Schedule effects. *Psychiatry Res* 141:91–93.

Room R, Greenfield T. (1993). Alcoholics Anonymous, other 12-step movements, and psychotherapy in the U.S. population, 1990. *Addiction* 88(4):555–562.

Roozen H, Boulogne J, van Tulder M, et al. (2004). A systematic review of the effectiveness of the community reinforcement approach in alcohol, cocaine, and opioid addiction. *Drug Alcohol Depend* 74:1–13.

Secades-Villa R, García-Rodríguez O, Higgins ST, et al. (2008). Community reinforcement approach plus vouchers for cocaine dependence in a community setting in Spain: Six-month outcomes. *J Subst Abuse Treat* 34(2):202–207.

Shearer J. (2007). Psychosocial approaches to psychostimulant dependence: A systematic review. *J Subst Abuse Treat* 32:41–52.

Shoptaw S, Reback CJ, Peck JA, et al. (2005a). Behavioral treatment approaches for methamphetamine dependence and HIV-related sexual risk behaviors among urban gay and bisexual men. *Drug Alcohol Depend* 78(2):125–134.

Shoptaw S, Reback CJ, Peck JA, et al. (2005b). *Getting off: A behavioral treatment manual for gay and bisexual methamphetamine users.* Retrieved October 9, 2007, from *www.uclaisap.org/assets/documents/Shoptawetal_2005_tx%20manual.pdf.*

Simon S, Dacey J, Glynn S, et al. (2004). The effect of relapse on cognitive in abstinent methamphetamine users. *J Subst Abuse Treat* 27:59–66.

Srisuraponont M, Sombatmai S, Boripuntakul T. (2007). Brief intervention for students with methamphetamine use disorders: A randomized controlled trial. *Am J Addict* 16:111–116.

Stotts A, Schmitz J, Rhoades H, et al. (2001). Motivational interviewing with cocaine-dependent patients: A pilot study. *J Consult Clin Psychology* 69:858–862.

Strona FV, McCright J, Hjord H, et al. (2006). The acceptability and feasibility of the Positive Reinforcement Opportunity Project, a community-based contingency management methamphetamine treatment program for gay and bisexual men in San Francisco. *J Psychoactive Drugs* (SARC Suppl. 3):377–383.

Thompson PM, Hayashi KM, Simon SL, et al. (2004). Structural abnormalities in the brains of humans who use methamphetamine. *J Neurosci* 24:6028–6036.

Volkow ND, Chang L, Wang G, et al. (2001). Higher cortical and lower subcortical metabolism in recently detoxified methamphetamine abusers. *Am J Psychiatry* 158:383–389.

Volpicelli JR, Pettinatti HM, McLellan AT, et al. (2001). *Combining medication and psychosocial treatment for addiction: The BRENDA approach.* New York: Guilford Press.

Whitlock EP, Polen MR, Green CA, et al. (2004). Behavioral counseling interventions in primary care to reduce risky/harmful alcohol use by adults: A summary of the evidence for the U.S. Preventive Services Task Force. *Ann Int Med* 140:557–568.

Zweben A, Zuckoff A. (2002). Motivational interviewing and treatment adherence. In W Miller, S Rollnick (Eds). *Motivational interviewing: Preparing people for change* (pp. 299–319). New York: Guilford Press.

Chapter 11

Pharmacological Treatment of Methamphetamine Addiction

Frank J. Vocci, Ahmed Elkashef, and Nathan M. Appel

A significant increase in methamphetamine (MA) abuse in the last decade has led to a significant increase in the number of individuals seeking treatment for MA dependence (Vocci & Appel, 2007; Rutkowski & Maxwell, Chapter 2, this volume). The National Institute on Drug Abuse (NIDA) has funded research toward developing behavioral, pharmacological, and immunological therapies to treat this disorder that has such grave impact on health care, social service, and criminal justice systems in the United States (Rawson & Condon, 2007). In this chapter we review the current pharmacological and immunological approaches that have been undertaken or are being proposed as potential therapeutic agents to moderate the appetitive drive of MA. The latter underlies the craving that makes maintaining abstinence so difficult for abstinent abusers and addicts. Next we review findings relating to MA-induced cognitive impairment and its potential impact on effectively treating MA abusers and addicts with pharmacotherapy. For the purposes of this chapter we are defining *appetitive drive* as a neuronal process that leads an organism (person) to approach or seek something in its environment.

Clinical Trials of Pharmacotherapies for MA Dependence

The NIDA Medications Development Program began to develop medications to treat MA dependence in 2000. Since that time, several studies have been conducted and completed, and three medications have shown some preliminary evidence of efficacy in reducing MA or amphetamine use.

Bupropion

The antidepressant bupropion is a mild stimulant that blocks dopamine uptake at the neuronal membrane dopamine transporter and is an effective treatment for nicotine dependence (Vocci & Appel, 2007). NIDA funded a multisite outpatient trial of bupropion following a clinical pharmacology study that showed bupropion reduced the subjective effects of intravenously administered MA (Newton et al., 2006). Subjects were randomized to bupropion or placebo using an adaptive "urn" randomization to balance treatment groups within sites on factors such as gender and self-report of baseline use ($\leq$18 days of use per month or >18 days per month). They received either sustained-release bupropion 150 mg (Zyban SR, GlaxoSmithKline) tablets or matching placebo doses that were film coated to preserve treatment masking (Elkashef et al., 2008). One hundred fifty-one subjects were enrolled at five sites.

Treatment consisted of 12 weeks of medication and thrice-weekly standardized, cognitive-behavioral therapy (90-minute sessions). Urines were collected three times per week to monitor compliance; positive urines were subjected to further analysis by gas chromatography/mass spectrometry. Each subject completed weekly self-reports of drug use and craving using the Brief Substance Craving Scale (BSCS). The Hamilton Rating Scale for Depression (Ham-D) and Addiction Severity Index (ASI-Lite, 2000 version) were conducted at baseline and completion of treatment. The primary outcome assessment was the percentage of participants who abstained from MA in a given treatment week. The weekly proportion of MA-free urines per treatment group was analyzed using generalized estimating equations (GEE). Other planned analyses were to evaluate use as a function of randomization factors and to analyze the BSCS, Ham-D, and ASI-Lite.

Seventy-nine patients (52%) completed the study. There was no differential completion rate across the treatment groups. The overall analysis revealed a trend favoring the bupropion group (GEE $p = .09$) in terms of using less MA during the study. The subgroup analysis revealed that the low-to-moderate MA baseline use group ($\leq$18 days per month) exhibited significant reduction of MA use ($p = .0001$). The quantitative urinalysis data from this group corroborated this finding (GEE, $p = .04$). The reduction in MA use was restricted to male subjects in the GEE analysis. Female subjects did not reduce their MA use (GEE, $p = .71$), possibly because the majority of females (54%) were in the high-baseline use group. A trend toward less MA use was seen in the bupropion subgroup with Ham-D scores lower than 12 ($p = .08$). No significant differences were noted across groups for the ASI-Lite and BSCS measures. As a follow-up, NIDA is funding further trials to confirm the effect of bupropion as a treatment for MA dependence.

Methylphenidate

Methylphenidate is a stimulant that, like bupropion, binds to the dopamine transporter and is often used to treat attention-deficit/hyperactivity disorder (Vocci & Appel, 2007). Tiihonen et al. (2007) randomized 53 subjects meeting DSM-IV criteria for intravenous amphetamine dependence to aripiprazole (15 mg/day), slow-release methylphenidate (54 mg/day), or placebo. The primary outcome measure was the proportion of amphetamine-positive urine samples. The trial was ended early because the interim analysis revealed that methylphenidate decreased amphetamine use (odds ratio = 0.46) compared with the placebo group. The outcome of the aripiprazole-treated group was less satisfactory in that the latter subjects returned more amphetamine-positive urine samples than did placebo controls (odds ratio = 3.77). NIDA is planning to follow up with additional trials.

Baclofen

Baclofen is considered the prototypic gamma-aminobutyric acid B ($GABA_B$) receptor agonist that has been reported to suppress the symptoms of alcohol withdrawal syndrome (Addolorato et al., 2006). Heinzerling et al. (2006) reported on a trial of baclofen (20 mg three times a day), gabapentin (800 mg three times a day), or placebo for treating MA dependence with 88 subjects randomized across the three groups. Study participants received thrice-weekly psychosocial counseling and were asked to provide urine specimens at each clinic visit so that compliance could be monitored. The primary outcome was MA use. Treatment retention, craving, depressive symptoms, and adverse events were recorded and analyzed as secondary outcome measures. Data were analyzed from the perspective of "intention to treat," with the GEE model used to analyze the primary data.

While there were no statistically significant differences in retention within the groups, retention in the baclofen group was 60% compared with 40.5% for the placebo group. Post hoc analysis showed that when medication compliance was considered in the analysis, baclofen increased the probability of a subject's providing an MA-free urine sample; however, neither baclofen nor gabapentin reduced MA use. Nevertheless, these results support a rationale for further exploring baclofen and other GABA-ergic medications in this context.

Topiramate

Topiramate is a sulphamate-substituted fructose derivative that was originally designed as an oral hypoglycemic (Vocci & Appel, 2007), but has approved indications as an anticonvulsant and for migraine prophylaxis. It increases brain GABA as well as antagonizes alpha-amino-3-hydroxy-5-methylisoxazole-4-propionic acid (AMPA)/kainate but not N-methyl-D-aspartate (NMDA) receptor-mediated currents (Vocci & Appel, 2007). Topiramate has shown preliminary evidence of efficacy in treating cocaine dependence (Kampman et al., 2004), efficacy in reducing drinking in alcohol dependent patients (Johnson, 2004), and has promoted abstinence from smoking in alcohol-dependent patients (Johnson et al., 2005). Johnson et al. (2007a) reported that 200 mg topiramate slightly increased the subjective effects of MA in an acute dosing interaction study. The effect was complex when these same subjects were also tested on a cognitive battery while on topiramate, MA, and the combination (Johnson et al., 2007b). Topiramate tended to improve attention and concentration, both alone and when administered with MA condition; however, psychomotor retardation worsened. A phase II outpatient study of 140 subjects to further investigate topiramate as an MA-abuse pharmacotherapy was completed in 2008 and is in the data analysis phase.

Lobeline

Lobeline is a natural product extracted from the dried leaves and tops of the Indian tobacco herb *Lobelina inflata* (Indian tobacco), which is a nicotinic receptor agonist as well as a membrane dopamine transporter and vesicular monoamine transporter 2 (VMAT2) inhibitor (see below). It is available over the counter as a supplement and was tested in clinical trials as a potential smoking cessation agent. It has a pharmacological profile in rodents like that of an MA antagonist. The pharmacological interactions of lobeline and MA are described elsewhere in this chapter.

Gamma-Vinyl-GABA (Vigabatrin)

Gamma-vinyl-GABA is a GABA transaminase inhibitor (Jung et al., 1977; Palfreyman et al., 1981; Nanavati & Silverman, 1989) with an approved indication as an anticonvulsant in Europe and Canada

(Vigabatrin, Sabril), but not in the United States. Preclinical studies suggested gamma-vinyl-GABA had therapeutic potential as an addiction pharmacotherapy in that it antagonized increases in nucleus accumbens dopamine in response to stimulants (cocaine and MA) as well as ethanol and heroin (Vocci & Appel, 2007). In a preliminary open-label clinical trial on volunteers with a history of cocaine abuse, a cohort of the participants were able to remain drug free for 28 days (Brodie et al., 2003). The investigators subsequently conducted another open-label clinical trial that included MA as well as cocaine abusers (Brodie et al., 2005). Eighteen of 30 participants completed the trial and tested negative for MA and cocaine at study completion. There have been reports that gamma-vinyl-GABA causes visual field defects (Wilton et al., 1999; Comaish et al., 2000). No adverse effects on visual field were noted in the cited human studies. Neither study included controls; thus, although the data are encouraging, one cannot conclude that the treatment itself accounted for the positive outcome.

Naltrexone

A preclinical study in rats revealed an effect of the opiate antagonist naltrexone to attenuate cue-induced MA seeking (Anggadiredja et al., 2004a, 2004b; Vocci & Appel, 2007). Jayaram-Lindstrom et al. (2004) administered naltrexone to healthy volunteers to ascertain its effects on the subjective responses to amphetamine. They reported that naltrexone antagonized the effects of 30 mg of oral *d*-amphetamine in an open-label trial of naltrexone in 20 amphetamine-dependent subjects. Compliant subjects had a significantly higher percentage of amphetamine-free urines (77% vs. 22% for the noncompliant group).

Modafinil

Modafinil is a nonamphetamine, weak psychostimulant that is effective for treating narcolepsy (Vocci & Appel, 2007). It has been suggested that modafinil may act via GABA-ergic or glutamatergic mechanisms, but definitive evidence is still lacking (Vocci & Appel, 2007). Dackis et al. (2005) reported an effect of modafinil to reduced cocaine consumption in cocaine-dependent users. No safety risks presented in a phase I clinical pharmacology trial to evaluate the combination of modafinil and MA (Jones & Mendelson, personal communication, 2007). An NIDA-funded multisite trial assessing modafinil for the treatment of MA dependence was initiated in 2008. With respect to MA, the mild stimulant effect of modafinil supports a rationale that it may improve concentration and daytime alertness and thereby improve cognitive functions in MA-dependent subjects, thereby allowing them to benefit from cognitive-behavioral therapy and other treatment compliance-enhancing forms of psychosocial therapy. A cognitive battery will be used to characterize the cognitive deficits at baseline and whether the amelioration of these deficits produces an enhanced treatment response.

Results from Basic and Clinical Science Studies

The development of pharmacotherapeutic and immunotherapeutic approaches to the treatment of MA dependence has been driven by the pharmacology of MA as currently understood and results from animal models. The latter are hoped to represent the expression of neurobiological processes that lead to progressively more intense drug use, addiction, and relapse. These processes presumably underlie the appetitive drive that leads the dependent or addicted person to seek the drug.

The pharmacology of MA has led to both similar and dissimilar approaches to developing medications. MA abusers self-administer the drug by ingestion, insufflation (nasal and smoking), and intravenous injection. It enters the bloodstream rapidly and, by virtue of its lipophilicity, crosses rapidly into the brain, where it becomes concentrated (Burchfield et al., 1991; Cook et al., 1993; Mendelson et al., 1995; Riviere et al., 2000; Harris et al., 2003).

Stimulants such as cocaine and the amphetamines are thought to initially elicit their rewarding effects by activating the brain mesolimbic dopamine system (Di et al., 2004; Pierce & Kumaresan, 2006), which subsequently affects other neurochemical-coded brain pathways (Everitt & Wolf, 2002). Unlike cocaine, amphetamines enter the neuron; in fact, cocaine blocks MA uptake (Zaczek et al., 1991a, 1991b; Pifl et al., 1995; Xie et al., 2000), which suggests that dopamine transporter inhibitors could affect the action of MA (see below). Once inside the neuron, it is widely accepted that the cardinal site via which MA ultimately affects synaptic dopamine is via VMAT2 (see below). VMAT2 is one of a class of mammalian "amine handling" proteins. It's expressed on intracellular secretory granules (vesicles) of dopaminergic as well as serotonergic, noradrenergic, adrenergic, and histaminergic neurons in the CNS and facilitates monoamine neurotransmitter storage in the neuron's secretory vesicles (Erickson et al., 1992; Weihe & Eiden, 2000). The reader is referred to the recent review by Fleckenstein et al. (2007) for a more comprehensive survey of the action of MA on dopaminergic neurons.

Behavioral pharmacologists have developed techniques that are thought to assess and reflect the underlying neurobiological processes that play a role in the development and maintenance of addiction. For an

excellent overview of animal models of addiction the reader is referred
to O'Brien & Gardner (2005). In the present review we concentrate on
three mechanisms that likely increase the appetitive drive that causes an
animal or person to seek and consume MA: conditioned cueing, drug
priming, and stress-induced reinstatement.

Conditioned Cueing

Conditioned cueing is a classical conditioning process whereby previously neutral stimuli become paired to drug experiences and develop
motivational significance (reviewed in Everitt & Robbins, 2000; Everitt
et al., 2001). Briefly, conditioned stimuli increase approach behavior,
facilitate Pavlovian to-instrument transfer, and become conditioned
reinforcers in their own right. Second-order schedules of drug reinforcement are used to study the influence of conditioned cues on the behavior
of interest. Lesioning studies in animals have implicated the basolateral
amygdala in the circuitry that is activated by conditioned cues. Human
imaging studies have reported that conditioned cues activate amygdala,
anterior cingulate, lateral orbitofrontal cortex, rhinal cortex, and right
hemispheric dorsolateral prefrontal cortex (Grant et al., 1996; Bonson
et al., 2002). The anatomical homology of conditioned cueing between
rodents and humans suggests rodent models may be of value in discover-
ing pharmacological agents that affect conditioned cues.

Several different pharmacological classes of potential medications
have been shown to modulate conditioned drug cues. There is evidence
suggesting that the endogenous opiate system may be involved in the conditioned cues associated with MA administration. In the Anggadiredja et
al. (2004b) study noted earlier, the investigators showed that in rats previously trained to self-administer MA upon association with simultane-
ous presentations of a light and a tone, the opiate antagonist naltrexone
attenuated cue-induced (but not drug-induced) MA-seeking behavior.

Similarly, there is also evidence that the brain endocannabinoid system may be involved in the subjective responses associated with MA.
The cannabinoid antagonist SR141716A (Rimonabant), attenuated both
cue- and MA-induced reinstatement behaviors in rats trained to self-
administer MA (Anggadiredja et al., 2004a). Furthermore, these authors
reported that diclofenac, a cyclooxygenase inhibitor, attenuated cue- and
drug-primed reinstatement in rats. These data provide a rationale for
evaluating cannabinoid antagonists in MA-dependent patient populations.

Several classes of compounds have been shown to antagonize conditioned cues associated with cocaine. It seems reasonable that these
classes of compounds should be investigated for their effects to antago-

nize cues associated with MA, as both drugs ostensibly produce their stimulant effects by increasing synaptic dopamine levels (Wise & Bozarth, 1987). The dopamine D_3 receptor antagonists SB277011A (Gal & Gyertyan, 2006; Cervo et al., 2007), NGB2904, and BP897 inhibit cocaine-cue-induced cocaine-seeking behavior (Gilbert et al., 2005), while the dopamine D_3 receptor antagonist SB277011A (Vorel et al., 2002) and the dopamine D_3 receptor partial agonist BP4.897 (Pilla et al., 1999), respectively, are reported to reduce the effects of conditioned cues on cocaine-induced place preference and cocaine-seeking behavior. SB277011A (Vorel et al., 2002) and NGB2904 (Xi et al., 2006) have also been shown to inhibit cocaine-primed drug-seeking behavior. Xi et al. (2004) also demonstrated that SB277011A inhibited foot-shock-induced reinstatement of cocaine-seeking behavior.

Glutamate antagonists have also been shown to affect response to conditioned cues. Specifically, AMPA antagonists can block cue-induced drug-seeking behavior (Di & Everitt, 2001; Backstrom & Hyytia, 2003).

Another approach to modulating conditioned cues is facilitating cue extinction. Pharmacological enhancement of extinction of a conditioned cue with D-cycloserine, a partial agonist at the NMDA receptor, has been demonstrated in rodents using conditioned fear (Walker et al., 2002; Ledgerwood et al., 2003). Moreover, D-cycloserine has been shown to facilitate fear extinction in patients who suffer from acrophobia (Ressler et al., 2004). D-Cycloserine has also been shown to decrease obsession-related distress in patients with obsessive–compulsive disorder (Kushner et al., 2007). To our knowledge, D-cycloserine has yet to be evaluated as an adjunct to cue extinction in an addicted human population. The utility of facilitating cue extinction in MA abusers may depend on the numbers of conditioned cues that the individuals develop during their years of MA abuse. Extinction of some conditioned cues may be helpful, but the magnitude of the effect may be limited if the individual has multiple specific and contextual cues.

Drug Priming

Drug priming can be operationally defined as the propensity of a drug to increase the drive to obtain it after only having received a single dose. The phenomenon is more robust in dependent or formerly dependent subjects and can be modeled in the animal laboratory by evaluating the effect of a noncontingent dose of drug on drug-seeking behavior or reinstatement.

The premise of altering the priming effects of MA is based on earlier preclinical research showing that decreasing the infusion rate of cocaine results in altered response rates similar to those seen when the unit dose is reduced (Balster & Schuster, 1973). It has been suggested that the pharmacokinetic–pharmacodynamic relationship between drug delivery rate and and reinforcement is an important variable in developing treatments for cocaine dependence (Gorelick, 1998). This hypothesis is just as valid for MA and is the basis for much of the research being funded in this area.

NIDA has funded many of the studies investigating the approach to reducing or eliminating the priming effect of MA by altering its pharmacokinetics, reducing its uptake into the neuron, or altering its interaction with the VMAT2. Altering the pharmacokinetics of MA can be accomplished by generating or administering anti-MA antibodies to bind the drug and thereby prevent it from entering the brain. Such a treatment could conceivably be administered in an emergency department to treat an intoxicated patient, or it could be used during periods of abstinence to prevent drug-induced relapse in a patient who is attempting to remain drug free. Two research groups are investigating immunotherapy to treat MA abuse (Danger et al., 2006; Kosten & Owens, 2005). They conceptualize abused drugs as toxins that must be blocked from accessing neural pathways in the brain and view immunotherapy as pharmacokinetic antagonism.

Mouse monoclonal anti-MA antibodies have been tested in animal models of MA overdose, stimulated locomotor activity, drug discrimination, and self-administration. Pretreatment with a high-affinity anti-MA antibody reduced brain exposure to intravenous MA (Laurenzana et al., 2003; Byrnes-Blake et al., 2003), decreased MA self-administration (McMillan et al., 2004), and reduced MA-induced locomotor activity in rats (Byrnes-Blake et al., 2003, 2005; Gentry et al., 2004). In addition, Daniels et al. (2006) reported that a mouse monoclonal anti-MA antibody blocked the discriminative stimulus effects of MA in pigeons. An interesting consideration is that an anti-MA antibody directed against the amphetamine moiety—that is, it doesn't differentiate between MA and amphetamine—may be useful in treating individuals who abuse designer drugs such as methylenedioxymethamphetamine (MDMA), methylenedioxyamphetamine (MDA), and methylenedioxy-N-ethylamphetamine (MDEA). This is in sharp contrast to the typical immunotherapeutic goal of raising the most highly selective antibody technically possible.

The outlook for immunotherapy as a treatment for abused substances is promising. In contrast to the aforementioned preclinical proof of concept studies for MA abuse, immunotherapy is currently being tested in clinical trials to prevent and treat nicotine addiction and as an aid to smoking cessation. NABI Biopharmaceuticals (Rockville, MD) and Xenova Group Ltd. (Slough, UK) are developing a nicotine conjugate vaccine to stimulate the immune system to produce antibodies that bind to nicotine to prevent it from entering the brain.

Aptamer therapy may provide an alternate approach to limiting brain exposure to abused MA (and other substances). Aptamers are synthetic strands of DNA or RNA with highly specific three-dimensional conformations. They can be designed to manifest appropriate binding affinities and specificities toward chosen target molecules (Patel et al., 1997). In contrast to antibodies, aptamers have very low immunogenicity themselves. The FDA recently approved the first aptamer-based drug to treat a form of age-related macular degeneration (Kourlas & Schiller, 2006).

The ultimate biophase for MA appears to be the VMAT2. Amphetamines enter the neuron via surface biogenic amine neurotransmitter transporters, where they appear to reverse transporter function and compete with endogenous neurotransmitters, as well as regulate their function and expression (Zahniser & Sorkin, 2004; Wilhelm et al., 2006). Once in the neuronal cytoplasm, amphetamines interact with the VMAT2, ultimately resulting in the contents of the neurotransmitter secretory vesicles being released into the neuronal cytoplasm. It has been suggested that this is accomplished by the effect of amphetamines to reverse VMAT2 transport, block VMAT2 transport, or disrupt the gradient between the vesicle and its surroundings (Sulzer & Rayport, 1990; Pifl et al., 1995; Wilhelm et al., 2004; Sulzer et al., 2005). Be that as it may, in dopaminergic neurons the ultimate outcome is an increase in dopamine concentration in the cytoplasm. Moreover, MA is an MAO inhibitor (Robinson, 1985). The increased dopamine can be released into the synaptic cleft via the membrane dopamine transporter (DAT) by reverse transport and thereby activate the mesolimbic brain reward system (Levi & Raiteri, 1993; Kitayama & Sogawa, 2005). Alternatively, it has been suggested that accumulated cytoplasmic dopamine underlies the neurotoxic effects of MA via its conversion to reactive oxygen species and quinones (Giovanni et al., 1995; LaVoie & Hastings, 1999; Fleckenstein & Hanson, 2003; Miyazaki et al., 2006). In that context, cognitive impairment can be considered a consequence of MA neurotoxicity.

In view of evidence that VMAT2 is the primary site of MA action, it would appear to be a logical target for a pharmacotherapeutic drug to treat MA abuse and dependence. Alpha-Lobeline (lobeline) is a nicotinic receptor agonist that has been tested in clinical trials as a smoking cessation agent (reviewed in Dwoskin & Crooks, 2002). Subsequent neurochemical studies revealed that lobeline inhibits dopamine uptake into synaptosomes and HEK-293 cells transfected with the human DAT and, furthermore, inhibits tetrabenazine binding to the VMAT2 (Teng et al., 1997, 1998; Miller et al., 2004). In view of these data, behavioral studies in animals have investigated whether lobeline might have potential as an MA abuse therapeutic. The results were encouraging. Lobeline attenuates MA-induced hyperactivity in mice and antagonized the discriminative stimulus properties of MA in rats (Miller et al., 2001). Lobeline selectively reduces MA self-administration in rats trained to self-administer the stimulant (Harrod et al., 2001). Furthermore, lobeline is not self-administered and does not substitute for MA in rats trained to self-administer the latter (Harrod et al., 2003). Lobeline may also be neuroprotective. Rats treated with lobeline prior to or after a neurotoxic MA dosing regimen showed reduced MA-induced decreases in VMAT2 the day after MA treatment. In addition, MA-induced decreases in dopamine and 5-HT content observed after 7 days were smaller than in rats that were not treated with lobeline. Moreover, these effects of lobeline were independent of effects on MA-induced hyperthermia (Eyerman & Yamamoto, 2005). Yaupon Therapeutics, Inc., (Radnor, PA) and the NIDA Medications Development Program are developing lobeline as a treatment for MA addiction; a phase I study has recently been completed.

Tetrabenazine is a benzoquinolizine derivative that is approved in Europe for treating dyskinesias (Asher & Aminoff, 1981; Jankovic & Orman, 1988). It is a competitive inhibitor at VMAT2 (Scherman & Henry, 1984; Howell et al., 1994; Peter et al., 1996; Thiriot & Ruoho, 2001). The NIDA Addiction Treatment Discovery Program (ATDP) is conducting proof-of-concept testing of tetrabenazine in animals to determine whether it may have potential as an MA abuse therapeutic. Tetrabenazine attenuates MA-stimulated locomotor activity in mice and, in addition, fully antagonizes the discriminative stimulus effects of MA in rats. Further studies are under way to characterize its anti-MA effects more fully. Prestwick Pharmaceuticals (Washington, DC) received approval of their New Drug Application in the United States to market tetrabenazine for Huntington's disease. Tetrabenazine is available for evaluation in a clinical trial for MA abuse.

The D_3 dopamine receptor antagonist SB277011A has been shown to reduce the functional connectivity between the ventral striatum and various brain regions (Schwarz et al., 2007). It follows that treatment of an MA-dependent patient with a D_3 dopamine antagonist might disrupt priming.

Stress-Induced Reinstatement

The foot-shock stress-induced reinstatement model that has been used to study the effect of stress on reinstatement to many drugs of abuse apparently has not been extensively tested with MA. There appeared to be only one paper on this subject in the literature at the time of writing this chapter. Shepard et al. (2004) compared the effects of foot-shock and yohimbine to reinstate MA drug-seeking behavior in rats previously trained to self-administer MA. No published studies were found in which putative pharmacotherapies that might block stress-induced MA-seeking behavior were tested.

MA Dependence Treatment and Cognitive Impairment

A multitude of cognitive deficits in domains that constitute or interact with executive function have been reported in MA users. In consideration of this effect of MA, we propose that cognitive impairments result in higher dropout rates, less effective therapy, and a greater propensity to relapse in abstinent users. An orderly relationship between cognitive impairments and treatment retention has been reported in cocaine users (Aharonovich et al., 2006); thus we postulate that the same relationship will be true for MA users. Moreover, our reading of the literature suggests that the greatest impairment occurs initially during early treatment, when therapy is the most intense (see below). The implication of this is that there may be a temporal mismatch between the learning expected of the patient during therapy and his or her ability to process and retain the new material that constitutes the therapeutic approach.

A comparison of 65 non-treatment-seeking MA users with 65 concurrent controls showed that the MA users had cognitive impairments in several domains (Simon et al., 2000). Specifically, MA users were impaired in word and picture recall, manipulation of information and psychomotor speed, ability to ignore irrelevant stimuli, and abstract thinking. No differences were noted in performance of the Wisconsin Card Sorting Test, however. A follow-up study in a separate cohort of 40 MA-using subjects reported, on average, that the MA users had poorer verbal recall, slower psychomotor speed, less ability to manipulate information, slight impairment on the Stroop Test, worse scores on the Shipley–Hartford tests of vocabulary and abstract thinking; and more errors, perseveration errors, and failure to maintain set on the Wisconsin Card Sorting Test (Simon et al., 2002). Another study of amphetamine users noted deficits in the Wisconsin Card Sorting Test, specifically performance impairment on the extradimensional set-shift task (Ornstein et al., 2000). Of note, a model of attentional set shifting has been developed in rodents. Rats administered an escalating dose regimen of amphetamine sulfate (intraperitoneally from 1 to 5 mg/kg for 5 weeks) demonstrated an inability to shift "rules" in an attentional set-shift paradigm. This acquired deficit in extradimensional set shifting suggests that amphetamine (and, by extension, MA) may produce this type of cognitive deficit (Fletcher et al., 2005, 2007).

A combined neuroimaging and neuropsychology study of 20 MA users and controls noted that the MA users had slower reaction times in tasks that required working memory, for example, sequential number (2-back) test (Chang et al., 2002). In a study where 27 abstinent non-treatment-seeking MA users were compared with controls, deficits in attention/psychomotor speed, learning and memory, verbal fluency, and nonverbal fluency were reported. Fifty-six percent of the MA-using subjects had fluency problems (Kalechstein et al., 2003). Another study compared 87 MA users with 71 controls on the Hopkins Verbal Learning Task—Revised. The MA users displayed deficient learning, recall, and utilization of semantic clustering and also showed higher rates of repetitions and intrusions (Woods et al., 2005). These results are consistent with inefficient strategic control of verbal encoding and retrieval. McKetin and Mattick (1998) also reported that amphetamine users performed worse than controls did on measures of verbal memory, attention/concentration, and delayed recall. A recent comparison of amphetamine users and healthy non-drug-using controls reported that the amphetamine users had significant impairments on the Tower of London test (a strategic thinking task), pattern recognition memory, and paired-association learning (Ersche et al., 2006). Although there was no difference in attentional extradimensional set shifting, the task was novel and the control group had a high failure rate (22%) on this portion of the test. This may have led to a reduced sensitivity to detect group differences.

The deficits in cognition may ameliorate over time. A longitudinal study of MA users has not been reported to date, but two cross-sectional studies of abstinent MA addicts have been. Deficits in psychomotor and verbal tasks performance improve somewhat with 3 to 14 months of abstinence (Volkow et al., 2001). MA users with a mean of 3 years of abstinence (range 3 months to 10 years) performed within the normal range on a neurocognitive battery, although they scored worse on 3 of 12 tasks (Johanson et al., 2006).

Deficits in attention and vigilance have also been reported in MA users. Poor performance on the Stroop Test (Salo et al., 2002), inability to ignore distracting information on a task-switching test (Salo et al., 2005), and impaired vigilance on a continuous performance-monitoring task have been reported (London et al., 2005). Salo et al. (2002) suggest that the inability to ignore irrelevant stimuli may account for the distractability seen in such patients.

Go/no-go tasks have been used to evaluate the effects of acute and chronic stimulant use on reaction time, and results imply inhibition of a prepotent stimulus. Acute administration of cocaine (Fillmore et al.,

2002) and *d*-amphetamine (Fillmore et al., 2003) have been shown to increase stop-signal reaction time (SSRT). Chronic cocaine users also showed a poorer ability to inhibit prepotent responses (Fillmore & Rush, 2002). Li et al. (2006) attribute the deficits in SSRT performance to diminished performance monitoring (which may be the mechanism of the increase in reaction time). Monterosso et al. (2005) also demonstrated that MA users were impaired on the SSRT task.

Cognition and subsequent decision making may be affected by the multifactorial nature of impulsivity. High impulsivity in cocaine-dependent patients, as measured by the Barratt Impulsivity Test, was associated with a higher dropout rate than patients with low impulsivity scores (Moeller et al., 2001). Similarly, in rats, MA administration increases impulsivity on performance tasks (Richards et al., 1999). Increased impulsivity also has been reported in clinical populations of MA users. Semple et al. (2005) reported high impulsivity in a group of 385 MA users that was correlated with moderate to severe depression scores in the Beck Depression Inventory. Impulsivity was associated with MA abuse in a second treatment group of 235 MA users (Simons et al., 2005). One construct recently evaluated is reflection cognition/impulsivity, defined as gathering and reflecting on information before making a decision. Impulsivity is expressed by inadequate reflection and increased errors. Amphetamine users use less information in this task than controls do and have a smaller chance of achieving a correct response (Clark et al., 2006). It seems reasonable to suggest that impulsivity in MA users would result in higher dropout rates and poorer treatment responses. Thus reducing impulsivity by increasing reflection may be a possible pharmacotherapy target for this patient group.

Another form of impulsivity is "delay discounting," that is, the choice of a small, immediate reinforcer versus a larger but temporally delayed reinforcer. Hoffman et al. (2006) reported that greater delay discounting occurred in a group of abstinent patients in treatment for MA dependence than in control subjects. This result was correlated with memory impairment in the MA users. A recent imaging study endeavored to demonstrate a neural basis of delay discounting in MA abusers (Monterosso et al., 2007). Although MA users exhibited the anticipated increase in "delay discounting," no related frontoparietal regional differences were found between the MA abusers and controls by functional magnetic resonance imaging (fMRI) to correlate responses to brain region activation patterns.

Altered decision-making capacity has been reported in MA-using populations. In fact, amphetamine users had similar decision-making deficits as patients with orbital prefrontal cortex lesions (Rogers et al., 1999). Both groups deliberated longer and made suboptimal decisions.

A positron emission tomography (PET) study of current and former amphetamine- and opiate-dependent subjects showed a different activation pattern than non-drug-using controls. Control subjects activated the right dorsolateral prefrontal cortex, whereas the drug users activated the left orbitofrontal cortex (Ersche et al., 2005). The Paulus laboratory has studied MA users in a variety of tasks while using fMRI to correlate responses to brain region activation patterns. MA-using subjects displayed less orbitofrontal, dorsolateral prefrontal, anterior cingulate, and parietal cortex activation during a task, which showed that the MA users were more influenced by previous decision success (Paulus et al., 2002). These investigators subsequently reported that the activation pattern in MA users (undergoing treatment) in a choice procedure was predictive of relapse; specifically, activation of the middle frontal gyrus, middle temporal gyrus, and posterior cingulate predicted time to relapse (Paulus et al., 2005). Another group, using a decision-making task known as the "gambling task," evaluated the performance of patients with ventromedial (VM) lesions, alcohol and stimulant abuse, and normal controls (Bechara et al., 2001). The VM patients had the worst performance relative to controls. The substance abusers were intermediate in their response, with 61% actually overlapping with the range of the VM patients. These results support the hypothesis that decision-making impairments in substance abusers may be associated with VM cortex dysfunction.

These aforementioned reports of neuropsychological effects of long-term amphetamine and MA use support the premise that this patient population may have deficits in multiple domains that would interfere with effective treatment (deficits in attention, working memory, recall, strategic thinking, impulsivity, and decision-making capacity). Perseveration errors (i.e., a deficit and inability to ignore irrelevant stimuli) have also been reported. In view of these data we are proposing the hypothesis that pharmacological remediation of cognitive deficits, improving attention, strengthening inhibitory circuits, enhancing extinction, and increasing ability to learn and retain material would increase retention and treatment efficacy of MA users undergoing treatment. The report by Dackis et al. (2005) in which modafinil was shown to reduce cocaine consumption in cocaine-addicted patient supports this hypothesis.

Modafinil affects multiple cognitive processes that may have salutary effects for treating MA users. Modafinil improved performance on digit span, visual recognition memory, spatial planning, and SSRT in normal volunteers at doses of 100 or 200 mg (Turner et al., 2003). These data suggest that modafinil may inhibit prepotent responses that are consistent with reducing impulsive responding. A follow-up double-blind, placebo-controlled, randomized study in 20 patients with attention-deficit/hyperactivity disorder (ADHD) noted that 200 mg of modafinil had similar effects to those seen in normal volunteers (Turner et al., 2004a). Working memory, visual memory, spatial planning, and SSRT improved; spatial planning accuracy was accompanied by increased response latency, suggesting that modafinil was increasing reflective cognition. In addition, modafinil increased sustained attention in the patients with ADHD. In a double-blind, placebo-controlled, randomized study of 200 mg of modafinil in patients with schizophrenia, increases in digit span and significant correction of the extradimensional set-shift deficit (characteristic of this patient group) were seen (Turner et al., 2004b). Thus modafinil may increase working memory and reflective cognition, sustain attention, correct extradimensional set-shift deficits and reduce impulsive responding. This constellation of provocative cognitive effects provides a strong rationale for evaluating modafinil in MA users.

Other targets may also provide opportunities for moderating attentional set-shifting deficits with pharmacotherapy. The dopamine D_1 receptor agonist SKF38393 reversed amphetamine-induced extradimensional set shifting in a food-seeking paradigm when it was infused into the medial prefrontal cortex of rats (Fletcher et al., 2005). Similarly, the dopamine D_4 receptor antagonist L745,870 improved set shifting in a visual-cue discrimination task when injected directly into the prefrontal cortex (Floresco et al., 2006). The $5\text{-}HT_6$ antagonists SB399885T and SB271046A improved set shifting in a food-seeking paradigm in rodents (Hatcher et al., 2005).

Extinction of conditioned stimuli is a cognitive target that involves strengthening an inhibitory system. Extinction is an active process that involves learning. D-Cycloserine, an NMDA receptor partial agonist, is an antimycobacterial medication that has been shown to enhance the learning process associated with extinction of fear in rats (Walker et al., 2002; Ledgerwood et al., 2003). Moreover, D-cycloserine enhanced extinction to fear of heights in acrophobics undergoing behavior exposure therapy for their phobia (Ressler et al., 2004). Thus, by analogy, medications that enhance NMDA-mediated glutamatergic activity may enhance extinction of conditioned cues to MA in MA users. NIDA is planning to test the utility of his approach. N-Acetylcysteine, a glatathione precursor that affects cystine/glutamate exchange, has been shown to restore glutamate levels in rodents (Baker et al., 2003). This restoration has been shown to both inhibit the self-administration of cocaine and to enhance the rate of extinction of self-administration of cocaine (Kalivas et al., 2005). It seems logical to extend this approach to MA self-administration in rodents to test the rationale for N-acetylcysteine testing in human MA users. Interestingly, N-acetylcysteine has been shown to reverse consolidation deficits in place preference learning in rats treated with MA (Achat-Mendes et al., 2007).

A more general approach to enhancing learning information presented during behavioral therapy could involve the concomitant use of cognitive enhancers during the initial months of therapy. Another approach toward the goal of enhancing learning may be by facilitating alpha-amino-3-hydroxy-5-methyl-4-isoxazolpropionate (AMPA) receptor–mediated transmission. CX516, an "ampakine" that increases glutamate potency at AMPA receptors, has been shown to enhance short-term memory in a delayed sample-to-matching test in rats (Hampson et al., 1998) and also enhance memory and cognition in humans (Danysz, 2002). In rodents, stimulation of AMPA receptors can lead to increased cocaine-seeking behavior on the one hand (Cornish et al., 1999), yet on the other hand AMPA receptor blockade can prevent cocaine-primed reinstatement of self-administration (Cornish & Kalivas, 2000). The utility of ampakines will depend on whether one might have beneficial effects on cognition without increasing MA drug seeking.

Other pharmacological approaches have been reported to enhance memory. Protein kinase C activators such as bryostatin enhance spatial learning in rats (Alkon et al., 2005). Other mechanisms that may find utility in enhancing memory might include carbonic anhydrase activators and selective inverse agonists targeting the alpha$_5$ subtype of GABA$_A$ receptors (reviewed in Amadio et al., 2004).

Compounds that selectively modulate impulsivity might also prove useful for treating MA dependence. The drug with the strongest evidence that supports utility in reducing impulsivity is modafinil (Turner et al., 2003). Quetiapine, a serotoninergic antidepressant, has been shown to reduce impulsivity in patients with borderline personality disorder (Villeneuve & Lemelin, 2005).

Conclusions

The NIDA has utilized a two-pronged strategy for the development of medication for the treatment of MA dependence. The first approach, using marketed medications, has yielded some encouraging positive results. NIDA will be following up on the initial results seen with bupropion and also will attempt to confirm the results of (Tiihonen et al., 2007) with methylphenidate. If confirmatory studies are positive for either medication, clinicians would have immediate access to a safe and well-known therapeutic drug that should be effective in low to moderate MA users as well as in daily users. In addition, immunological and other approaches to altering the pharmacokinetics and distribution of MA have the promise to change the emergency treatment of acute reactions as well as outpatient therapy.

Scientists and clinicians endeavoring to develop medications to treat MA users have surveyed possibilities that arise from modulating the effects of MA directly, to modulating appetitive drives increased by its use, to employing medications that may affect cognitive remediation and improve treatment retention and efficacy. A logical extension of the pharmacotherapeutic approach would involve combining medications that address different mechanisms to determine whether additive effects can be attained.

The interactions of pharmacotherapies and behavioral therapies should be appreciated and approached in a systematic way. The determination of whether a cognitive enhancer improves learning and retention of a behavioral therapy is a natural starting point for such an approach. Assuming that the cognitive enhancer actually helps patients retain material, the next step will be to document the gain in treatment efficacy that would be assumed by the enhancement. Moreover, it is conceivable that a medication may interact selectively with a certain type of behavioral therapy. This has been shown in cocaine users (Poling et al., 2006) and alcohol-dependent patients in clinical trials with naltrexone (O'Malley, 1996). As contingency management has been shown to reduce MA use, it will be of interest to see whether bupropion, which may be effective in its own right, increases the efficacy of the behavioral treatment.

The second approach used by NIDA has been to develop molecular targets from discoveries in the neuropharmacology of MA. This approach has yielded numerous rational medication targets. Assuming that some of these targets will yield useful effective medications, the next challenge will be to determine which medications work most efficiently in which patients. This will likely be accomplished by genotyping and phenotyping patients and determining the correlation of these approaches to treatment response. Hypothesis-driven trials can determine whether changes in the appetitive or cognitive target of interest have a relationship to the proposed reduction or elimination of MA use. Four outcomes are possible. The first is that the medication has the proposed effect but does not reduce MA use. The second is that the medication does not have the proposed effect and does not reduce MA use. The third is that the medication does not have the proposed effect and yet it reduces MA use. The fourth possibility is that the medication has the proposed effect and reduces MA use. Assuming that a temporal or coincidental relationship is found between modulation of some process and efficacy, confirmatory trials will attempt to solidify the utility of matching the patient to the medications. The future prescribing of medications for management of MA abuse, dependence, and its sequelae will then rest on an evidentiary basis.

Medications development for the treatment of MA dependence has progressed rapidly in a short period of time. Confirmatory clinical studies are ongoing for the most promising medications development candidates, bupropion and methylphenidate. Immunologically based therapies may be tested within the next several years. Multiple molecular targets have been discovered that could affect the appetitive processes of cueing, priming, and stress-related increases in drug use. The challenge is to now move the best medication candidates forward that affect these processes and test them in patient populations. Finally, cognitive remediation offers the promise of restoring an individual to a different level of behavior and functioning.

Conflict-of-Interest Declaration

Sources of funding: None. *Connection with tobacco, alcohol, pharmaceutical, or gaming industry:* Frank J. Vocci owns pharmaceutical company stocks that are within the allowable ethical limits of the National Institutes of Health. *Constraints on publishing:* None.

References

Achat-Mendes C, Anderson KL, Itzhak Y. (2007). Impairment in consolidation of learned place preference following dopaminergic neurotoxicity in mice is ameliorated by N-acetylcysteine but not D_1 and D_2 dopamine receptor agonists. *Neuropsychopharmacology* 32:531–541.

Addolorato G, Leggio L, Agabio R, et al. (2006). Baclofen: A new drug for the treatment of alcohol dependence. *Int J Clin Pract* 60:1003–1008.

Aharonovich E, Hasin DS, Brooks AC, et al. (2006). Cognitive deficits predict low treatment retention in cocaine-dependent patients. *Drug Alcohol Depend* 81:313–322.

Alkon DL, Epstein H, Kuzirian A, et al. (2005). Protein synthesis required for long-term memory is induced by PKC activation on days before associative learning. *Proc Natl Acad Sci U.S.A.* 102:16432–16437.

Amadio M, Govoni S, Alkon DL, et al. (2004). Emerging targets for the pharmacology of learning and memory. *Pharmacol Res* 50:111–122.

Anggadiredja K, Nakamichi M, Hiranita T, et al. (2004a). Endocannabinoid system modulates relapse to methamphetamine seeking: Possible mediation by the arachidonic acid cascade. *Neuropsychopharmacology* 29:1470–1478.

Anggadiredja K, Sakimura K, Hiranita T, et al. (2004b). Naltrexone attenuates cue- but not drug-induced methamphetamine seeking: A possible mechanism for the dissociation of primary and secondary reward. *Brain Res* 1021:272–276.

Asher SW, Aminoff MJ. (1981). Tetrabenazine and movement disorders. *Neurology* 31:1051–1054.

Backstrom P, Hyytia P. (2003). Attenuation of cocaine-seeking behavior by the AMPA/kainate receptor antagonist CNQX in rats. *Psychopharmacology* 166:69–76.

Baker DA, McFarland K, Lake RW, et al. (2003). Neuroadaptations in cystine–glutamate exchange underlie cocaine relapse. *Nat Neurosci* 6:743–749.

Balster RL, Schuster CR. (1973). Fixed-interval schedule of cocaine reinforcement: Effect of dose and infusion duration. *J Exp Anal Behav* 20:119–129.

Bechara A, Dolan S, Denburg N, et al. (2001). Decision-making deficits, linked to a dysfunctional ventromedial prefrontal cortex, revealed in alcohol and stimulant abusers. *Neuropsychologia* 39:376–389.

Bonson KR, Grant SJ, Contoreggi CS, et al. (2002). Neural systems and cue-induced cocaine craving. *Neuropsychopharmacology* 26:376–386.

Brodie JD, Figueroa E, Dewey SL. (2003). Treating cocaine addiction: From preclinical to clinical trial experience with gamma-vinyl-GABA. *Synapse* 50:261–265.

Brodie JD, Figueroa E, Laska EM., et al. (2005). Safety and efficacy of gamma-vinyl-GABA (GVG) for the treatment of methamphetamine and/or cocaine addiction. *Synapse* 55:122–125.

Burchfield DJ, Lucas VW, Abrams RM, et al. (1991). Disposition and pharmacodynamics of methamphetamine in pregnant sheep. *JAMA* 265:1968–1973.

Byrnes-Blake KA, Laurenzana EM, Carroll FI, et al. (2003). Pharmacodynamic mechanisms of monoclonal antibody-based antagonism of (+)-methamphetamine in rats. *Eur J Pharmacol* 461:119–128.

Byrnes-Blake KA, Laurenzana EM, Landes RD, et al. (2005). Monoclonal IgG affinity and treatment time alters antagonism of (+)-methamphetamine effects in rats. *Eur J Pharmacol* 521:86–94.

Cervo L, Cocco A, Petrella C, et al. (2007). Selective antagonism at dopamine D_3 receptors attenuates cocaine-seeking behaviour in the rat. *Int J Neuropsychopharmacol* 10:167–181.

Chang L, Ernst T, Speck O, et al. (2002). Perfusion MRI and computerized cognitive test abnormalities in abstinent methamphetamine users. *Psychiatry Res* 114:65–79.

Clark L, Robbins TW, Ersche KD, et al. (2006). Reflection impulsivity in current and former substance users. *Biol Psychiatry* 60:515–522.

Comaish IF, Gorman C, Galloway NR. (2000). Visual field defect associated with vigabatrin: Many more patients may be affected than were found in study. *BMJ* 320:1403.

Cook CE, Jeffcoat AR, Hill JM, et al. (1993). Pharmacokinetics of methamphetamine self-administered to human subjects by smoking S-(+)-methamphetamine hydrochloride. *Drug Metab Dispos* 21:717–723.

Cornish JL, Duffy P, Kalivas PW. (1999). A role for nucleus accumbens gluta-mate transmission in the relapse to cocaine-seeking behavior. *Neurosci-ence* 93:1359–1367.

Cornish JL, Kalivas PW. (2000). Glutamate transmission in the nucleus accum-bens mediates relapse in cocaine addiction. *J Neurosci* 20:RC89.

Dackis CA, Kampman KM, Lynch KG, et al. (2005). A double-blind, placebo-controlled trial of modafinil for cocaine dependence. *Neuropsychophar-macology* 30:205–211.

Danger Y, Gadjou C, Devys A, et al. (2006). Development of murine monoclo-nal antibodies to methamphetamine and methamphetamine analogues. *J Immunol Methods* 309:1–10.

Daniels JR, Wessinger WD, Hardwick WC, et al. (2006). Effects of anti-phen-cyclidine and anti-(+)-methamphetamine monoclonal antibodies alone and in combination on the discrimination of phencyclidine and (+)-metham-phetamine by pigeons. *Psychopharmacology* 185:36–44.

Danysz W. (2002). CX-516 Cortex pharmaceuticals. *Curr Opin Investig Drugs* 3:1081–1088.

Di CG, Bassareo V, Fenu S, et al. (2004). Dopamine and drug addiction: The nucleus accumbens shell connection. *Neuropharmacology* 47(Suppl. 1):227–241.

Di CP, Everitt BJ. (2001). Dissociable effects of antagonism of NMDA and AMPA/KA receptors in the nucleus accumbens core and shell on cocaine-seeking behavior. *Neuropsychopharmacology* 25:341–360.

Dwoskin LP, Crooks PA. (2002). A novel mechanism of action and potential use for lobeline as a treatment for psychostimulant abuse. *Biochem Pharmacol* 63:89–98.

Elkashef AM, Rawson RA, Anderson AL, et al. (2008). Bupropion for the treatment of methamphetamine dependence. *Neuropsychopharmacology* 33:1162–1170.

Erickson JD, Eiden LE, Hoffman BJ. (1992). Expression cloning of a reserpine-sensitive vesicular monoamine transporter. *Proc Natl Acad Sci U.S.A.* 89:10993–10997.

Ersche KD, Clark L, London M, et al. (2006). Profile of executive and memory function associated with amphetamine and opiate dependence. *Neuropsy-chopharmacology* 31:1036–1047.

Ersche KD, Fletcher PC, Lewis SJ, et al. (2005). Abnormal frontal activations related to decision making in current and former amphetamine and opiate dependent individuals. *Psychopharmacology* 180:612–623.

Everitt BJ, Dickinson A, Robbins TW. (2001). The neuropsychological basis of addictive behavior. *Brain Res Brain Res Rev* 36:129–138.

Everitt BJ, Robbins TW. (2000). Second-order schedules of drug reinforcement in rats and monkeys: Measurement of reinforcing efficacy and drug-seek-ing behaviour. *Psychopharmacology* 153:17–30.

Everitt BJ, Wolf ME. (2002). Psychomotor stimulant addiction: A neural sys-tems perspective. *J Neurosci* 22:3312–3320.

Eyerman DJ, Yamamoto BK. (2005). Lobeline attenuates methamphetamine-induced changes in vesicular monoamine transporter 2 immunoreactivity and monoamine depletions in the striatum. *J Pharmacol Exp Ther* 312:160–169.

Fillmore MT, Rush CR. (2002). Impaired inhibitory control of behavior in chronic cocaine users. *Drug Alcohol Depend* 66:265–273.

Fillmore MT, Rush CR, Hays L. (2002). Acute effects of oral cocaine on inhibitory control of behavior in humans. *Drug Alcohol Depend* 67:157–167.

Fillmore MT, Rush CR, Marczinski CA. (2003). Effects of *d*-amphetamine on behavioral control in stimulant abusers: The role of prepotent response tendencies. *Drug Alcohol Depend* 71:143–152.

Fleckenstein AE, Hanson GR. (2003). Impact of psychostimulants on vesicular monoamine transporter function. *Eur J Pharmacol* 479:283–289.

Fleckenstein AE, Volz TJ, Riddle EL, et al. (2007). New insights into the mechanism of action of amphetamines. *Ann Rev Pharmacol Toxicol* 47:681–698.

Fletcher PJ, Tenn CC, Rizos Z, et al. (2005). Sensitization to amphetamine, but not PCP, impairs attentional set shifting: Reversal by a D_1 receptor agonist injected into the medial prefrontal cortex. *Psychopharmacology* 183:190–200.

Fletcher PJ, Tenn CC, Sinyard J, et al. (2007). A sensitizing regimen of amphetamine impairs visual attention in the 5-choice serial reaction time test: Reversal by a D_1 receptor agonist injected into the medial prefrontal cortex. *Neuropsychopharmacology* 32:1122–1132.

Floresco SB, Magyar O, Ghods-Sharifi S, et al. (2006). Multiple dopamine receptor subtypes in the medial prefrontal cortex of the rat regulate set shifting. *Neuropsychopharmacology* 31:297–309.

Gal K, Gyertyan I. (2006). Dopamine D_3 as well as D_2 receptor ligands attenuate the cue-induced cocaine-seeking in a relapse model in rats. *Drug Alcohol Depend* 81:63–70.

Gentry WB, Ghafoor AU, Wessinger WD, et al. (2004). (+)-Methamphetamine-induced spontaneous behavior in rats depends on route of (+)METH administration. *Pharmacol Biochem Behav* 79:751–760.

Gilbert JG, Newman AH, Gardner EL, et al. (2005). Acute administration of SB-277011A, NGB 2904, or BP 897 inhibits cocaine cue-induced reinstatement of drug-seeking behavior in rats: Role of dopamine D_3 receptors. *Synapse* 57:17–28.

Giovanni A, Liang LP, Hastings TG, et al. (1995). Estimating hydroxyl radical content in rat brain using systemic and intraventricular salicylate: Impact of methamphetamine. *J Neurochem* 64:1819–1825.

Gorelick DA. (1998). The rate hypothesis and agonist substitution approaches to cocaine abuse treatment. *Adv Pharmacol* 42:995–997.

Grant S, London ED, Newlin DB, et al. (1996). Activation of memory circuits during cue-elicited cocaine craving. *Proc Natl Acad Sci U.S.A.* 93:12040–12045.

Hampson RE, Rogers G, Lynch G, et al. (1998). Facilitative effects of the ampakine CX516 on short-term memory in rats: Correlations with hippocampal neuronal activity. *J Neurosci* 18:2748–2763.

Harris DS, Boxenbaum H, Everhart ET, et al. (2003). The bioavailability of intranasal and smoked methamphetamine. *Clin Pharmacol Ther* 74:475–486.

Harrod SB, Dwoskin LP, Crooks PA, et al. (2001). Lobeline attenuates *d*-methamphetamine self-administration in rats. *J Pharmacol Exp Ther* 298:172–179.

Harrod SB, Dwoskin LP, Green TA, et al. (2003). Lobeline does not serve as a reinforcer in rats. *Psychopharmacology* 165:397–404.

Hatcher PD, Brown VJ, Tait DS, et al. (2005). 5-HT$_6$ receptor antagonists improve performance in an attentional set-shifting task in rats. *Psychopharmacology* 181:253–259.

Heinzerling KG, Shoptaw S, Peck JA, et al. (2006). Randomized, placebo-controlled trial of baclofen and gabapentin for the treatment of methamphetamine dependence. *Drug Alcohol Depend* 85:177–184.

Hoffman WF, Moore M, Templin R, et al. (2006). Neuropsychological function and delay discounting in methamphetamine-dependent individuals. *Psychopharmacology* 188:162–170.

Howell M, Shirvan A, Stern-Bach Y, et al. (1994). Cloning and functional expression of a tetrabenazine sensitive vesicular monoamine transporter from bovine chromaffin granules. *FEBS Lett* 338:16–22.

Jankovic J, Orman J. (1988). Tetrabenazine therapy of dystonia, chorea, tics, and other dyskinesias. *Neurology* 38:391–394.

Jayaram-Lindstrom N, Wennberg P, Hurd YL, et al. (2004). Effects of naltrexone on the subjective response to amphetamine in healthy volunteers. *J Clin Psychopharmacol* 24:665–669.

Johanson CE, Frey KA, Lundahl LH, et al. (2006). Cognitive function and nigrostriatal markers in abstinent methamphetamine abusers. *Psychopharmacology* 185(3):327–338.

Johnson BA. (2004). Uses of topiramate in the treatment of alcohol dependence. *Expert Rev Neurother* 4:751–758.

Johnson BA, Ait-Daoud N, Akhtar FZ, et al. (2005). Use of oral topiramate to promote smoking abstinence among alcohol-dependent smokers: A randomized controlled trial. *Arch Intern Med* 165:1600–1605.

Johnson BA, Roache JD, Ait-Daoud N, et al. (2007a). Effects of acute topiramate dosing on methamphetamine-induced subjective mood. *Int J Neuropsychopharmacol* 10:85–98.

Johnson BA, Roache JD, Ait-Daoud N, et al. (2007b). Effects of topiramate on methamphetamine-induced changes in attentional and perceptual-motor skills of cognition in recently abstinent methamphetamine-dependent individuals. *Prog Neuropsychopharmacol Biol Psychiatry* 31:123–130.

Jung MJ, Lippert B, Metcalf BW, et al. (1977). gamma-Vinyl-GABA (4-aminohex-5-enoic acid), a new selective irreversible inhibitor of GABA-T: Effects on brain GABA metabolism in mice. *J Neurochem* 29:797–802.

Kalechstein AD, Newton TF, Green M. (2003). Methamphetamine dependence is associated with neurocognitive impairment in the initial phases of abstinence. *J Neuropsychiatry Clin Neurosci* 15:215–220.

Kalivas P, Moran M, Melendez R, et al. (2005, December). Regulating glu-tamate homeostasis in treating cocaine addiction. Paper presented at the annual ACNP meeting, Waikoloa, Hawaii.

Kampman KM, Pettinati H, Lynch KG, et al. (2004). A pilot trial of topiramate for the treatment of cocaine dependence. *Drug Alcohol Depend* 75:233–240.

Kitayama S, Sogawa C. (2005). Regulated expression and function of the soma-todendritic catecholamine neurotransmitter transporters. *J Pharmacol Sci* 99:121–127.

Kosten T, Owens SM. (2005). Immunotherapy for the treatment of drug abuse. *Pharmacol Ther* 108:76–85.

Kourlas H, Schiller DS. (2006). Pegaptanib sodium for the treatment of neo-vascular age-related macular degeneration: A review. *Clin Ther* 28:36–44.

Kushner MG, Kim SW, Donahue C, et al. (2007). D-Cycloserine augmented exposure therapy for obsessive–compulsive disorder. *Biol Psychiatry* 62:833–838.

Laurenzana EM, Byrnes-Blake KA, Milesi-Halle A, et al. (2003). Use of anti-(+)-methamphetamine monoclonal antibody to significantly alter (+)-meth-amphetamine and (+)-amphetamine disposition in rats. *Drug Metab Dis-pos* 31:1320–1326.

LaVoie MJ, Hastings TG. (1999). Dopamine quinone formation and protein modification associated with the striatal neurotoxicity of methamphet-amine: Evidence against a role for extracellular dopamine. *J Neurosci* 19:1484–1491.

Ledgerwood L, Richardson R, Cranney J. (2003). Effects of D-cycloserine on extinction of conditioned freezing. *Behav Neurosci* 117:341–349.

Levi G, Raiteri M. (1993). Carrier-mediated release of neurotransmitters. *Trends Neurosci* 16:415–419.

Li CS, Milivojevic V, Kemp K, et al. (2006). Performance monitoring and stop-signal inhibition in abstinent patients with cocaine dependence. *Drug Alcohol Depend* 85:205–212.

London ED, Berman SM, Voytek B, et al. (2005). Cerebral metabolic dysfunc-tion and impaired vigilance in recently abstinent methamphetamine abus-ers. *Biol Psychiatry* 58:770–778.

McKetin R, Mattick RP. (1998). Attention and memory in illicit amphetamine users: Comparison with non-drug-using controls. *Drug Alcohol Depend* 50:181–184.

McMillan DE, Hardwick WC, Li M, et al. (2004). Effects of murine-derived anti-methamphetamine monoclonal antibodies on (+)-methamphetamine self-administration in the rat. *J Pharmacol Exp Ther* 309:1248–1255.

Mendelson J, Jones RT, Upton R, et al. (1995). Methamphetamine and ethanol interactions in humans. *Clin Pharmacol Ther* 57:559–568.

Miller DK, Crooks PA, Teng L, et al. (2001). Lobeline inhibits the neuro-chemical and behavioral effects of amphetamine. *J Pharmacol Exp Ther* 296:1023–1034.

Miller DK, Crooks PA, Zheng G, et al. (2004). Lobeline analogs with enhanced affinity and selectivity for plasmalemma and vesicular monoamine transporters. *J Pharmacol Exp Ther* 310:1035–1045.

Miyazaki I, Asanuma M, Diaz-Corrales FJ, et al. (2006). Methamphetamine-induced dopaminergic neurotoxicity is regulated by quinone-formation-related molecules. *FASEB J* 20:571–573.

Moeller FG, Dougherty DM, Barratt ES, et al. (2001). The impact of impulsivity on cocaine use and retention in treatment. *J Subst Abuse Treat* 21:193–198.

Monterosso JR, Ainslie G, Xu J, et al. (2007). Frontoparietal cortical activity of methamphetamine-dependent and comparison subjects performing a delay discounting task. *Hum Brain Mapp* 28:383–393.

Monterosso JR, Aron AR, Cordova X, et al. (2005). Deficits in response inhibition associated with chronic methamphetamine abuse. *Drug Alcohol Depend* 79:273–277.

Nanavati SM, Silverman RB. (1989). Design of potential anticonvulsant agents: Mechanistic classification of GABA aminotransferase inactivators. *J Med Chem* 32:2413–2421.

Newton TF, Roache JD, De La GR, et al. (2006). Bupropion reduces methamphetamine-induced subjective effects and cue-induced craving. *Neuropsychopharmacology* 31:1537–1544.

O'Brien CP, Gardner EL. (2005). Critical assessment of how to study addiction and its treatment: Human and non-human animal models. *Pharmacol Ther* 108:18–58.

O'Malley SS. (1996). Opioid antagonists in the treatment of alcohol dependence: Clinical efficacy and prevention of relapse. *Alcohol Alcohol Suppl* 31(Suppl. 1):77–81.

Ornstein TJ, Iddon JL, Baldacchino AM, et al. (2000). Profiles of cognitive dysfunction in chronic amphetamine and heroin abusers. *Neuropsychopharmacology* 23:113–126.

Palfreyman MG, Schechter PJ, Buckett WR, et al. (1981). The pharmacology of GABA-transaminase inhibitors. *Biochem Pharmacol* 30:817–824.

Patel DJ, Suri AK, Jiang F, et al. (1997). Structure, recognition, and adaptive binding in RNA aptamer complexes. *J Mol Biol* 272:645–664.

Paulus MP, Hozack NE, Zauscher BE, et al. (2002). Behavioral and functional neuroimaging evidence for prefrontal dysfunction in methamphetamine-dependent subjects. *Neuropsychopharmacology* 26:53–63.

Paulus MP, Tapert SF, Schuckit MA. (2005). Neural activation patterns of methamphetamine-dependent subjects during decision making predict relapse. *Arch Gen Psychiatry* 62:761–768.

Peter D, Vu T, Edwards RH. (1996). Chimeric vesicular monoamine transporters identify structural domains that influence substrate affinity and sensitivity to tetrabenazine. *J Biol Chem* 271:2979–2986.

Pierce RC, Kumaresan V. (2006). The mesolimbic dopamine system: The final common pathway for the reinforcing effect of drugs of abuse? *Neurosci Biobehav Rev* 30:215–238.

Pifl C, Drobny H, Reither H, et al. (1995). Mechanism of the dopamine-releasing actions of amphetamine and cocaine: Plasmalemmal dopamine transporter versus vesicular monoamine transporter. *Mol Pharmacol* 47:368–373.

Pilla M, Perachon S, Sautel F, et al. (1999). Selective inhibition of cocaine-seeking behaviour by a partial dopamine D_3 receptor agonist. *Nature* 400:371–375.

Poling J, Oliveto A, Petry N, et al. (2006). Six-month trial of bupropion with contingency management for cocaine dependence in a methadone-maintained population. *Arch Gen Psychiatry* 63:219–228.

Rawson RA, Condon TP. (2007). Why do we need an *Addiction* supplement focused on methamphetamine? *Addiction* 102(Suppl. 1):1–4.

Ressler KJ, Rothbaum BO, Tannenbaum L, et al. (2004). Cognitive enhancers as adjuncts to psychotherapy: Use of D-cycloserine in phobic individuals to facilitate extinction of fear. *Arch Gen Psychiatry* 61:1136–1144.

Richards JB, Sabol KE, de Wit H. (1999). Effects of methamphetamine on the adjusting amount procedure: A model of impulsive behavior in rats. *Psychopharmacology* 146:432–439.

Riviere GJ, Gentry WB, Owens SM. (2000). Disposition of methamphetamine and its metabolite amphetamine in brain and other tissues in rats after intravenous administration. *J Pharmacol Exp Ther* 292:1042–1047.

Robinson JB. (1985). Stereoselectivity and isoenzyme selectivity of monoamine oxidase inhibitors: Enantiomers of amphetamine, N-methylamphetamine and deprenyl. *Biochem Pharmacol* 34:4105–4108.

Rogers RD, Everitt BJ, Baldacchino A, et al. (1999). Dissociable deficits in the decision-making cognition of chronic amphetamine abusers, opiate abusers, patients with focal damage to prefrontal cortex, and tryptophan-depleted normal volunteers: Evidence for monoaminergic mechanisms. *Neuropsychopharmacology* 20:322–339.

Salo R, Nordahl TE, Moore C, et al. (2005). A dissociation in attentional control: Evidence from methamphetamine dependence. *Biol Psychiatry* 57:310–313.

Salo R, Nordahl TE, Possin K, et al. (2002). Preliminary evidence of reduced cognitive inhibition in methamphetamine-dependent individuals. *Psychiatry Res* 111:65–74.

Scherman D, Henry JP. (1984). Reserpine binding to bovine chromaffin granule membranes: Characterization and comparison with dihydrotetrabenazine binding. *Mol Pharmacol* 25:113–122.

Schwarz AJ, Gozzi A, Reese T, et al. (2007). Pharmacological modulation of functional connectivity: The correlation structure underlying the phMRI response to d-amphetamine modified by selective dopamine D_3 receptor antagonist SB277011A. *Magn Reson Imaging* 25:811–820.

Semple SJ, Zians J, Grant I, et al. (2005). Impulsivity and methamphetamine use. *J Subst Abuse Treat* 29:85–93.

Shepard JD, Bossert JM, Liu SY, et al. (2004). The anxiogenic drug yohimbine reinstates methamphetamine seeking in a rat model of drug relapse. *Biol Psychiatry* 55:1082–1089.

Simon SL, Domier C, Carnell J, et al. (2000). Cognitive impairment in individuals currently using methamphetamine. *Am J Addict* 9:222–231.

Simon SL, Domier CP, Sim T, et al. (2002). Cognitive performance of current methamphetamine and cocaine abusers. *J Addict Dis* 21:61–74.

Simons JS, Oliver MN, Gaher RM, et al. (2005). Methamphetamine and alcohol abuse and dependence symptoms: Associations with affect lability and impulsivity in a rural treatment population. *Addict Behav* 30:1370–1381.

Sulzer D, Rayport, S. (1990). Amphetamine and other psychostimulants reduce pH gradients in midbrain dopaminergic neurons and chromaffin granules: A mechanism of action. *Neuron* 5:797–808.

Sulzer D, Sonders MS, Poulsen NW, et al. (2005). Mechanisms of neurotransmitter release by amphetamines: A review. *Prog Neurobiol* 75:406–433.

Teng L, Crooks PA, Dwoskin LP. (1998). Lobeline displaces [^{3}H]dihydrotetrabenazine binding and releases [^{3}H]dopamine from rat striatal synaptic vesicles: Comparison with *d*-amphetamine. *J Neurochem* 71:258–265.

Teng L, Crooks PA, Sonsalla PK, et al. (1997). Lobeline and nicotine evoke [^{3}H] overflow from rat striatal slices preloaded with [^{3}H]dopamine: Differential inhibition of synaptosomal and vesicular [^{3}H]dopamine uptake. *J Pharmacol Exp Ther* 280:1432–1444.

Thiriot DS, Ruoho AE. (2001). Mutagenesis and derivatization of human vesicle monoamine transporter 2 (VMAT2) cysteines identifies transporter domains involved in tetrabenazine binding and substrate transport. *J Biol Chem* 276:27304–27315.

Tiihonen J, Kuoppasalmi K, Fohr J, et al. (2007). A comparison of aripiprazole, methylphenidate, and placebo for amphetamine dependence. *Am J Psychiatry* 164:160–162.

Turner DC, Clark L, Dowson J, et al. (2004a). Modafinil improves cognition and response inhibition in adult attention-deficit/hyperactivity disorder. *Biol Psychiatry* 55:1031–1040.

Turner DC, Clark L, Pomarol-Clotet E, et al. (2004b). Modafinil improves cognition and attentional set shifting in patients with chronic schizophrenia. *Neuropsychopharmacology* 29:1363–1373.

Turner DC, Robbins TW, Clark L, et al. (2003). Cognitive enhancing effects of modafinil in healthy volunteers. *Psychopharmacology* 165:260–269.

Villeneuve E, Lemelin S. (2005). Open-label study of atypical neuroleptic quetiapine for treatment of borderline personality disorder: impulsivity as main target. *J Clin Psychiatry* 66:1298–1303.

Vocci FJ, Appel NM. (2007). Approaches to the development of medications for the treatment of methamphetamine dependence. *Addiction* 102(Suppl. 1):96–106.

Volkow ND, Chang L, Wang GJ, et al. (2001). Loss of dopamine transporters in methamphetamine abusers recovers with protracted abstinence. *J Neurosci* 21:9414–9418.

Vorel SR, Ashby CR, Jr, Paul M, et al. (2002). Dopamine D$_3$ receptor antagonism inhibits cocaine-seeking and cocaine-enhanced brain reward in rats. *J Neurosci* 22:9595–9603.

Walker DL, Ressler KJ, Lu KT, et al. (2002). Facilitation of conditioned fear extinction by systemic administration or intra-amygdala infusions of D-cycloserine as assessed with fear-potentiated startle in rats. *J Neurosci* 22:2343–2351.

Weihe E, Eiden LE. (2000). Chemical neuroanatomy of the vesicular amine transporters. *FASEB J* 14:2435–2449.

Wilhelm CJ, Johnson RA, Eshleman AJ, et al. (2006). Hydrogen ion concentration differentiates effects of methamphetamine and dopamine on transporter-mediated efflux. *J Neurochem* 96:1149–1159.

Wilhelm CJ, Johnson RA, Lysko PG, et al. (2004). Effects of methamphetamine and lobeline on vesicular monoamine and dopamine transporter-mediated dopamine release in a cotransfected model system. *J Pharmacol Exp Ther* 310:1142–1151.

Wilton LV, Stephens MD, Mann RD. (1999). Visual field defect associated with vigabatrin: Observational cohort study. *BMJ* 319:1165–1166.

Wise RA, Bozarth MA. (1987). A psychomotor stimulant theory of addiction. *Psychol Rev* 94:469–492.

Woods SP, Rippeth JD, Conover E, et al. (2005). Deficient strategic control of verbal encoding and retrieval in individuals with methamphetamine dependence. *Neuropsychology* 19:35–43.

Xi ZX, Gilbert J, Campos AC, et al. (2004). Blockade of mesolimbic dopamine D_3 receptors inhibits stress-induced reinstatement of cocaine-seeking in rats. *Psychopharmacology* 176:57–65.

Xi ZX, Newman AH, Gilbert JG, et al. (2006). The novel dopamine D_3 receptor antagonist NGB2904 inhibits cocaine's rewarding effects and cocaine-induced reinstatement of drug-seeking behavior in rats. *Neuropsychopharmacology* 31:1393–1405.

Xie T, McCann UD, Kim S, et al. (2000). Effect of temperature on dopamine transporter function and intracellular accumulation of methamphetamine: Implications for methamphetamine-induced dopaminergic neurotoxicity. *J Neurosci* 20:7838–7845.

Zaczek R, Culp S, De Souza EB. (1991a). Interactions of [³H]amphetamine with rat brain synaptosomes: II. Active transport. *J Pharmacol Exp Ther* 257:830–835.

Zaczek R, Culp S, Goldberg H, et al. (1991b). Interactions of [³H]amphetamine with rat brain synaptosomes: I. Saturable sequestration. *J Pharmacol Exp Ther* 257:820–829.

Zahniser NR, Sorkin A. (2004). Rapid regulation of the dopamine transporter: Role in stimulant addiction? *Neuropharmacology* 47(Suppl. 1)80–91.

Chapter 12

Treatment of Methamphetamine Addiction That Co-Occurs with Serious Mental Illness

Jagoda Pasic and Richard Ries

Co-occurring severe mental illness and substance abuse is a major public health problem. From the late 1970s clinicians have recognized that the presence of substance abuse/dependence in combination with mental illness had profound implications for patients, health care systems, and social and treatment outcomes. The treatment of co-occurring substance and mental disorders is challenging, and the integration of substance abuse treatment and mental health services for persons with co-occurring disorders has become a major treatment initiative (U.S. Department of Health and Human Services, 2005). There are special challenges when severely mentally ill persons abuse psychostimulants since these substances are so potent in causing or amplifying major psychiatric symptoms, thus confounding both diagnosis and treatment. The Center for Substance Abuse Treatment's (CSAT) Treatment Improvement Protocol (U.S. Department of Health and Human Services, 1998) has outlined the knowledge about treatment effectiveness in stimulant users, including methamphetamine (MA) users; however, the clinical presentation and treatment of MA addiction and co-occurring severe mental illness have not been well studied or described. This chapter summarizes the limited research available as well as its implications.

Serious mental illness (SMI) generally refers to the psychiatric diagnoses of schizophrenia, schizoaffective disorder, bipolar disorder, and recurrent major depression, and further implies that these illnesses are persistent or recurrent and cause functional impairment. Co-occurrence between drug abuse/dependence and SMI is very common. Estimates from different sources suggest that 20–65% of persons suffering from SMI are currently using, or have recently used, recreational drugs (Bellack & DiClemente, 1999). Approximately 50% of individuals with SMI suffer from a diagnosable substance abuse disorder at some point during their lives (Regier et al., 1990). In addition, almost half of the individuals who have a current addictive disorder have a co-occurring mental disorder. As discussed by Kessler at al. (1996), some of the co-occurring disorders are considered to be organic brain syndromes caused by the effects of substances. However, they argue that the temporal relationships between these disorders suggest that most of them are primary independent disorders that did not cause one another.

Patients with co-occurring disorders have been observed in both mental health treatment settings and addiction treatment settings (U.S. Department of Health and Human Services, 2002, 2005). It has often been assumed that the substance abuse problems of psychiatric patients are less severe than those of patients in substance abuse treatment and, similarly, that the mental disorders of patients receiving substance abuse treatment are less severe than those of psychiatric patients. However, Havassy et al. (2004) compared the patients with comorbid illness in mental health and drug treatment settings and found high prevalence of SMI in drug treatment clients and serious drug problems in mental health patients. They reported one diagnostic difference between the groups: schizophrenia spectrum disorders were more common among mental health patients than among drug treatment patients (43 vs. 31%).

Prevalence of MA and SMI has not been well delineated in the literature. There are no epidemiological data on the prevalence of MA and SMI since the recent MA epidemic. Our small sample study of MA users in the psychiatric emergency services showed high rates (43%) of previous psychiatric diagnoses: depression (23%), bipolar disorder (13%), and schizophrenia 6%) (Pasic et al., 2007). An Australian Emergency Department study reported comorbidity of depression (17%) and schizophrenia (8%) in their sample of patients with amphetamine-related presentations (Gray et al., 2007). Havassy et al. (2004) reported no difference in prevalence of comorbid mental disorder and amphetamine use disorders in the mental health treatment centers (25%) compared with substance abuse treatment settings (15%, OR = 0.60, 95% CI 0.30–1.19). High rates of psychiatric comorbidity were reported in a forensic sample of MA-dependent individuals (Kalechstein et al., 2000). In particular, the authors reported that MA-dependent individuals were more likely to endorse a syndrome consisting of depression (57%) and suicidal ideations (49%) in the 12 months prior to their interview. Data from the Methamphetamine Treatment Project also reported that MA users had high levels of depression, anxiety, and psychotic symptoms, and 27% of the sample attempted suicide in their lifetime (Zweben et al., 2004). However, in this study the authors used a Brief Symptom Inventory instrument rather than a specific DSM-IVTR diagnosis. Although there are no data exploring the association between MA use and bipolar disorder, a number of studies found that depression was both a symptom and a syndrome among MA abusers during active use, withdrawal, early abstinence, and prolonged abstinence (Simon et al., 2000; Cho & Melega, 2002). A strong relationship between major depression disorder was found in female adolescents with methamphetamine use; however, the association was not demonstrated in multivariate analysis (Yen & Chong, 2006). There were no reports on comorbidity with bipolar disorder or schizophrenia. Data from a Taiwanese sample of incarcerated MA abusers showed similar rates of mood disorders between male (9%) and female (11%) subjects (Lin et al., 2004).

Individuals who suffer from both debilitating substance use disorders and serious mental illnesses are typically more difficult to treat than those suffering from only one of these disorders (Bellack & DiClemente, 1999; Dixon, 1999; Drake & Mueser, 2001). Relative to non-substance-abusing persons with SMI, persons suffering from substance use disorders and comorbid SMI tend to have increased psychotic symptoms (Dixon, 1999), poorer treatment compliance (Bennett et al., 2001), poorer medication adherence (Hudson et al., 2004), poorer response to antipsychotic treatment (Green et al., 2004), diminished abilities to manage their financial resources (Ries & Dyck, 1997), increased cognitive impairment (Jackson et al., 2001), poor housing circumstances (Galanter et al., 1998), high rates of HIV infection (RachBiesel et al., 1999) and related risk behaviors (Carey et al., 1997), and to be both perpetrators and victims of violence (Bennett et al., 2001). They also make greater use of community medical services such as emergency rooms (Dixon, 1999) and are more likely to leave an inpatient setting against medical advice (Pages et al., 1998). As an unfortunate aside, being female tends to further exacerbate the observed relationship between substance abuse and SMI. Females are more likely to be victimized and have more medical complaints, including HIV, than do males (Brunette & Drake, 1997). We can extrapolate the above negative outcomes to individuals with MA addiction and co-occurring SMI because the above studies did not specifically address this population. Some insight can be gained from the research involving cocaine use and SMI. For example cocaine use has been found to worsen the clinical course of schizophrenia by exacerbating many of the symptoms of the disorder resulting in relapse and increased need for hospitalization (Brady et al., 1990). Future studies will show whether adding treatment programs in metal health centers with a specific focus on individuals with MA addiction and co-occurring SMI will have a more desirable outcome on individual health and psychosocial issues.

Individuals with both substance use disorders and schizophrenia spectrum diagnoses, while being admitted with higher levels of symptoms, seem to stabilize more quickly than those with schizophrenia alone during acute hospitalizations (Ries et al., 2000). The authors hypothesized this was likely due to (1) an interruption of these patients' supply of substances (i.e., rapid decrease in substance-induced or amplified psychotic symptoms) and (2) the possibility that patients with both schizophrenia and substance use disorders may have better-prognosis-type schizophrenia in the first place. This suggests that treating the substance abuse of this population may have significant recovery benefit for both substance abuse and schizophrenic or other SMI, an observation also made by Dixon et al. (1998) more broadly in substance use disorders and SMI outpatients.

Empirical Review
of the Co-Occurring Disorder Treatments with Reference to MA

Most individuals who have co-occurring disorders need treatment for both their mental illness and their substance use problems. The delivery of appropriate treatment has been a challenge. Individuals with dual diagnosis use mental health and substance abuse treatment services more frequently than persons with only one disorder. However, most report having received no mental health or substance abuse treatment in the previous year (Narrow et al., 1993). According to a national survey of care for persons with co-occurring mental health and substance use disorders despite available and effective treatment options, most individuals do not receive effective treatment (Watkins et al., 2001). The primary modality of treatment of MA-use disorders is behavioral; most data focus on the effectiveness of community-based treatment programs utilizing the matrix model (Rawson et al., 2002a). Recently preliminary data have been published on the use of contingency management techniques for the treatment of MA-use disorders (Roll et al., 2006; Rawson et al., 2006; Shoptaw et al., 2006). Although contingency management, which is based on the principles of operant conditioning, has a long history of use in the treatment of individuals with SMI, to date there are no published data on the use of behavioral or psychosocial modes for the treatment of MA addiction and co-occurring SMI. Our research group has recently received a grant to study contingency management intervention in SMI patients with comorbid MA abuse/addiction. Other studies are likely to be developed in the near future as the research in this field continues to grow.

Pharmacological Agents

Data are limited with regard to pharmacological interventions in the treatment of MA-use disorders. Currently there are no FDA-approved medications for the treatment of MA dependence. As discussed in Chapter 11, a number of different compounds are being tested, such as recent trials with selegeline (Newton et al., 2005), bupropion (Newton et al., 2006), baclofen (Heinzerling et al., 2006), modafinil (Ling et al., 2006), rivastigmine (National Institute on Drug Abuse [NIDA], 2006b), and topiramate (Johnson et al., 2007). These and other clinical trials included individuals without comorbid mental illness; however, if the medications prove to be beneficial, they may find their use in MA users with co-occurring SMI.

Although there are no FDA-approved medications for the treatment of MA-use disorders and SMI, clinicians tend to use available psychotropic agents to reduce symptoms of underlying mental disorders. Given that comorbidity of major depression and MA addiction has the highest prevalence, it would be reasonable to consider antidepressants, particularly those that have shown promising results in the treatment of MA addiction, such as selegeline (Newton et al., 2005), an MAO-B inhibitor that increases dopaminergic neurotransmission, which is thought to be impaired in MA addiction. Mirtazapine, a noradrenergic and specific serotonergic antidepressant, is another candidate. A phase II clinical trial is under way to test the efficacy of mirtazapine in reducing MA use in homosexual men (NIDA, 2007). If it proves to be helpful, mirtazapine might be an option for the treatment of MA addiction comorbid with major depression or depressive disorders. A theoretical approach might involve using bupropion both for treating depression and for its possible effectiveness in treating attention-deficit/hyperactivity disorder (ADHD) (Levin et al., 2002). Bupropion is an antidepressant that inhibits the reuptake of dopamine and norepinephrine and enhances dopamine neurotransmission, effects that may ameliorate addiction, depression, and concentration in chronic MA use. Currently, an NIDA-sponsored pilot study is under way on citicholine, a supplement, for the treatment of depression in bipolar disorder or major depression and comorbid amphetamine abuse/dependence (NIDA, 2006a).

Second-generation antipsychotics are often used in clinical practice for the treatment of schizophrenia comorbid with MA addiction, although there are no FDA-approved agents. Case studies have shown that olanzapine (Misra et al., 2000) and risperidone (Misra & Kofoed, 1997) are effective in reducing symptoms of MA-induced psychosis, suggesting that they may be useful in the treatment of patients with schizophrenia and comorbid MA addiction. In our study of MA users in psychiatric emergency services we found that acutely MA-intoxicated patients who were treated with orally disintegrating tablets (ODT), most often olanzapine, accepted the care and referral to outpatient chemical dependency next-day appointment (Pasic et al., 2007). This procedure suggests that medicating acutely MA-intoxicated patients with antipsychotic medications, such as ODT, may be viewed as the first step in a needed chemical dependency treatment. Given that 19% of patients in this sample had comorbid bipolar disorder and schizophrenia, we might speculate that this treatment would benefit the patients with MA intoxication and SMI. However, future placebo-controlled studies would need to confirm this. An NIDA-sponsored study is currently under way with aripiprazole (NIDA, 2005a), and risperidone and quetiapine are being tested for MA-use disorders comorbid with both schizophrenia (NIDA, 2006c) and bipolar disorder (NIDA, 2005b). In addition, atypical antipsychotics have been shown to improve cognitive function in schizophrenia, so there is a potential for future studies to investigate whether cognitive deficits that arise from chronic MA abuse can be improved in individuals with SMI (Wieckert et al., 2003).

In a recent publication, Camacho and Akiskal (2005)proposed a bipolar–stimulant spectrum in which subthreshold bipolar traits are complicated by stimulant abuse, eventually leading to pathology characteristic of both disorders. They argue that the contribution of bipolarity to this spectrum is supported by premorbid cyclothymic and hyperthymic traits, familial bipolarity, and presence of subthreshold bipolar signs and symptoms during protracted sobriety, and that anticonvulsants/mood stabilizers in this spectrum treat the acute escalation of activated and mixed depressive states, withdrawal symptoms, and craving for the stimulant. This is an interesting and provocative proposal, but until evidence-based data are available, it justifies the rationale for off-label use of anticonvulsants such as lamotrigine, oxcarbazepine, topiramate, and valproate for the treatment of MA-use disorders and comorbid bipolar disorder(s). The initial data on the use of gabapentin for the treatment of MA dependence showed disappointing results (Ling et al., 2006), so it is less promising that gabapentin would be beneficial in treating patients with bipolar disorder and MA addiction.

Information regarding the treatment of MA addiction that might apply to the treatment of co-occurring disorders may be gained from cocaine treatment and trials with pharmacological agents. Case reports and uncontrolled studies suggest that clozapine (Yovell & Opler, 1994; Drake et al., 2000), olanzapine (Tsuang et al., 2002), and risperidone (Smelson et al., 2002) reduce craving and use of cocaine in patients with schizophrenia. Other agents that have been identified as potentially useful in reducing cocaine use include disulfiram, naltraxone, baclofen, topiramate, and modafinil (Vocci et al., 2002), and future studies will determine their applicability for the treatment of MA addiction in individuals with SMI.

Psychosocial Interventions

Although in this section we discuss in more detail pharmacological interventions, summarized in Table 12.1, psychosocial interventions are necessary to provide complete and effective treatment for patients with substance use and SMI. Some insight into treatment of MA addiction and co-occurring SMI might be gained from existing treatment models for MA addiction. For example, the matrix model (Rawson et al., 2002a), which integrates several interventions such as individual psychotherapy, relapse prevention, family education, urine testing, and participation in 12-step programs, might be adapted for individuals with SMI. Contingency management, which has recently proven successful

TABLE 12.1. Off-Label Medication Options for MA Addiction and Co-Occurring Severe Mental Illness

Symptom/diagnosis	Pharmacological agent
Depression/dysphoria/major depression	Bupropion Mirtazapine Selegeline Modafinil
Cognitive deficits	Bupropion Modafinil
Psychosis/schizophrenia/ schizoaffective disorder/bipolar mania with psychosis	Aripiprazole Olanzapine Quetiapine Risperidone
Bipolar disorder	Gabapentin (less promising) Lamotrigine Oxcarbazepine Quetiapine Risperidone Topiramate Valproate

in reducing MA use and retaining users in treatment (Roll et al., 2006), could be tailored for SMI. Also, successful treatment techniques for treating SMI and co-occurring substance use disorders can be applied for the treatment of MA addiction in individuals with SMI. Several well-developed and successful strategies, including motivational interviewing, cognitive-behavioral therapy (Barrowclough et al., 2001), and contingency management have been adopted for the treatment of substance use disorders in individuals with SMI. Contingency management in particular has been demonstrated in several feasibility studies to be successful at reducing the drug use of persons suffering from SMI (Roll et al., 2004). Further support for the use of contingency management techniques in individuals with SMI comes from studies of managing disability benefits among patients with substance dependence and SMI. The patients with contingently managed disability benefits used significantly less alcohol and drugs and showed much better money management than those with noncontingent management (Drake et al., 1998). In this study cocaine was the most common drug of choice in individuals with SMI; hence, the benefits of contingency management could be extrapolated to a useful strategy for the treatment of MA addiction and co-occurring SMI.

Ultimately, an integrated treatment approach whereby one treatment team can deliver medication management as well as substance abuse and psychosocial treatment services (Drake et al., 1998) would be most desirable. In addition, the success of the treatment options for individuals dually diagnosed with MA addiction will likely improve by addressing population-specific issues for various patient groups, such as homosexual or bisexual men, pregnant women, and young adults, to name a few.

Current Controversies

Diagnostic Considerations

Intoxication and withdrawal from substances of abuse can mimic psychiatric symptoms, or amplify them in a person with a preexisting major psychiatric disorder, and complicate treatment, as well as making specific diagnoses in these patients difficult to confirm when they are using substances (Drake et al., 1998). Comorbidity of SMI and MA-use diagnoses are easier to distinguish when a person was diagnosed with SMI prior to MA use. However, it becomes a diagnostic challenge to distinguish, for example, in an individual with symptoms of depression or psychosis during prolonged MA abstinence, whether his or her symptoms of depression/psychosis are considered to be substance induced (perhaps due to irreversible neurotoxicity of dopaminergic circuits) or whether at some point the individual has an independent depressive/psychotic disorder.

Ontogeny of the Comorbid Disorder

Much effort has gone into trying to understand the nature of the relationship between substance use disorders and SMI (Phillips & Johnson, 2001). Theoretical accounts have been put forth that address the issue from the level of the neuron to the environment. Many have noted the similar neurochemical involvement in schizophrenia and substance abuse, with the preponderance of the work to date being on dopaminergic, serotonergic, and nicotinic systems (Cooper et al., 1991). Suggestions have been made that drugs are abused to try to compensate for the disordered neurochemistry found in schizophrenia (Scheller-Gilkey et al., 2003; Chen et al., 1998). Namely, individuals with schizophrenia— which is described as a state of prefrontal dopamine hypofunction— take MA and other stimulants that are dopamine agonists to counteract their negative symptoms or attention deficit. Similarly, it has been suggested that drugs are abused to counteract the side effects of many of the medications, such as cognitive blunting and dysphoria associated with conventional antipsychotics used to treat schizophrenia. Both of these instances would fall under the rubric of self-medication theories. Others have suggested that prolonged, heavy use of drugs of abuse (especially amphetamines) may lead to the presentation of schizophrenia-like, depressive, or bipolar-type symptoms as a result of neurochemical alteration (Chen et al., 1998). In addition, an association between MA abuse and ADHD has recently been identified. Between 33 and 71% of adult MA abusers have a presumptive childhood ADHD (Sim et al., 2002; Jaffe et al., 2005). ADHD is considered to be a state of relative prefrontal dopamine hypoactivity, and the mainstream pharmacological treatment of ADHD includes treatment with stimulants such as methylphenidate and amphetamine. Hence, individuals with childhood or adult ADHD may be at risk of using MA as a way of dealing with their neurochemical deficits.

Undoubtedly, the above issues do occur, and when they do they complicate the clinician's ability to make an accurate diagnosis. Finally, others have implied that persons with SMI are more likely than the general population to develop substance abuse problems because drugs are often an easily obtainable yet powerful source of reinforcement that they are less able to satisfactorily obtain from their environment (Gearon et al., 2001). We suspect all of these accounts are correct, and that comorbid substance abuse/dependence, including MA, by those with SMI is most likely multiply determined.

Treatment-Related Issues

Most treatments for MA disorders investigated so far have used only an addiction treatment model, and individuals with comorbid SMI have most often been excluded. There are no established treatment guidelines for MA disorders and co-occurring SMI, yet there are a number of treatment-related challenges to consider.

Limited data are available on treatment outcomes among MA users. The only long-term follow-up study of MA users available in the literature was reported by Rawson et al. (2002b). In this study the authors examined the outcome for MA users 2 to 5 years after outpatient treatment and found a significant reduction in self-reported MA use during the follow-up. Although there is currently a rapidly emerging research on MA addiction with best empirical support for psychosocial and behavioral treatments, little is known about the long-term effects of medications in MA-related disorders.

In addition, long-term integrated treatment programs for MA users do not discuss anything about emergency room presentations, detoxification facilities, inpatient units, and mental health centers where individuals with comorbid MA addiction and co-occurring SMI commonly present. There are no guidelines on whether individuals with co-occurring SMI who are actively using MA should be treated for their underlying mental disorder. In our experience, individuals who present in emergency room benefit from rapidly dissolvable atypical antipsychotics. Despite a perceived benefit, it is controversial whether treating acutely MA-intoxicated individuals would reinforce their use once they know that they can receive a temporary relief in the emergency room. In our experience that has not been the case. It is also controversial whether acutely MA-intoxicated individuals with prominent psychiatric symptoms such as dysphoria and psychosis should be referred to detoxification facilities or managed on inpatient psychiatric units. Presumably, those who are a danger to self or others or are gravely disabled do need to be hospitalized, although less often on a voluntary basis.

Unanswered Questions

Clearly, there are many important unanswered questions in the field of MA addiction and co-occurring SMI. For example should acutely MA-intoxicated individuals be aggressively treated with either antipsychotics or antidepressants, or both, to prevent the development of persistent psychosis, triggering of schizophrenia (as some think MA does), or persistent depression during abstinence? Should MA addiction in individuals with co-occurring SMI, particularly schizophrenia and major depression, be treated with agonist-like replacement pharmacotherapies similar to opiate–methadone model? Options could include dextroamphetamine and a number of currently approved long-acting agents such as dexmethilphenidate chloride (Focalin XR), lisdexamphetamine dimesylate (Vyvanse), methylphenidate extended release (Concerta SR), and methylphenidate transdermal patch (Daytrana). Would agents such as atomoxetine (Straterra), a norepinephrine reuptake inhibitor and non-stimulant medication approved for treating ADHD, be beneficial for the treatment of symptoms of depression and cognitive deficits in MA users? A clear benefit of Straterra in an addicted population would be its low addiction potential (Heil et al., 2002). However, we do not know whether administering stimulants to individuals who are already vulnerable to psychotic symptoms would ultimately make them more psychotic. It is also unknown whether treating individuals with co-occurring SMI and MA addiction with antidepressants would be beneficial, given that the current literature provides weak evidence for their effectiveness in treating depression in patients with schizophrenia spectrum disorders (Whitehead et al., 2003). Likewise, we don't know whether interventions such as the matrix model, contingency management, or other psychological interventions will work in SMI with MA addiction. Other unanswered questions pertain to the duration of treatment of psychiatric symptoms in individuals with MA addiction.

Conclusion

Although there have been recent efforts initiated by the NIDA to conduct research on pharmacological treatments and a real world applicability of new treatments by establishing the Methamphetamine Clinical Trials Group (Elkashef et al., 2007), it is evident that further research is required to develop protocols and treatment programs utilizing pharmacological agents in integrated treatment programs for MA addiction and co-occurring SMI.

References

Barrowclough C, Haddock G, Tarrier N, et al. (2001). Randomized controlled trial of motivational interviewing, cognitive behavior therapy, and family intervention for patients with comorbid schizophrenia and substance use disorders. *Am J Psychiatry* 158:1706–1713.
Bellack AS, DiClemente CC. (1999). Treating substance abuse among patients with schizophrenia. *Psychiatric Services* 50:75–80.

Bennett ME, Bellack AS, Gearon JS. (2001). Treating substance abuse in schizo-phrenia. An initial report. *J Subst Abuse Treat* 20:163–175.

Brady K, Anton R, Ballenger J, et al. (1990). Cocaine abuse among schizo-phrenic patients. *Am J Psychiatry* 147:1164–1167.

Brunette MF, Drake RE. (1997). Gender differences in patients with schizo-phrenia and substance abuse. *Comprehensive Psychiatr* 38:109–116.

Camacho A, Akiskal HS. (2005). Propolas for a bipolar-stimulant spectrum: Temperament, diagnostic validation and therapeutic outcomes with mood stabilizers. *J Affective Disorder* 85:217–230.

Carey MP, Carey KB, Kalichman SC. (1997). Risk for human immunodefi-ciency virus (HIV) infection among persons with severe mental illness. *Clin Psychol Res* 17:271–291.

Chen YR, Swann AC, Johnson BA. (1998). Stability of diagnosis in bipolar dis-order. *J Nerv Ment Dis* 186:17–23.

Cho AK, Melega WP. (2002). Patterns of methamphetamine abuse and their consequences. *J Addict Dis* 21:21–34.

Cooper JR, Bloom FE, Roth RH. (1991). *The Biochemical Basis of Behavior.* NY: Oxford University Press.

Dixon L. (1999). Dual diagnosis of substance abuse in schizophrenia: Preva-lence and impact on outcomes. *Schizophr Res* 35(Suppl. S):93–100.

Dixon L, McNary S, Lehman AF. (1998). Remission of substance use disor-der among psychiatric inpatients with mental illness. *Am J Psychiatry* 155:239–243.

Drake RE, Mercer-McFadden C, Mueser KT, et al. (1998). A review of inte-grated mental health and substance abuse treatment for patients with dual disorders. *Schizophr Bull* 24:589–608.

Drake RE, Xie H, McHuto GJ, et al. (2000). The effects of clozapine on alcohol and drug use disorders among patients with schizophrenia. *Schizophr Bull* 26:441–449.

Drake RE, Mueser KT. (2001). Managing comorbid schizophrenia and sub-stance abuse. *Curr Psychiatry Rep* 3:418–422.

Elkashef A, Rawson RA, Smith E, et al. (2007). The NIDA Methamphetamine Clinical Trials Group: A strategy to increase clinical trials research capac-ity. *Addiction* 102(Suppl. 1):107–113.

Galanter M, Dermatis H, Egelko S, et al. (1998). Homelessness and mental ill-ness in a professional- and peer-led cocaine treatment clinic. *Psychiatr Serv* 49:533–535.

Gearon JS, Bellack AS, Rachbeisel J, et al. (2001). Drug-use behavior and cor-relates in people with schizophrenia. *Addict Behav* 26:51–61.

Gray SD, Fatovich DM, McCoubrie DL, et al. (2007). Amphetamine-related presentations to an inner-city tertiary emergency department: A prospec-tive evaluation. *Med J Australia* 186:336–339.

Green A, Tohen M, Hamer R, et al. (2004). First episode of schizophrenia-related psychosis and substance use disorders: Acute response to olanzap-ine and haloperidol. *Schizophr Res* 66:125–135.

Havassy BE, Alvidrez J, Owen KK. (2004). Comparisons of Patients with

Comorbid Psychiatric and Substance Use Disorders: Implications for Treatment and Service Delivery. *Am J Psychiatry* 161:139–145.

Heil SH, Holmes HW, Bickel WK, et al. (2002). Comparison of the subjective, physiological, and psychomotor effects of amoxetine and methylphenidate in light drug users. *Drug Alcohol Depend* 67:149–156.

Heinzerling KG, Shoptaw S, Peck JA, et al. (2006). Randomized, placebo-controlled trial of baclofen and gabapentin for the treatment of methamphetamine dependence. *Drug Alcohol Depend* 85:177–184.

Hudson TJ, Owen RR, Thrush CR, et al. (2004). A pilot study of barriers to medication adherence in schizophrenia. *J Clin Psychiatry* 65:211–216.

Jackson CT, Fein D, Essock SM, et al. (2001). The effects of cognitive impairment and substance abuse on psychiatric hospitalizations. *Community Ment Health J* 37:303–312.

Jaffe C, Bush KR, Straits-Troster K, et al. (2005). A comparison of methamphetamine-dependent inpatients childhood attention deficit hyperactivity disorder symptomatology. *J Addict Dis* 24:133–152.

Johnson BA, Roache JD, Ait-Daoud N, et al. (2007). Effects of acute topiramate dosing on methamphetamine-induced subjective mood. *Int J Neuropsychopharmacol* 10:85–98.

Kalechstein A, Newton TF, Longshore D, et al. (2000). Psychiatric comorbidity of methamphetamine dependence in a forensic sample. *J Neuropsychiatry Clin Neurosci* 12:480–484.

Kessler RC, Nelson CB, McGonagle KA, et al. (1996). The epidemiology of co-occurring addictive and mental disorders: Implications for prevention and service utilization. *American J Orthopsychiatry* 66:17–31.

Levin FR, Evans SM, McDowell DM, et al. (2002). Bupropion treatment for cocaine abuse and adult attention deficit/hyperactivity disorder. *J Addict Dis* 21:1–16.

Lin S-K, Ball D, Hsiao C-C, et al. (2004). Psychiatric comorbidity and gender differences of persons incarcerated for methamphetamine abuse in Taiwan. *Psychiatry Clin Neurosci* 58:206–212.

Ling W, Rawson RA, Shoptaw S, et al. (2006). Management of methamphetamine abuse and dependence. *Curr Psychiatry Rep* 8(5):345–354.

Misra L, Kofoed L. (1997). Risperidone treatment of methamphetamine psychosis. [Letter]. *Am J Psychiatry* 154:1170.

Misra L, Kofoed L, Oesterheld JR, et al. (2000). Olanzapine treatment of methamphetamine psychosis. [Letter]. *J Clin Psychopharmacol* 20:393–394.

Narrow WE, Regier DA, Rae DS, et al. (1993). Use of services by persons with mental and addictive disorders. Findings from the National Institute of Mental Health Epidemiologic Catchment Area Program. *Arch Gen Psychiatry* 50:95–107.

National Institute of Drug Abuse. (2005a). *Assessment of interactions between methamphetamine and aripiprazole.* Retrieved August 29, 2007, from *www.clinicaltrials.gov/ct/show/NCT00208143.*

National Institute of Drug Abuse. (2005b). *A randomized control trial comparing quetiapine to risperidone in bipolar disorder with stimulant depen-*

dence. Retrieved August 29, 2007, from *www.clinicaltrials.gov/ct/show/NCT00227123*.

National Institute of Drug Abuse. (2006a). *A pilot study of citicoline add-on therapy in patients with bipolar disorder or major depressive disorder and amphetamine abuse or dependence*. Retrieved September 20, 2007, from *www.clinicaltrials.gov/ct/show/NCT00377299*.

National Institute of Drug Abuse. (2006b). *Rivastigmine for methamphetamine-dependent individuals*. Retrieved September 20, 2007, from *www. clinicaltrials.gov/ct/show?NCT00158210*.

National Institute of Drug Abuse. (2006c). *Seroquel therapy for substance use disorders comorbid with schizophrenia*. Retrieved August 29, 2007, from *www.clinicaltrials.gov/ct/show/NCT00208143*.

National Institute of Drug Abuse. (2007). *Mirtazapine to reduce methamphetamine use among MSM with high-risk HIV behaviors*. Retrieved August 29, 2007, from *www.clinicaltrials.gov/ct/show/NCT00497081*.

Newton TF, DeLaGarza II R, Fong T, et al. (2005). A comprehensive assessment of the safety of intravenous methamphetamine administration during treatment with selegeline. *Pharmacolo Biochem Behav* 82:704–711.

Newton TF, Roache JD, DeLaGarza II R, et al. (2006). Bupropion reduces methamphetamine-induced subjective effects and cue-induced craving. *Neuropsychopharmacology* 31:1537–1544.

Pages K, Russo J, Wingerson D, et al. (1998). Predictors and outcome of discharge against medical advice from the psychiatric units of a general hospital. *Psychiatr Serv* 49:1182–1192.

Pasic J, Russo J, Ries R, et al. (2007). Methamphetamine users in the psychiatric emergency services: A case-control study. *Am J Drug Alcohol Abuse* 33(5):675–686.

Phillips P, Johnson S. (2001). How does drug and alcohol misuse develop among people with psychotic illness? A literature review. *Soc Psychiatry Psychiatr Epidemiol* 36:269–276.

RachBeisel J, Scott J, Dixon L. (1999). Co-occurring severe mental illness and substance use disorders: A review of recent research. *Psychiatric Serv* 50:1427–1434.

Rawson RA, Gonzales R, Brethen P. (2002a). Treatment of methamphetamine use disorders: An update. *J Subst Abuse Treat* 23:145–150.

Rawson RA, Huber A, Brethen P, et al. (2002b). Status of methamphetamine users 2–5 years after outpatient treatment. *J Addict Dis* 21:107–119.

Rawson RA, McCann MJ, Flammino F, et al. (2006). A comparison of contingency management and cognitive-behavioral approaches for stimulant-dependent individuals. *Addiction* 101:267–274.

Regier DA, Farmer ME, Rae DS, et al. (1990). Comorbidity of mental disorders with alcohol and other drug abuse: Results from the Epidemiological Catchment Area (ECA) study. *JAMA* 264:2511–2518.

Ries RK, Dyck DG. (1997). Representative payee practice of community mental health centers in Washington State. *Psychiatr Serv* 48:811–814.

Ries RK, Dyck DG, Short R, et al. (2004). Outcomes of managing disability benefits among patients with substance dependence and severe mental illness. *Psychiatr Serv* 55:445–447.

Ries RK, Russo J, Wingerson D, et al. (2000). Shorter hospital stays and more rapid improvement among patients with schizophrenia and substance disorders. *Psychiatr Serv* 51:210–215.

Roll JM, Chermack ST, Chudzynski JE. (2004). Investigating the use of contingency management in the treatment of cocaine abuse among individuals with schizophrenia: A feasibility study. *Psychiatry Res* 125:61–64.

Roll JM, Petry NM, Stitzer ML, et al. (2006). Contingency management for the treatment of methamphetamine use disorders. *Am J Psychiatry* 163:1993–1999.

Scheller-Gilkey G, Woolwine BJ, Cooper I, et al. (2003). Relationship of clinical symptoms and substance use in schizophrenia patients on conventional versus atypical antipsychotics. *Am J Drug Alcohol Abuse* 29:553–566.

Shoptaw S, Klausner JD, Reback CJ, et al. (2006). A public health response to the methamphetamine epidemic: The implementation of contingency management to treat methamphetamine dependence. *BMC Public Health* 6:214.

Sim T, Simon SL, Comier CP, et al. (2002). Cognitive deficits among methamphetamine users with attention deficit hyperactive disorder symptomatology. *J Addict Dis* 21:75–89.

Simon SL, Domier C, Carnell J, et al. (2000). Cognitive impairment in methamphetamine abusers. *A J Drug Alcohol Dep* 9:222–232.

Smelson DA, Losonezy MF, Davis CW, et al. (2002). Risperidone decreases craving and relapse in individuals with schizophrenia and cocaine. *Can J Psychiatry* 47:671–675.

Tsuang J, Marder SR, Han A, et al. (2002). Olanzapine treatment for patients with schizophrenia and cocaine abuse. *J Clin Psychiatry* 63:1180–1181.

US Department of Health and Human Services. (1998). *Treatment for stimulant use disorders: TIP 33*. DHHS Publication No. (SMA) 99-3296 Rockville, MD: SAMHSA.

US Department of Health and Human Services. (2002). *Report to Congress on the prevention and treatment of co-occurring substance abuse and mental disorders*. Available at: *www.samhsa.gov/reports/congress2002/index.html*.

US Department of Health and Human Services. (2005). *Substance abuse treatment for persons with co-occurring disorders. A treatment improvement protocol. TIP 42*. DHHS Publication No. (SMA) 05-3992. Rockville, MD: SAMHSA.

Vocci FJ, Arci J, Elkashef A. (2002). Medication development for addictive disorders: The state of the science. *Am J Psychiatry* 162:1432–1440.

Watkins WE, Burnam A, Kung FY, et al. (2001). A national survey of care for persons with co-occurring mental and substance use disorders. *Psychiatr Serv* 52:1062–1068.

Weickert TW, Goldberg TE, Marenco S, et al. (2003). Comparison of cognitive performance during a placebo period and an atypical antipsychotic treatment period in schizophrenia: Critical examination of confounds. *Neuropsychopharmacology* 28:1491–1500.

Whitehead C, Moss S, Cadno A, et al. (2003). Antidepressants for the treatment of depression in people with schizophrenia: A systematic review. *Psychol Med* 33:589–599.

Yen CF, Chong MF. (2006). Comorbid psychiatric disorders, sex, and methamphetamine use in adolescents: A case-control study. *Comp Psychiatry* 47:215–220.

Yovell Y, Opler LA. (1994). Clozapine reverses cocaine craving in a treatment-resistant mentally ill chemical abuser: A case report and hypothesis. *J Nerv Ment Dis* 182:591–592.

Zweben JE, Cohen JB, Christian D, et al. (2004). Psychiatric symptoms in methamphetamine users. *Am J Addict* 13:181–190.

Chapter 13

Conclusion

Charles R. Schuster, Chris-Ellyn Johanson, and John M. Roll

This book brings together contributions from scholars working at all levels of analysis to understand and eliminate methamphetamine (MA) addiction. The co-location of these contributions in one book greatly simplifies the process of learning about MA. As the editors suggest in their introductory chapter, the individual who has read this book in its entirety will have a good grasp of our current understanding of MA addiction. This should help the reader formulate new questions to explore, develop sound policy, and understand the plight of those addicted to MA.

Moreover, the book is a hopeful one. It provides the reader with an inspiring message that, while MA addiction is an undeniably terrible affliction for an individual and a seemingly insurmountable burden for their families and communities, recovery from the affliction is absolutely possible, although certainly not easy.

Taken as a whole, the book also nicely illustrates that MA addiction, like other drug addictions, is an entirely predictable result of the three-way interaction among our human physiology, the drug's pharmacology, and the environments in which we live. These three factors set the stage for MA to function as a powerful positive reinforcer in the same way that cocaine, heroin, nicotine, and alcohol become positive reinforcers and abused drugs. The foregoing should not be taken as relieving addicts from personal responsibility for their addiction. Indeed, we are all responsible for our actions, which are largely displayed to our fellow human beings by the choices we make. We choose to have one more drink, to smoke a cigarette, to inject heroin, or to snort MA. However, years of rigorous science in the field of the experimental analysis of behavior have yielded myriad examples demonstrating that our behavior and our choices are orderly outcomes that can be predicted from our current and past environments and that can be controlled by altering our current and future environments. Once it is realized that drug-taking behavior is largely a product of our environment, which enhances or diminishes the probability of our electing to take a drug repeatedly by raising and lowering the drug's reinforcing efficacy, it becomes much easier to engineer successful prevention and treatment strategies.

It is interesting that MA has received so much press and public attention. It is not a new drug, nor is this the first serious "epidemic" of MA addiction (e.g., Karch, 2002). Unfortunately, much of the press surrounding MA addiction has been incorrect. The authors of the various chapters in this book have gone a long way toward correcting the misconceptions of MA as "a super reinforcer" and of MA addiction as an "untreatable" malady. Although it is beyond our scope to delve too deeply into the reason for these misperceptions about MA, it does seem likely that they are related to the current widespread addiction to MA observed in certain areas of the United States. The widespread use in these locales suggests that, for individuals in certain environments, MA's reinforcing efficacy is very high. This is likely the result of these individuals' inability to access other sources of reinforcement on a regular basis because of educational and economic deficits.

A person who has no money and consequently cannot provide for his or her family, who lacks the educational requirements for a well-paying job, and who lives in an area where an abundant labor source is readily available to meet the demands for menial work, is likely to find it difficult to obtain much reinforcement for positive behavior as he or she navigates a sterile existence. People may initially use MA to enhance their ability to acquire other sources of positive reinforcement; for example, a young woman might initially take it to control her weight in order to make herself more attractive to a mate. Or a laborer may take it to enhance his ability to work long periods without sleep to earn more money to provide for his family. When they take the drug, users undeniably feel a euphoric sense of well-being that transports them from their current state of despair, at least temporarily. This good feeling and relief from feeling bad combine to make the drug a powerful source of reinforcement that is returned to more frequently as the person becomes better acquainted with its reinforcing effects. Unfortunately, human physiology leads to behavioral habituation to the drug's effects, and pharmacology leads to tolerance of the drug's effects. This in turn requires the neophyte addict to take more and more of the drug until his or her use becomes the compulsive use characterizing dependence. Gone are thoughts of the original reason the drug was used. These individuals are consumed with acquiring and taking the drug without regard for themselves, their families, or those with whom they share a community. Of course, this is only one way addiction may start, but we believe it is a common pathway for the development of MA addiction.

On the other hand, others may initially take the drug to enhance sexual experiences as a result of peer pressure, or merely through adolescent experimentation. Most of these individuals will be able to stop taking it before they hold their futures hostage to addiction. A very fruitful area of research would be to develop a better understanding of the strategies used by those who experiment with the drug but don't become addicted to it. It seems likely that these individuals are better able to moderate MA's reinforcing efficacy via juxtaposing its use with other salient sources of reinforcement in their environment. For instance, quality time spent with families or friends or pursuit of a career or hobbies all are likely to compete with MA addiction by providing alternative salient sources of positive reinforcement.

The exciting basic science findings presented in these chapters are important because they help us understand not only MA addiction but also how our brains work and how behavior is produced. The basic science chapters also demonstrate the use of state-of-the-art technology to address socially meaningful problems and to produce results that can be built upon by researchers developing treatments and providers delivering those treatments. This results in a translational approach to scientific inquiry in which basic science informs applied science; this approach has always held the very best promise for addressing socially important problems.

The chapters on treatment are interesting and demonstrate cutting-edge pharmacological and behavioral methodology for reducing MA's reinforcing efficacy, which is the hallmark of successful treatment. The search for pharmacotherapeutic agents to treat MA addiction is an exciting endeavor and one we believe holds great promise. As illustrated in the various chapters, the combination of a pharmacotheraputic agent with a behavioral treatment may hold the best chance for success. Currently, though, the behavioral treatments that have proven effective in treating cocaine addiction seem to be the frontline for treating MA addiction.

There is a paucity of knowledge available on preventing MA addiction. However, we suspect that an approach to prevention that borrows the treatment strategy of lowering MA's reinforcing efficacy could be quite effective. By providing youth and at-risk individuals with the skills and opportunities to acquire salient reinforcement from non-drug-related activities (e.g., interactions with families and friends, work, hobbies) before they become addicted to MA, it should be possible to prevent, or greatly reduce, the likelihood of the individual becoming addicted.

The field also needs to do much more work on the teratology of MA, particularly because the drug is often used by young women. Although some excellent work is being done on the topic (e.g., Smith et al., 2006), much remains to be learned. It is our hope that sound science will inform policy surrounding this issue. For instance, we hope individuals do not confuse the effects of poor prenatal care with MA exposure. Fetal effects of drugs are often subtle and need to be carefully studied and parsed before definitive statements are made. On a related topic, we are generally opposed to the criminalization of a mother who exposes her neonate to MA. Certainly, this is dangerous and irresponsible behavior, but punishing the mother for the behavior is unlikely to help the unborn child. Instead we would suggest that, as has been done for other drugs often abused by expecting mothers, specific treatment strategies be devised to assist expecting mothers in terminating their MA use (e.g., Heil et al., 2008; Svikis et al., 2007).

Drug addiction is not a new phenomenon. The current MA "epidemic" will not be the last drug "epidemic" faced. However, for those affected by MA addiction, the work described in these chapters holds great promise.

References

Heil SH, Higgins ST, Bernstein IM, et al. (2008). Effects of voucher-based incentives on abstinence from cigarette smoking and fetal growth among pregnant women. *Addiction* 103:1009–1018.

Karch SB. (2002). *Pathology of drug abuse.* New York: CRC Press.

Smith LM, LaGasse LL, Derauf C, et al. (2006). The infant development, environment, and lifestyle study: Effects of prenatal methamphetamine exposure, polydrug exposure, and poverty on intrauterine growth. *Pediatrics* 118:1149–1156.

Svikis DS, Silverman K, Haug NA, et al. (2007). Behavioral strategies to improve treatment participation and retention by pregnant drug-dependent women. *Subst Use Misuse* 42:1527–1535.

Index